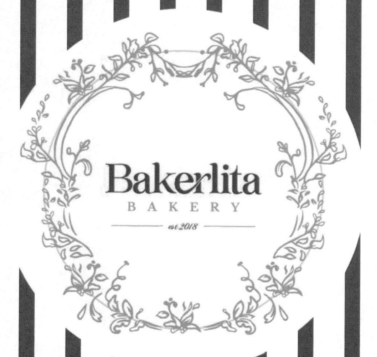

Bakerlita

BAKERY

est. 2018

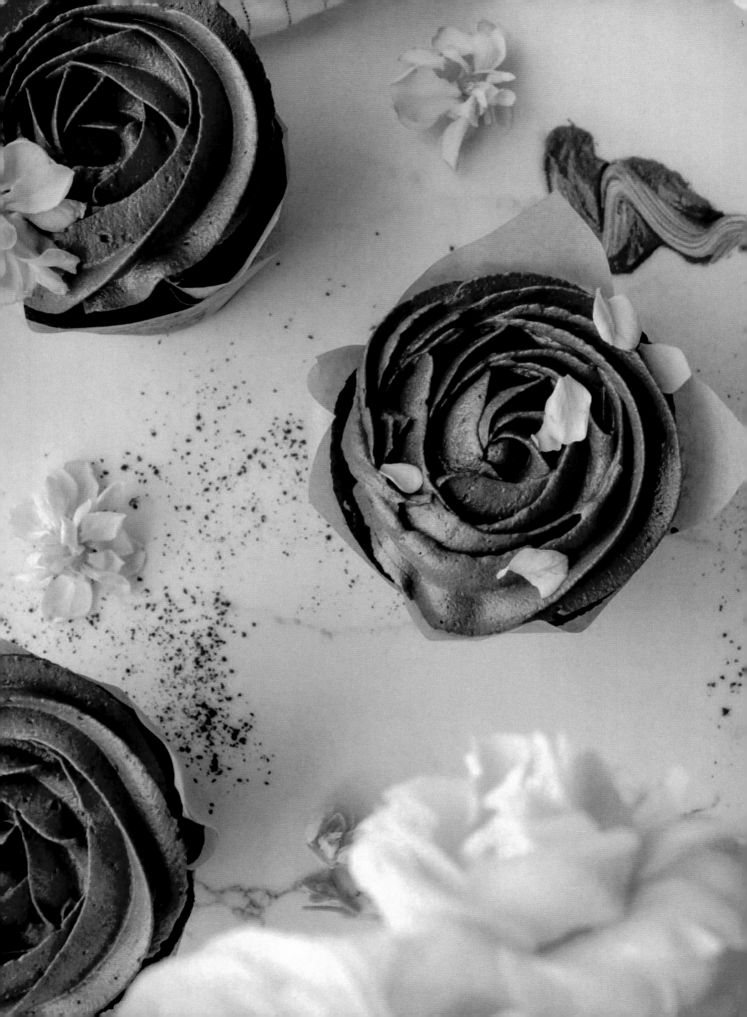

Bakerlita

BAKERY

a collection of guilt-free recipes that will bless you from the inside out

SUGAR-FREE | GLUTEN-FREE | GRAIN-FREE | PALEO | KETO

Andrea Witthoeft

WRITTEN & PHOTOGRAPHY BY ANDREA WITTHOEFT

Edited by Ami Ulici

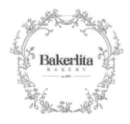

To my Beloveds

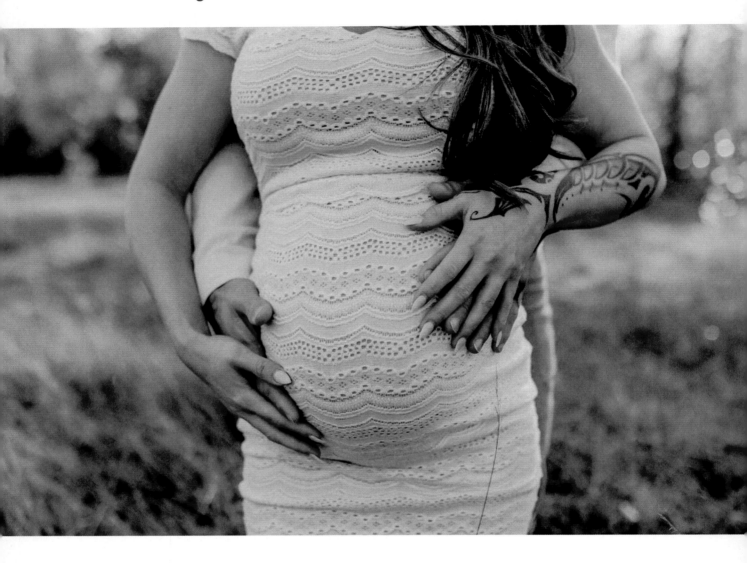

To my husband, my one flesh! You, my precious husband, are the greatest earthly gift I could ever imagine receiving. The endless praises you continually speak over me have given me the confidence I needed to believe in my God-given ability to write this book. Your unconditional and sacrificial love and support towards me as your wife have an eternal seal on my spirit. I thank God for you every day, always praying for me, washing me in the Word, that I may grow in the grace and knowledge of our Lord.

To my baby bundle that is on the way! You have brought me into this new and restful season which has given me the priceless time to bundle my favourite recipes and create this book... I am waiting with eager anticipation to bake for you and, in the years to come, make it a family tradition to bond and bake with you. *"For this child, I prayed, and the LORD has granted me my petition which I asked of Him."*

To my God, lover of my soul. My heavenly Father, You have given me the grace and joy to do everything I do! You have taught me that, above all, I need to use the gifts and talents You have given me to serve not myself but to bless others. May I strive to do everything I do for Your glory.

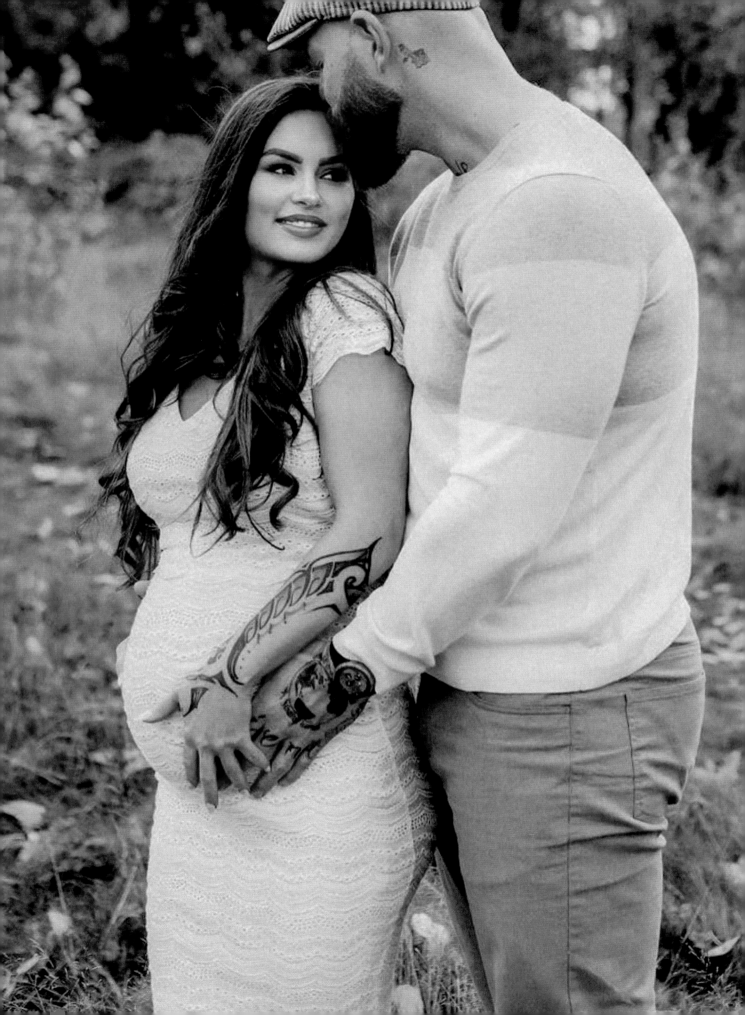

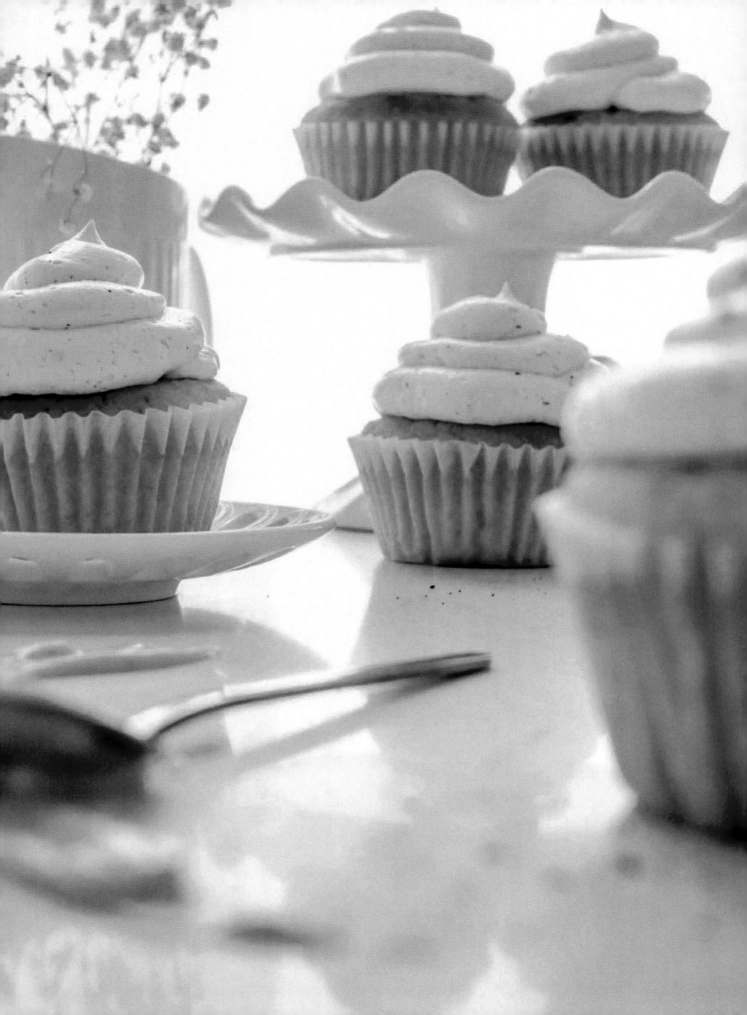

Contents

I have a sweet, festive surprise for you at the end of each chapter.

When I decided to write my *Bakerlita Bakery Cookbook,* I wanted to get it into your hands before my child was born and before the Christmas baking spirit began. I longed to celebrate the birth of my first baby during this beautiful and blessed season. I will be receiving the most precious gift I could see this Christmas, and I wanted to share my most cherished Christmas recipes with you as an expression of the joy and gratitude in my heart!

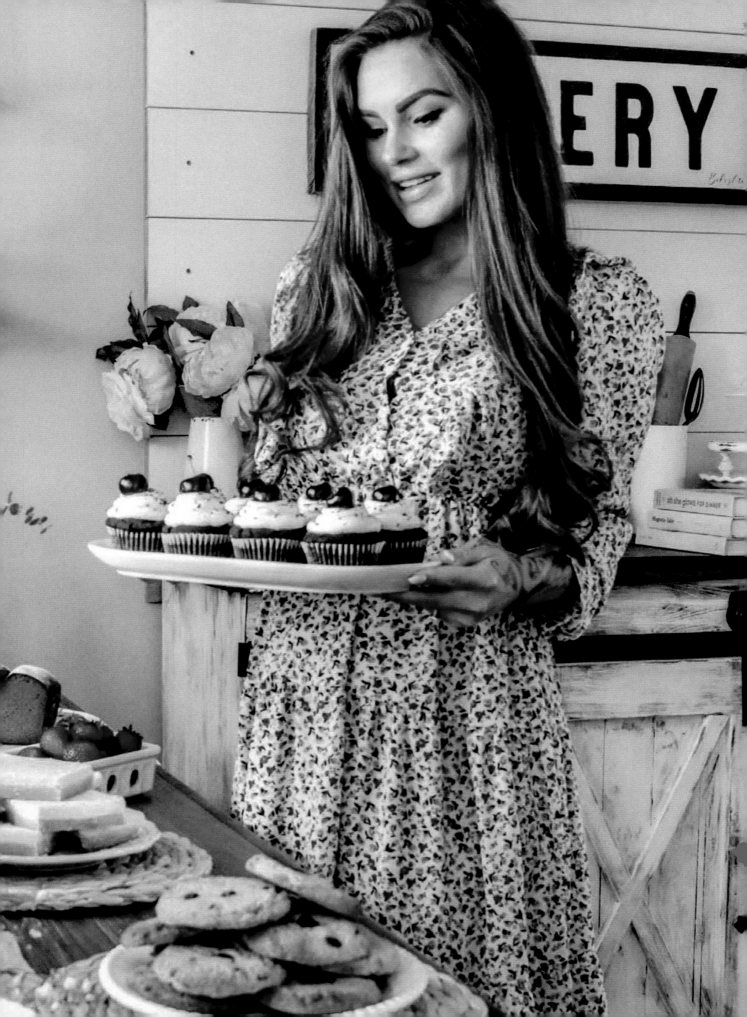

Introduction

Great suffering and a deep emptiness in my heart led me to find my identity and my passion and love for baking.

As a little girl, I found joy in the kitchen - watching the amazing things my stepmom created from simple ingredients like flour, sugar, butter, and eggs... I still remember how my sisters and I gathered around the table with sheer JOY on our faces as we indulged in the dozen freshly baked, homemade chocolate chip cookies. Right then and there, I knew something wonderfully unique about homemade baking made everyone gather around the table to enjoy such a simple and sweet delight.

Unfortunately, I did not have the healthiest diet growing up since money was short. I often had stomach/digestive issues; I struggled with tummy aches, constipation, and bloating - you name it! And they seemed to get worse as I got older, especially in the season of my life that unfolded next.

As life took its course, it brought about trials and hard times... which led to stress and tension as I have never experienced before, leading to the most horrific stomach issues I have ever had... My innocent, childish laughter quickly transformed into sobbing.

My family's struggles with various addictions and separations only grew; these were the most challenging and trying times of my life. Sorrow, sadness, and survival became my new way of life.

Purpose, success, beauty & money. This was what I decided *a perfect life* was supposed to look like when I was 16 years old. I was so motivated that I was determined to reach all my goals regarding the ideal body, health, wealth and prosperity. Achieving all this is what the world told me would lead me to fulfilment, satisfaction and happiness. But the opposite happened. Striving to find a way out without any direction or positive guidance led me to seek satisfaction in what the world had to offer me...

I cannot describe the emptiness that overcame me the closer I reached the "ideal life." The more I strived for perfection, the emptier and emptier I became.

By my outer appearance, you would have believed that I had everything a girl could ever want. However, on the inside, I was still that little girl sobbing with deep pains in her soul and her body. As time passed, my stomach issues became the number one pain point I could not figure out. It seemed that the more I tried to eat healthily *(well, what I thought was healthy at the time)*, the worse it became. I was without hope: empty on the inside - while pursuing what was supposed to fill me with satisfaction and deep physical pain. All I could do was to keep going, keep striving in the hope of finding the healing and sweet happiness my soul was longing for.

Then one day, God made Himself known to me. He showed me my true worth and identity through His great grace and love. It was not found in what I looked like or what I achieved but purely in whom God designed and desired me to be. I did not have to strive to be perfect anymore. I was made to be perfected in Him, in His image and likeness.

The turning point of my life was when I realized and acknowledged that I was living for myself alone. I guess you can call that being selfish, and yes, I honestly was selfish indeed! I had cut off from my life so many friends and family because they hindered me and my goals. I finally saw that they were also lost and without hope. Jesus opened my blind eyes. I saw the pain I caused others. I saw all I cared about what I could get in life. Jesus Christ died for all of my sins. He has forgiven my past and has graciously filled me with compassion and an ability to forgive my family for the hard times I faced in my childhood. I rejoice now; I count it all a blessing - because, having endured the pain myself, I now have a new love and understanding for others facing difficulties.

As I grew in the knowledge of God, I also started to understand the true meaning of life and my purpose. I saw the world in a new way. My passions began to change as I understood what brought true healing and harmony in the world and my longing soul. I still loved being in the kitchen, especially baking. However, knowing the havoc, traditional baking caused in my tummy made me believe I would have to kiss that dream goodbye. I desperately wanted to find a way to use my love of baking and talents to not just temporarily satisfy people's tastebuds but also to bring healing to their bodies.

I genuinely believe this because He created all the beautiful ingredients and helped me see all the potential in the ingredients I needed to bake to heal, nourish and restore all my stomach issues, and I hope yours too! Also, as my customers will happily attest, *"Baking The Bakerlita Way"* tastes even better than traditional baking! With God, all things are possible.

I am honoured to serve a lovely and loyal local customer base I bake for weekly. I am beyond grateful for this opportunity to share my love for baking with you!

"Remembering the words the Lord Jesus himself said:
'It is more blessed to give than to receive.' "

ACTS 20:35

Bakerlita

The meaning behind the name

"BAKERLITA" emerged from a burning passion to see lives transformed by using an innovative approach in baking-to-bless one's inner self, not just the taste buds!

"BAKER" to bake is to be co-partners/co-creators with God; it is not only my great passion, but it is also the opportunity to educate, inspire and influence my community through the creativity of combining wholesome and natural ingredients, to nourish and heal your body, soul & spirit.

"LITA" means JOY! Baking brings me abundant joy and gladness, especially knowing that it blesses my customers, friends and family.

"Bake The Bakerlita Way. Bake To Bless!"

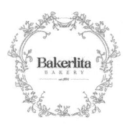

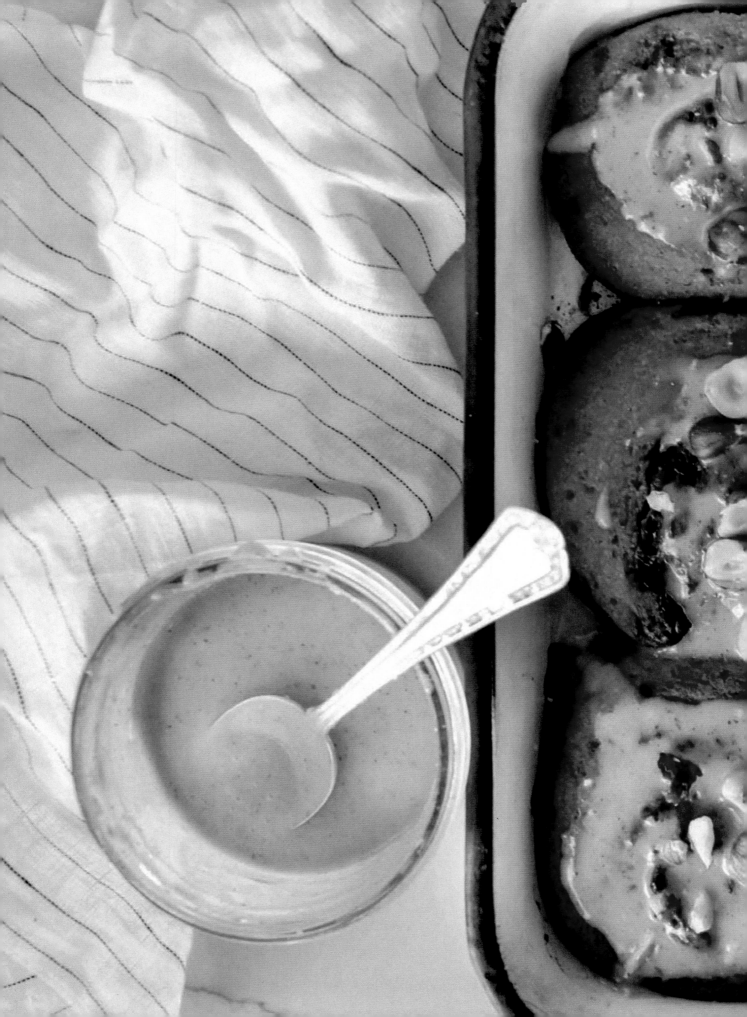

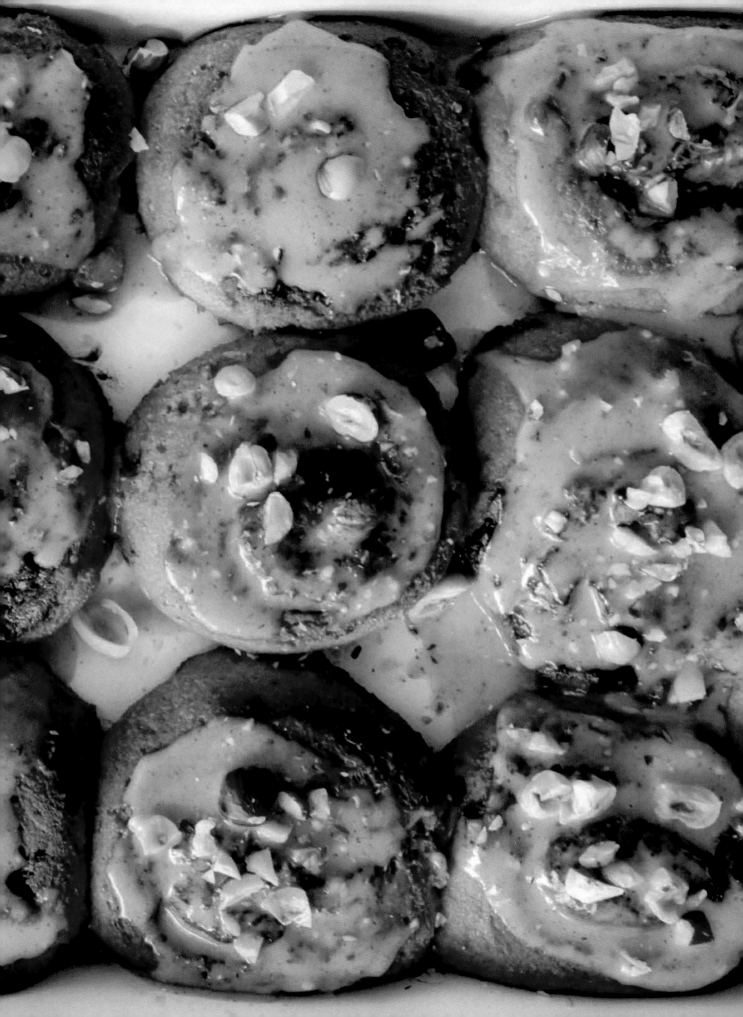

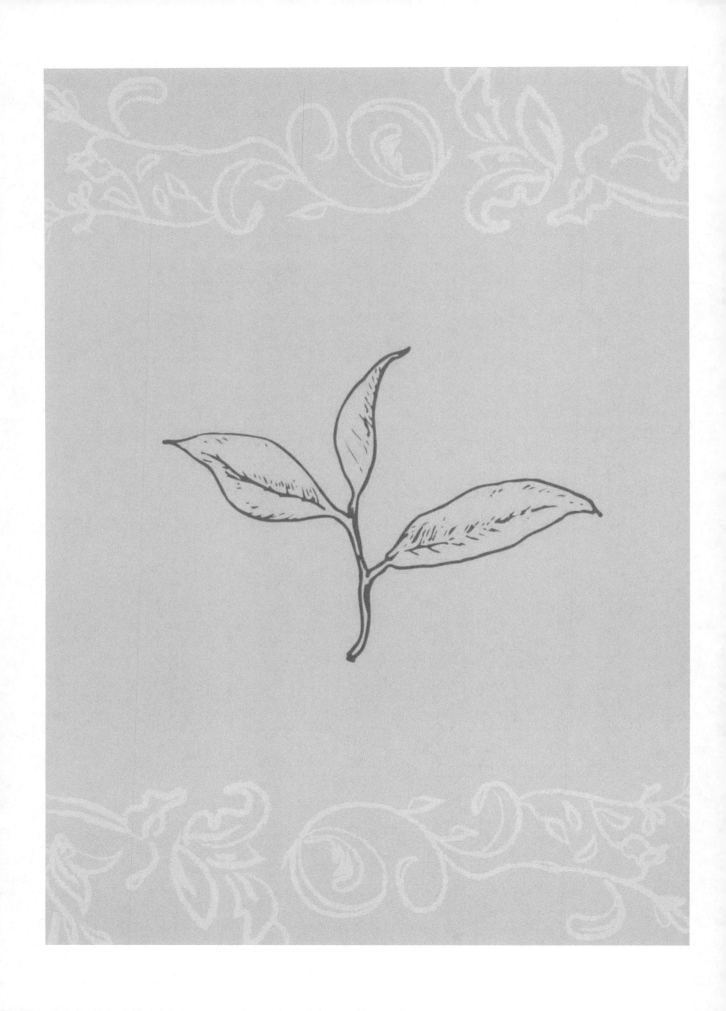

The Art of Baking

I love my baked goods, and I love baking too. I guess that is pretty obvious... But, what I love even more than baking, is using the art of cultivating God's wholesome, nutritious ingredients and transforming them into a light and lovely piece of CAKE, and then sharing it with others. Nothing is more satisfying to me than blessing others with a package of my baked goodies! Homemade baking is always a great gift to others, even more so when it is delicious and healing for their body, soul and spirit! And that is the secret I want to share with you in my Bakerlita Bakery cookbook. I can't wait for you to dive in and dig into a piece of cake too - *"guilt-free, of course"*!

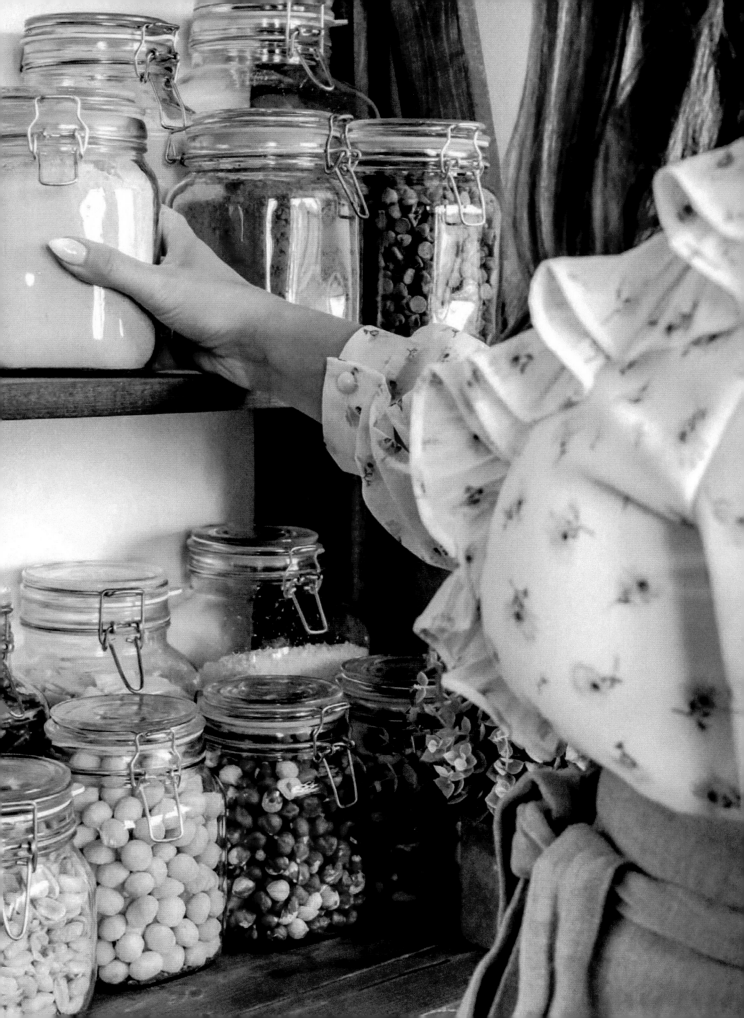

Bake the Bakerlita Way!

Baking the Bakerlita way is quite simple. Baking can be very complex, yet, using wholesome, organic and nutrient-packed ingredients makes it easier to master the art of great baking. Not only will these anti-inflammatory and holistic ingredients taste amazing, but they also serve the most crucial role: to bless your body with the health and energy it needs to thrive daily. Wouldn't it be amazing to eat a piece of cake and feel great after - not tired, inflamed and guilty? Yep, it is possible - you can enjoy all your favourite baked goods again, and I can't wait to show you how!

The Bakerlita Method

The Bakerlita baking method is a low-carb, low-inflammation, paleo, and ketogenic approach. When learning how to bake this way, something extraordinary happens to you on a physiological level. You see, when your body takes in even small amounts of carbs/sugars, your body has extra glucose levels to burn, which end up being stored in your liver, which insulin transforms into fats. *Baking the Bakerlita Way* means your body can now BURN body fat as fuel - not store it in your liver! YES! ~ even while eating your most loved baked goods, you will still stay in a state of ketosis! Once you're in ketosis, your liver produces those powerful ketones.

When ketones are present in the body, you don't crave sugar & carbs because your body is so satisfied with the perfect fuel source, HEALTHY FATS! These ketones bless your brain with fantastic brain clarity and provide your body with endless clean energy. Also, eating this way keeps unwanted body fat off while you still get to eat delicious goodies.

Being on a keto diet should never leave you unsatisfied, hungry and deprived. On special occasions and during the holidays, it is easy to overindulge in unhealthy foods and afterward feel overwhelmed at the realization that you now have 5-10lbs you need to lose; not anymore! The goal is to keep your crabs under 50g a day to reap all the blessings ketosis has to offer your body.

One of my favourite times to have a bake-athon *(baking marathon)* is around the holiday season. Treat yourself, your family and your friends this holiday with the wholesome gift of Christmas goodies - you will find these at the end of each chapter to satisfy your sweet festive cravings!

I believe that no one should miss out on delicious baked goodies at Christmas or any special occasion. Saying NO to every treat or feeling guilty about eating baked goods will not be your reality anymore! This year you will fill up on your most loved baked goods guilt-free! **It's time you experience baking in a whole new way -** *Bake The Bakerlita Way* **- my sweet gift. In the following chapters, I will show you how to do just that.**

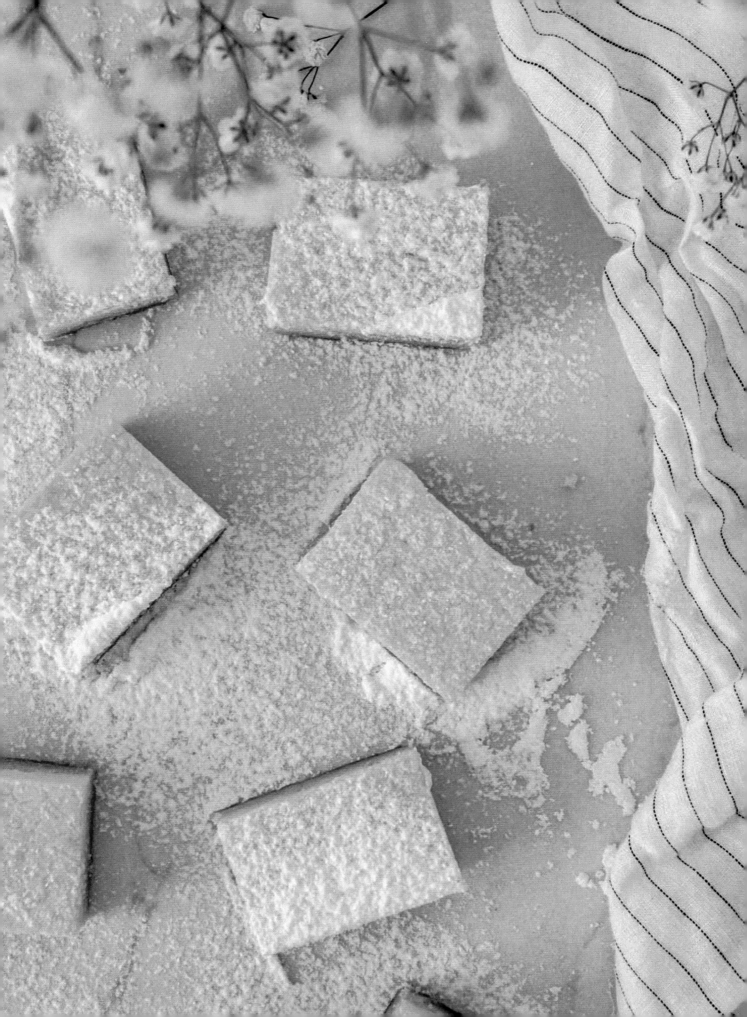

Why go sugar-free?

EATING TOO MUCH SUGAR & CARBS CAN CAUSE THESE SIDE EFFECTS, SICKNESSES & DISEASES!

- sugar/carb cravings
- irritability
- diabetes 1 & 2
- obesity
- autoimmune diseases
- low thyroid
- alzheimer's
- candida/fungal overgrowth

- hormonal imbalances
- weight gain/belly fat
- inflammation
- brain fog/lack of focus
- IBS *(irritable bowels syndrome)*
- skin problems
- low energy/energy crashes
- sleep disorders

What's in the Bakerlita pantry?

It can become overwhelming when you're out searching for all the great ingredients in this cookbook. So I wanted to help you get into the kitchen & bake - not drive around town for days trying to find the best ingredients and brands I use to create all my recipes. As a result, I have made a page on my website, sourced from Amazon.ca, to quickly source out all your ingredients with the click of a button!

bakerlita.market/collections/bake-pantry

ALMOND FLOUR

Almond flour is my number one most used ingredient for most of my baking. Not only are almonds very low in carbs *(among the lowest out of all nuts)*, but they are also highly alkalizing to the body and provide an abundance of amazing vitamins and minerals. Another reason I love using almond flour in almost all of my recipes is that it is rich in fibre, protein, and healthy monounsaturated fats leading to a much more moist and delicious dessert. As for the ground type, I always try to find: ***fine ground blanched.*** However, if you cannot use almonds due to an almond allergy, try sunflower seed flour or cashew flour for a lower-carb option. Cassava flour can also be a beautiful substitution, however, it is a bit higher in carbs.

COCONUT FLOUR

Coconut flour has far fewer healthy fats than almond flour. However, it has far more fibre, which will satisfy you and your tummy for hours. I typically combine a small amount of coconut flour in most of my baking recipes to balance out the almond flour, soak up any extra liquid/moisture, and give the end product a beautiful balance of structure and depth. For example, if you were to bake cookies just with almond flour, instead of one dozen cookies, you would obtain ONE giant cookie as big as the baking sheet because there would be no structure/fibre ingredient to hold the individual cookies together. Coconut flour provides the needed structure.

MONK FRUIT

Mont fruit is a naturally occurring sweetener. It acts just like sugar, with a 1-to-1 ratio for any recipe. Unlike stevia, monk fruit has zero aftertastes and tastes exactly like sugar. Monk fruit comes from a small round fruit in the gourd family, also known as Luo Han Guo, named after the Luo Han monks who discovered it. The best part about this sweet goodness is that it has zero calories and zero negative effects on your glycemic index. Subbing monk fruit even for the popular paleo options of coconut sugar, honey, and maple syrup will dramatically help you control your overall carb/sugar intake. I could not imagine baking without this glorious sweetener, and it will surely become your favourite too! My number one recommended brand for monk fruit is **Lakanto.** You can purchase it on my website:
bakerlita.market/pages/bake-pantry

GRANULATED MONK FRUIT

Granulated monk fruit is my absolute favourite. Just as sugar has the option of a granular texture, you can also find that in many brands of monk fruit. This type of sweetener is my staple sweetener for all my recipes. You will not be able to tell the difference between monk fruit and traditional sugar - it is that good!

POWDERED MONK FRUIT

Powdered monk fruit acts as icing sugar *(yet sugar-fee, and good for you)*. It is a must for any frostings, icings, glazes, and in anything, you don't want the grittiness from the granulated version.

OTHER SWEETENERS

There are other sugar-free natural sweeteners out there. However, monk fruit does not only taste the best, but it also has the most health benefits. The following are also potential sugar substitutes. Please note, however, that they could cause some stomach issues *(diarrhea/tummy discomfort)*.

- Erythritol
- Xylitol

BUTTER *(grass-fed)*

Truthfully, I have always been anti-dairy until I met my new favourite sidekick for my baking, grass-fed butter. It is called grass-fed butter because the cows eat grass, making their butter high in unsaturated omega-3 fatty acids. Not only does grass-fed butter have impressive health and gut benefits, but it also hardly has any lactose.

Grass-fed butter usually comes from cows that do not eat any grains. This is important because cows that eat grains tend to have more unwanted saturated omega-6 & 9 fatty acids. One of my favourite gut-healing properties in grass-fed butter is high in butyric acid *(for which butter is named).* Butyric is considered anti-inflammatory. Studies have shown that butyric acid has helped heal Crohn's disease. Butyric acid is actually the preferred food for the cells of the colon. Grass-fed butter is one of the best fats to bake and cook with since it has an extremely high smoke *(heat)* point of 485° F, which makes it the perfect baking pantry staple.

So butter up, buttercup! It is a no-brainer that baking with butter minimizes fat oxidation and maximizes flavour. Grass-fed butter contains high amounts of vitamin A, K2, and CLA-conjugated linoleic acid *(which may help burn stubborn body fat and may help prevent certain chronic diseases, such as type 2 diabetes, heart disease, and even certain cancers).*

GHEE *(grass-fed)*

For all who are lactose and casein sensitive, you may find that ghee is a great substitute for grass-fed butter. Ghee is grass-fed butter that has gone through a clarifying process. This process heats the butter until the liquid fat and milk solids have separated, which eliminates almost all the digestive upsets caused by milk solids from dairy proteins, lactose and casein.

COLLAGEN *(grass-fed)*

Collagen is what made my baked goods truly stand out from most other keto and paleo bakeries. Collagen is by far my biggest secret when it comes to creating a chewy texture in my baking - especially when making cookies, brownies and blondies. And it's even great for making a sticky caramel sauce! Collagen has been a huge contribution to the healing of my stomach over the past seven years. Believe it or not, you can source this miracle protein from cows, fish and even plants. I typically use organic grass-fed beef collagen; it has almost zero flavours and dissolves beautifully. The list of benefits of adding collagen to our diet is endless. As I mentioned above, it heals the digestive tract and intestines by rebuilding the walls. Collagen also builds and restores muscles, ligaments, and tendons. And a few of my favourite natural beauty-boosting benefits are that it helps grow strong and luscious hair, adds a healthy, youthful glow and firmness to your skin, reduces fine lines and wrinkles, and reduces the appearance of fine lines and wrinkles, strengthens your skin and nails. Okay, I can keep going on and on - but when it comes to baking, it is the only heat-resistant protein that doesn't get damaged when used in baking/cooking. Once heated, other proteins create toxins, leading to more inflammation once ingested. My number one recommended brand for collagen is **Organika.** You can purchase it on my website: *bakerlita.market/pages/bake-pantry*

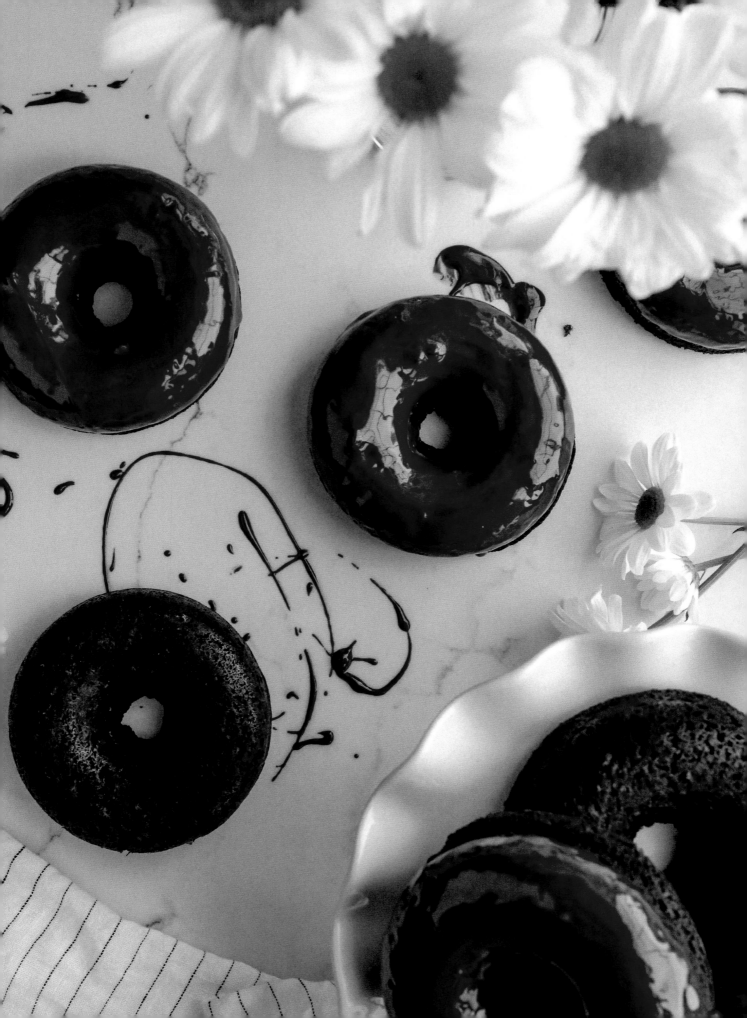

PALM SHORTENING

If you absolutely cannot do any dairy, I found that high-quality, organic palm shortening makes a fantastic substitution for butter. However, keep in mind that shortening has more fat than butter, so if you are baking cookies, you may need to add a few extra tablespoons of coconut flour to compensate for the excess moisture and maintain its structure. Palm shortening is an excellent substitute for vegan and dairy-free frosting.

EGGS -FREE RUN

I always choose farm-fresh, local, organic free-run eggs when sourcing eggs. I guess you could also call them *happy eggs from happy chicken!* Eggs are an excellent complete source of high-quality protein and are rich in Omega-3 fatty acids. Eggs contain a good dose of selenium, choline, vitamin D & B12, riboflavin, and phosphorus. Eggs are the best binders for baking, bringing together all the beautiful ingredients and flavours as one perfect baked good. Eggs are also fantastic for creating that desired fluffy, light, airy structure, especially in gluten-free baking.

AVOCADO OIL

Baking the Bakerlita Way is all about healthy fats. Avocado oil was a game-changer when I started incorporating it into my cakes, cupcakes, muffins, and donut recipes. Usually, when you look up a traditional cake recipe, it typically calls for canola oil, which is highly unhealthy for you. Yet, it does create a perfectly moist and decadent dessert.

I tried many oil alternatives and found that avocado oil simulated the same effect as canola oil, adding all the healthy nutrients I was looking for. Like grass-fed butter and coconut oil, avocado has a high smoke point *(the temperature at which oil begins to degrade and become toxic under heat),* making it an optimal choice for high-heat baking and cooking without jeopardizing any of the health benefits this lovely oil has to give.

Top 7 Health Benefits
- *lowers (LDL) bad cholesterol*
- *lowers blood pressure*
- *detoxes toxins in your body*
- *fights fine lines & wrinkles*
- *thicker & faster-growing hair*
- *helps burn body fat*
- *boosts nutrient absorption*

COCONUT OIL

Coconut oil, like avocado oil, has many health qualities. I love the flavour of coconut oil when creating a coconut dessert. One of the unique features of coconut oil is that it is made up of medium-chained saturated fatty acids *(MCFAs,* also known as MCT oil), which are used highly efficiently as clean, long-lasting energy for the body.

COCONUT CREAM/MILK

Coconut cream is such an excellent dairy-free alternative. One of my favourite uses of coconut cream is to make a lovely fluffy, and coconut whipped cream. Make sure you always read the labels to make sure it is BPA-free.

PSYLLIUM HUSK POWDER

Psyllium husk powder is an excellent ingredient when baking keto and paleo-friendly recipes. There isn't a better alternative to this high-fibre flour to create a glutenous *(without-the gluten)* texture. Psyllium works wonders for quick bread recipes, like donuts, bread and cinnamon buns. It also works great when added in small amounts to cupcakes and cakes, adding more structure to the cake base. Also, adding psyllium to your diet will keep you regular and more satisfied between meals or desserts!

CACAO/COCOA POWDER

Eat chocolate! Raw, unsweetened cacao has incredible, health-boosting benefits. However, I like combining it with less nutritious, dutch processed cocoa to add depth and richness to any decadent chocolate dessert. Look for organic, unsweetened cacao & dutch processed cocoa.

Do you know the happy feeling of Serotonin in your brain when you indulge in chocolate? It comes from the lovely, natural contents of cacao, not sugar! When your brain produces Serotonin, it acts as a natural antidepressant & reduces emotional stress. Many of these beautiful benefits result from cacao's blessed polyphenols, which are micronutrients and a natural compound with powerful antioxidant properties.

Eat Cacao & reap the rewards
- *reduces inflammation*
- *lowers risks of chronic disease*
- *prevents aging*
- *powerhouse antioxidant*
- *reduces blood pressure*
- *reduces stress*
- *reduces levels of glucose*
- *increases testosterone*

CACAO BUTTER

When making homemade chocolate bars or chocolate chips, you will need high-quality cocoa butter. This glorious fat comes directly from cocoa beans. Just like cacao powder, it has an impressive profile of health benefits and is delicious!

CHOCOLATE BARS & CHIPS

You will notice that a good portion of Bakerlita recipes will use some chocolate chips and bars. Finding a high-quality, organic, sugar-free, and dairy-free chocolate bar or chips can be hard to come by. However, I have my most loved brands in my Amazon shop **(link can be found on page 9).**

I created a fantastic **chocolate bar and chocolate chip recipe on page 223** if you are looking to make it yourself. However, buying my recommended brands can make your baking experience much less time-consuming. If you have the extra time, I suggest bulk-producing your chocolate to have a large backup stock ready to go.

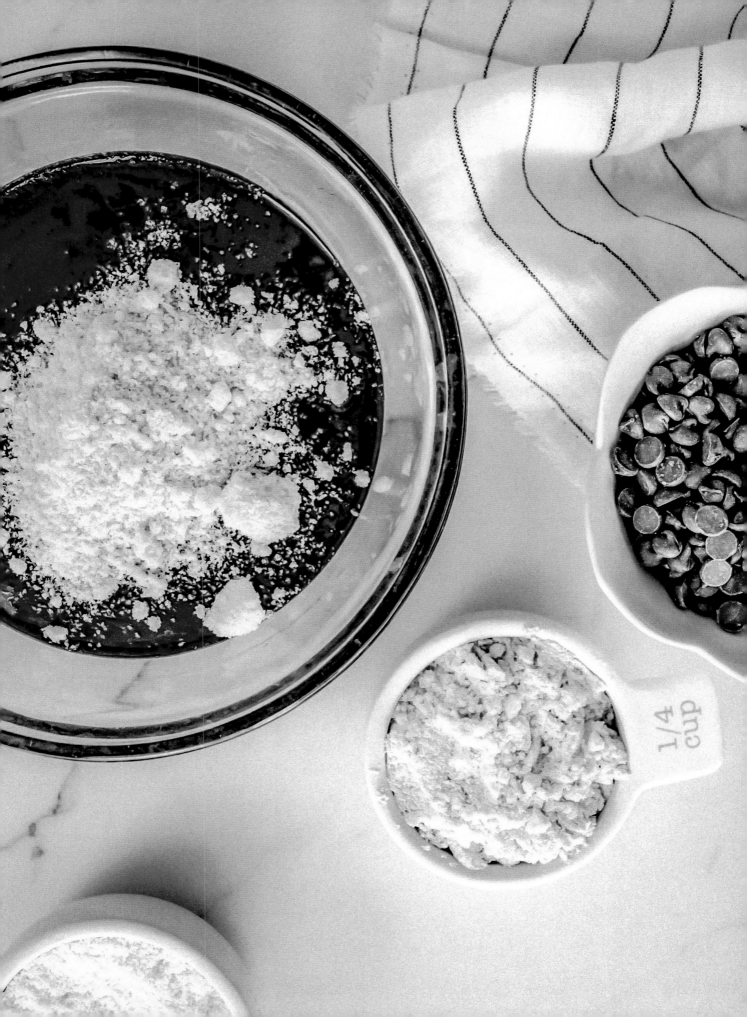

GELATIN (grass-fed)

Like the glorious collagen protein, gelatin is a beautiful binder with just as many beauty-boosting benefits as collagen. It works wonders for thickening custards and jams! I don't use it often, but for suitable recipes, it works wonders! I only use grass-fed, organic cow collagen.

ARROWROOT FLOUR

Arrowroot or tapioca flour is a natural-flavoured flour used extensively in Paleo baking. However, it is high in carbs, so I use it sparingly. My primary use is dusting the top of my artesian homemade bread. Arrowroot flour is a great thickener alternative as well.

BAKING POWDER

Baking powder is always a must in baking and especially in gluten-free baking. Look for brands that are free of cornstarch and aluminum.

BAKING SODA

Baking soda and baking powder are both used for leavening. One way to help your baking get extra fluffy and light are to add acid ingredients (such as lemon juice and apple cider) to your baking soda.

LEMON JUICE

As mentioned above, I typically use lemon juice in my vanilla-based cakes and cupcakes - it's a great way to fluff up your cake to the next level! Always get 100% pure lemon juice.

APPLE CIDER VINEGAR

Apple cider vinegar is a fermented apple juice. Like lemon juice, it is a great leavening agent. More importantly, apple cider kills *harmful & bad* bacteria, and it helps the growth of *good* bacteria. I have used apple cider for years to help add those much-needed gut-healing bacteria and enzymes. I especially love using apple cider vinegar in my quick bread recipes.

HIMALAYAN SEA SALT

Salt enhances flavours, especially the fantastic ph-balancing Himalayan sea salt. Yes, even in your sweets. When my baking is lacking in the salt department, it tastes like it is missing something fundamental. Himalayan sea salt is the most stunning salt, and it is loaded with 84 marvellous minerals.

HONEY/ MAPLE SYRUP

There are endless health benefits to adding raw honey and pure maple syrup to your diet. However, Baking The Bakerlita Way is all about reducing the overall intake of sugars and overall carbs. Using honey or maple syrup as your primary sweetener *(even if it's paleo approved)* will not allow your body to use your fabulous long-lasting fat as fuel, nor your stored sugars and carbohydrates as energy. I only use the "healthy," unrefined, natural sugars to activate my yeast recipes. I only use honey/maple syrup when I want to activate the yeast. Typically you only need 1-2 tablespoons to activate the yeast to make a batch of fluffy, delicious cinnamon buns or donuts *(or any quick bread recipe)*.

VANILLA EXTRACT

Of course, any baker knows the delightful aroma of good quality, pure vanilla extract. And most of you know how expensive it is! But it is worth every penny since there is nothing like a batch of freshly baked vanilla cupcakes with a lovely natural hint of vanilla. Try finding a gluten-free source.

NUTS/ NUT BUTTERS

Who isn't nuts for nut butter? Adding slightly roasted & salted nuts into or onto any recipe calls for a gathering. Nuts have so many unique flavours that they can completely transform a recipe into wide, excellent varieties just by changing what nut you use. This is especially true when making it into flour for the recipe's base. Nuts, of course, are packed full of healthy fats, proteins, and a small number of carbs. Like any ingredient, always choose fresh, raw, and, if possible organic. The flavour will always add an extra edge to your baking. Nut recipe example: *Raw Strawberry Cashew Cheese Cake* or *Creamy Cashew Cheese*. They are both so simple to make and contain mainly nuts!

BLACKSTRAP MOLASSES

Blackstrap molasses is the healthiest molasses of all because it contains the most vitamins and minerals. It is also the thickest and darkest of molasses. A little of this glorious *"black nectar"* goes a long way, and your cookies will thank you for it.

Adding one teaspoon to a batch of cookies will replicate the perfect homemade cookies without the brown sugar!

FRESH BERRIES/FRUIT

Buying fresh local fruit is the best, but for many of us, spring and summer are the only *"fruit seasons," and they* only come once a year. Making the most of those short seasons can mean getting up extra early to hit your local farmers' markets. Fruits, with their natural bright colours and flavours, are an easy and perfect addition to decorating or garnishing cakes, cupcakes, pies, etc. This is a great way to get the best quality fruits and support your local community. One way to save money is to check your natural grocery store for frozen berries since they are great for jams and fillings. Just make sure you look for organic since berries are highly sprayed. Berries are your best bet when it comes to low carbs and sugars. I also like to incorporate small amounts of apples and bananas into some of my recipes to give them those loved flavours that you can't live without!

SPICES & HERBS

Sugar and spice, and everything nice. There are just a few spices that you should not go without in your pantry. Cinnamon stands out the most - it is used in many combinations to add warmth and a festive feel. You will notice other spices throughout the recipes. Like always, choose organic for the best quality and flavour.

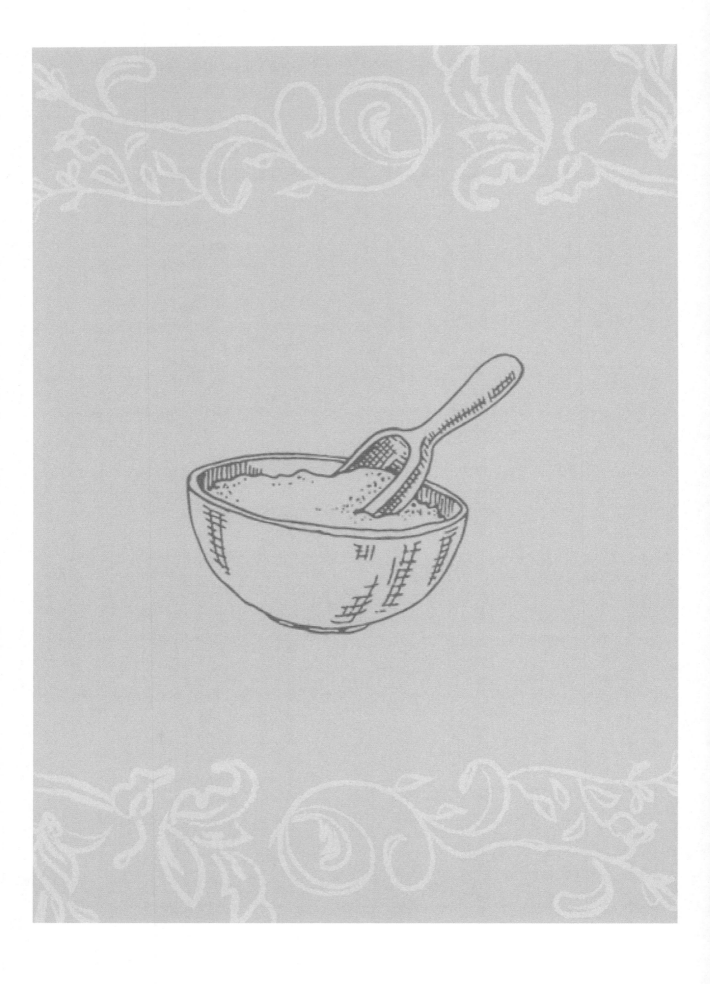

Essential Baking Tools

You don't need many baking tools to make most of these beautiful baked goods. However, I believe in investing in some more expensive pieces of equipment to make the baking experience a blissful delight.

Basics to bake the Bakerlita way

Like the ingredients, when you want to get the most bang for your buck on some essential baking tools, it can seem exhausting to research what the best brands are. I have made another page on my website, sourced from Amazon.ca, to quickly source out all your essential tools with the click of a button.

bakerlita.market/collections/bake-ware

STAND MIXER

A stand mixer can make the job of whipping up a beautiful batch of buttercream, coconut whipped cream, cookies, or even just mixing a thicker dough/batter *(like my beauty bombs)* much more manageable. I use the stand mixer's beater blade and whisk attachment daily. However, if you can't afford a good stand mixer, invest in a less expensive, handheld electric mixer. My favourite brand is KitchenAid.

BOWLS AND WHISKS

Yes, you can almost get away with using just these two tools for all of the Bakerlita recipes. You will most definitely need plenty of bowls in a variety of sizes. I would also recommend purchasing some glass, heat-proof bowls for melting chocolate.

KITCHEN SCALE

I use my scale to weigh all my ingredients, even the wet/liquid ones. Kitchen scales do a much more accurate job than measuring the ingredients with cups. Purchase one ASAP!

RUBBER SPATULA

There is no better baking tool for getting every last drop of your cherished ingredients. With a rubber spatula, you can scrap the last bit of dough, batter, or icing out of your bowl. Also, I find them a perfect tool for mixing and folding. Look for a few different sizes; small ones are great for getting into those tight spaces, like blenders.

COOKIE SCOOPS

Cookie scoops are a must. Invest in three to four different sizes of high-quality cookie scoops. Scoops also work wonders for portioning out cupcakes and donut batter.

Small size: 1.5 Tbsp/ 23 ml/ 0.8 oz
Medium size: 2.8 Tbsp/ 42 ml/ 1.4 oz
Large size: 5.4 Tbsp/ 81 ml/ 2.7 oz

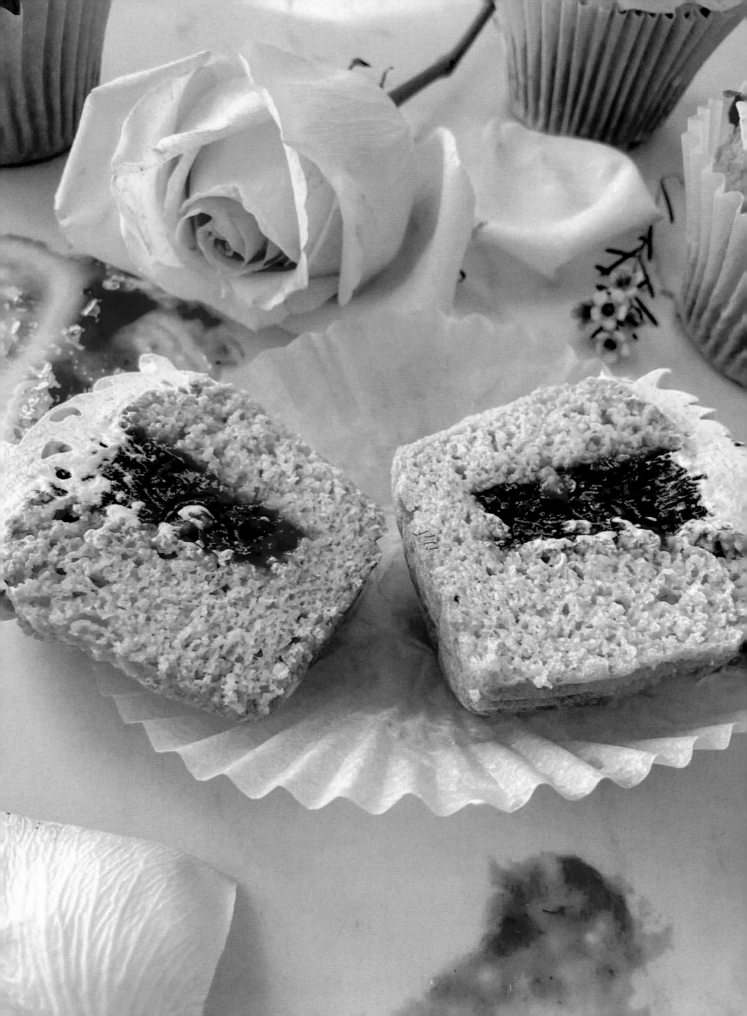

HIGH SPEED BLENDER

Having a high-quality blender is one piece of equipment I highly recommend purchasing. My most recommended blender is a Vitamix. Nothing is quite as efficient when it comes to making a creamy, silky and smooth cashew cheese, cashew cheesecake batter, and nut butter.

FOOD PROCESSOR

A food processor can also get ingredients processed/blended into a silky smooth state, much like a blender. However, food processors work wonders for making homemade nut flours *(almonds, hazelnuts, and even macadamia)*. Most food processors also come with graters, so grating up carrots or zucchini can drastically cut down your prep time.

BAKING/COOKIE SHEETS

You will want to have at least 2-4 cookie sheets on hand at all times. Invest in a few regular sizes and one larger pan. A half-sheet pan is lovely to have on hand to make a batch of two dozen cookies when you have extra company coming over.

OFFSET SPATULA

Spreading the icing layers onto the cake, decorating your cake by making those beautiful simple curves, or levelling out the brownie batter before popping them into the oven calls for an offset spatula. Offset spatulas look like a flat butter knife with a little bend on the end. If possible, look for a smaller one; it's much easier to get into tight corners when spreading.

BAKING/LOAF PAN

Making brownies, blondies, lemon squares, crumble bars, bread and loaf cakes (to name a few) will require baking/loaf pans. I would suggest getting a couple of 8 inches by 8 inches or 8 inches by 12 inches pans to double recipes if you're hosting any gatherings. Also, a good loaf pan size is 4 inches by 8 inches.

SPRINGFORM CAKE PAN

I don't think I will ever again bake 6 or 9-inch cakes without a springform cake pan. Once I tried it and saw how easy it is to get cakes to come out of the pan, I never looked back. The bottom is removable and has an easy-release buckle, making the cake base come out effortlessly!

PARCHMENT PAPER

I use parchment paper in almost every recipe when lining cookie sheets, cake pans, and loaf pans. Plus, it makes clean-up time *(washing your sheets & pans)* a piece of cake.

PIPING TIPS

The wonderful thing about piping tips is that you don't need to be a great baker to make a gorgeous rose cupcake! I typically use only three piping tips for all of my cupcakes and cakes:

- Making that sweet swirl is the **Ateco 805 tip** *(large round)*.
- The irresistible rose is the **Ateco 823 tip** *(Large star)*.
- The beautiful, elegant ruffle is the **Wilton 190** *(open star)*.

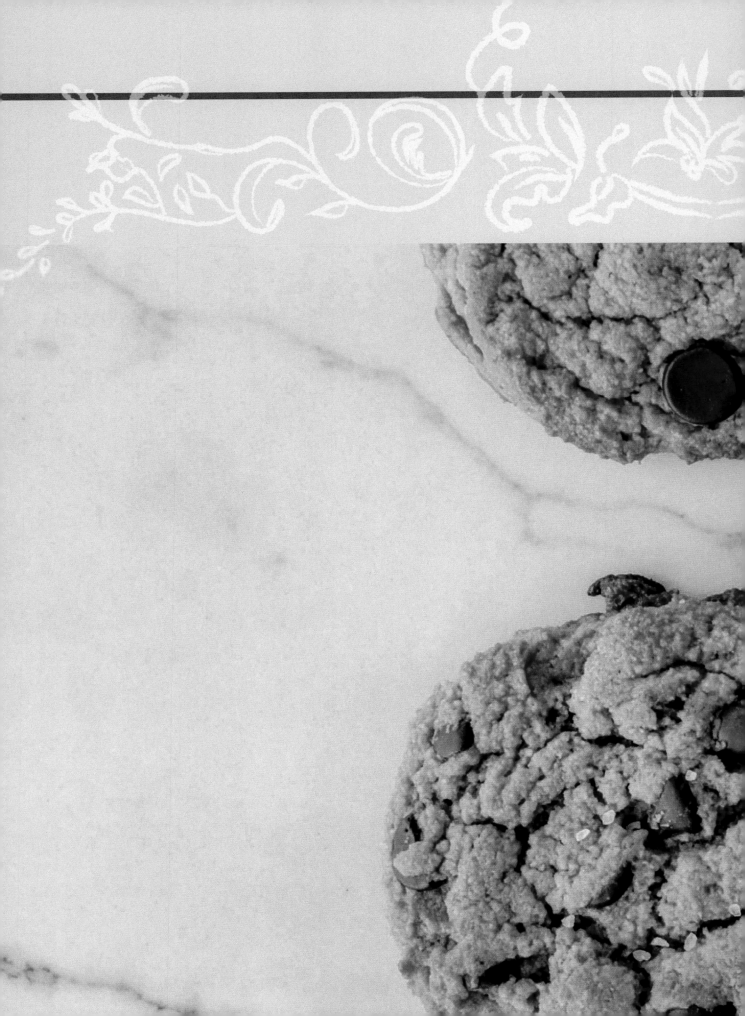

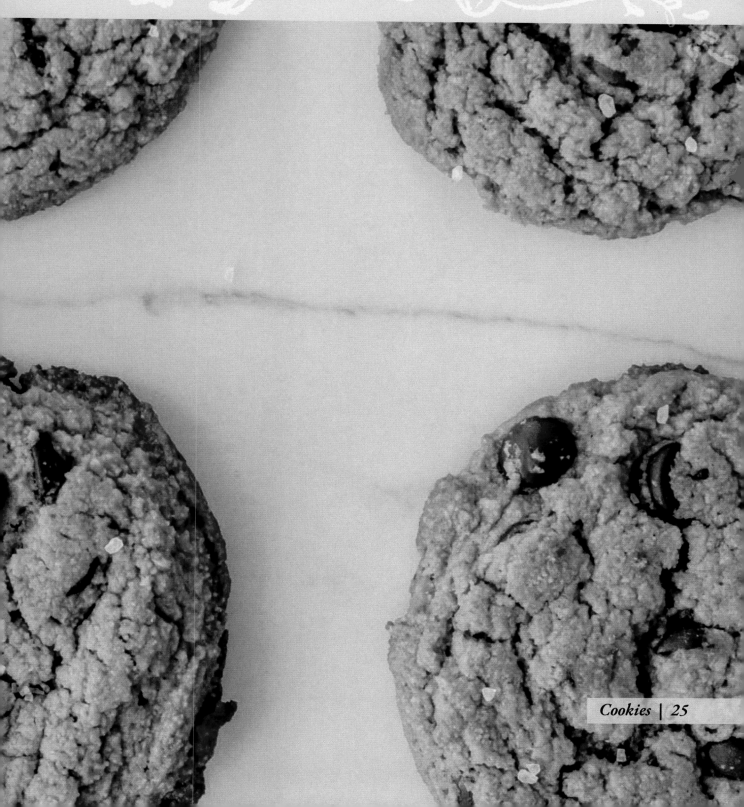

Chapter One COOKIES

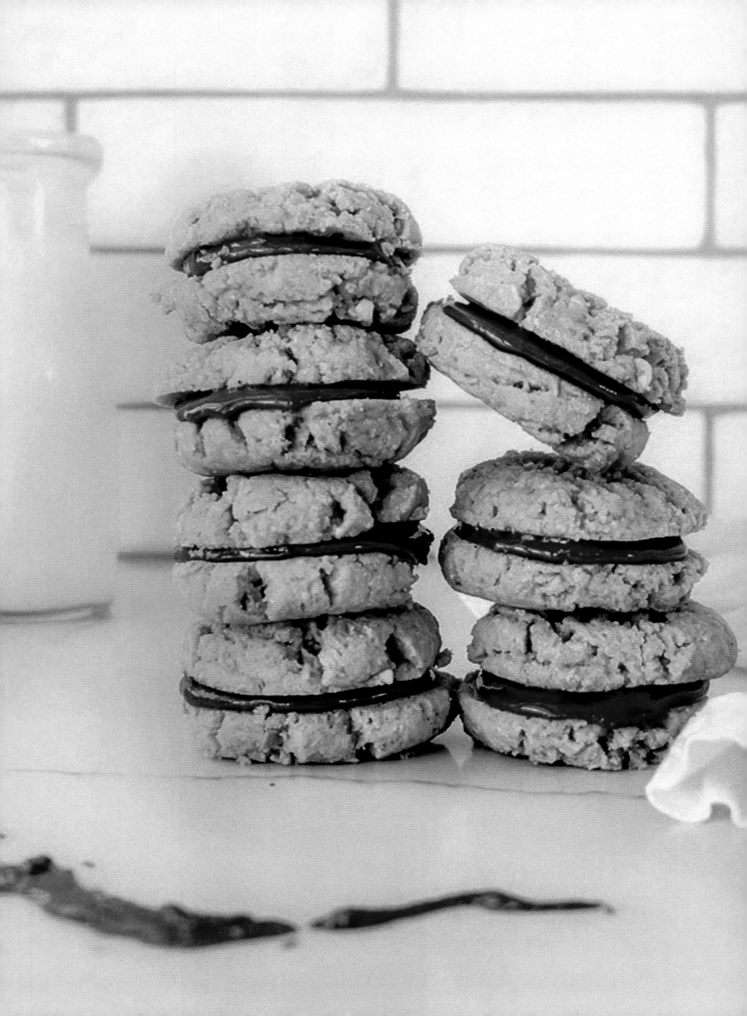

Reversed Reese's

prep: *19 min* **bake:** *7-9 min* **cool:** *5-10 min* **serves:** *14-18 cookies*

I have never met a person who didn't adore the intelligent combination of chocolate and peanut butter. I believe God knew that these two ingredients were meant to go together to bring us joy. Oh, how they complement one another. These cute little reversed Reese's cookies are so deliciously heavenly.

Dry ingredients
- 168g *(1½ cups)* almond flour
- 46g *(1/2 cup)* coconut flour
- 56g *(1/2 cup)* organic collagen *grass-fed*
- 152g *(3/4 cup)* sweetener
  monk fruit, erythritol, xylitol
- 1 teaspoon sea salt
- 1 teaspoon baking soda

Wet ingredients
- 1 free-run egg *room temp*
- 113g *(1/2 cup)* grass-fed butter *room temp*
  sub for palm shortening to make **DF**
- 57g *(1/2 cup)* peanut butter *natural*
- 10mL *(2 teaspoons)* blackstrap molasses
- 10mL *(2 teaspoons)* pure vanilla extract

Chocolate ganache filling
- 120g *(1/2 cup)* peanut butter *natural*
- 110g *(1/2cup)* chocolate chip
  the recipe is found on page 223
- 14g *(1 tablespoon)* coconut oil extra virgin
- 60g *(1/2 cup)* powdered sweetener
  monk fruit, erythritol, xylitol

Instructions
1. Mix all dry ingredients into a medium bowl; whisk until combined, and set aside.
2. Cream butter, peanut butter & sweetener in a stand mixer bowl with a beater blade/paddle attachment or an electric hand mixer. Beat until softened, 3-4 minutes. The butter should become lighter and almost double in volume.
3. Add the egg, vanilla, and molasses to the butter, and continue to cream for another 5 minutes.
4. Add all the dry ingredients to the butter mixture and beat until incorporated.
5. Prepare a baking sheet with parchment paper using a **small-size 1.85-inch scoop**; scoop out cookies on a baking sheet *(about 14-18 cookies)*.
6. Using the palm of your hand, slightly press down the cookie.
7. Place cookies in the fridge for 20min to allow them to chill.
8. **Preheat oven to 350°F/180°C.**
9. Bake for 7-9 minutes.
10. Allow the cookies to cool completely on the tray while making chocolate PB filling.
11. **PB chocolate ganache:** In a small heatproof bowl, melt chocolate chips with coconut oil in the microwave for 10-sec intervals, stirring between intervals; repeat 3-5 times until completely melted.
12. Add peanut butter and powdered sweetener. Mix until well incorporated, and it becomes a thick paste.
13. Add a heaping ½ tablespoon of PB chocolate filling on each cookie's flipped bottom sides.
14. Sandwich them together by adding the top to each cookie.
15. Store in an airtight container for five to six days and freeze for up to three months.

Note

- Make sure your butter is soft to the touch and at room temperature
- Let the egg sit out at room temperature for a few hours before using it
- The cookies will spread somewhat during baking, but you still need to pre-shape them. The more you pre-flatten them, the more they'll spread.

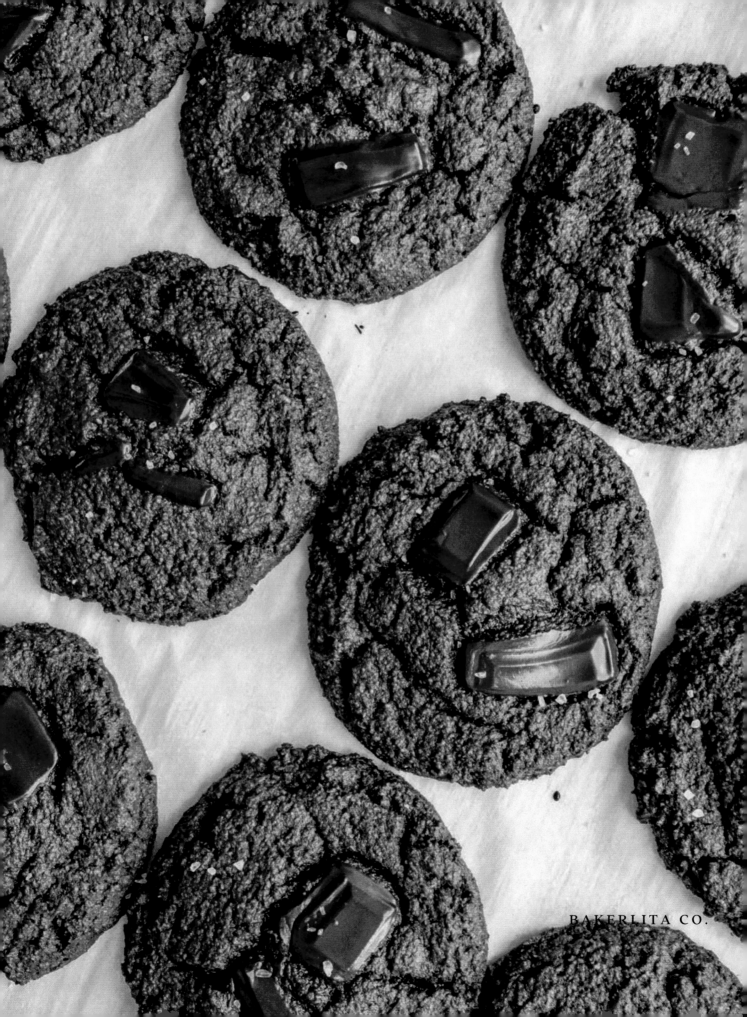

Double Chocolate Chunk

prep: *12 min*   **bake:** *9-11 min*   **cool:** *5-10 min*   **serves:** *12 cookies*

Ever since I was a little girl, my sister and I LOVED double chocolate chunk cookies. I am sure not only will you love them, but your kiddos will enjoy them just as much and not even know they are healthy for them too! These cookies taste like the real deal - actually even better.

Dry ingredients

- 168g *(1½ cups)* almond flour
- 56g *(1/2 cup)* cocoa powder
- 34g *(1/4 cup)* coconut flour
- 56g *(1/2 cup)* organic collagen *grass-fed*
- 152g *(3/4 cup)* sweetener
  monk fruit, erythritol, xylitol
- 1 teaspoon sea salt
- 1 teaspoon baking soda
- 80g *(1 full bar)* chocolate bar
  the recipe is found on page 223
- flaky sea salt - *to garnish*

Wet ingredients

- 113g *(1/2 cup)* grass-fed butter *room temp*
  sub for palm shortening to make **DF**
- 1 free-run egg *room temp*
- 2 teaspoons blackstrap molasses
- 10mL *(2 teaspoons)* pure vanilla extract

Instructions

1. Mix all dry ingredients into a medium bowl; whisk until combined and set aside.
2. Cream butter & sweetener in a stand mixer bowl with a beater blade/paddle attachment or an electric hand mixer. Beat until softened, 3-4 minutes. The butter should become lighter and almost double in volume.
3. Add the egg, vanilla, and molasses to the butter, and continue to cream for another 5 minutes.
4. Add all the dry ingredients to the butter mixture, and beat again until incorporated.
5. Prepare a baking sheet with parchment paper. Using a **medium-size 1.97-inch** scoop, scoop cookies onto the baking sheet. This recipe will yield 9 jumbo cookies or 12 medium cookies.
6. Using the palm of your hand, slightly press down the cookies.
7. Chop up the chocolate bar in chunks, and press down two chocolate chunks on top of each cookie.
8. Place cookies in the fridge for 20min to allow them time to chill.
9. **Preheat oven to 350°F/180°C.**
10. Bake for 9-10 minutes for the medium cookies and 12-13 minutes for the jumbo ones. Remove from oven.
11. Garnish with flaky sea salt, allow the cookies to cool completely on the trays & enjoy with a cup of coffee!
12. Store in an airtight container for five to six days and freeze for up to three months.

Note

- Make sure your butter is soft to the touch and at room temperature
- Let the egg sit out at room temperature for a few hours before using it
- The cookies will spread somewhat during baking, but you still need to pre-shape them. The more you pre-flatten them, the more they'll spread. The more they spread, the crispier they'll be, so if you like them cakier, don't flatten them too much!

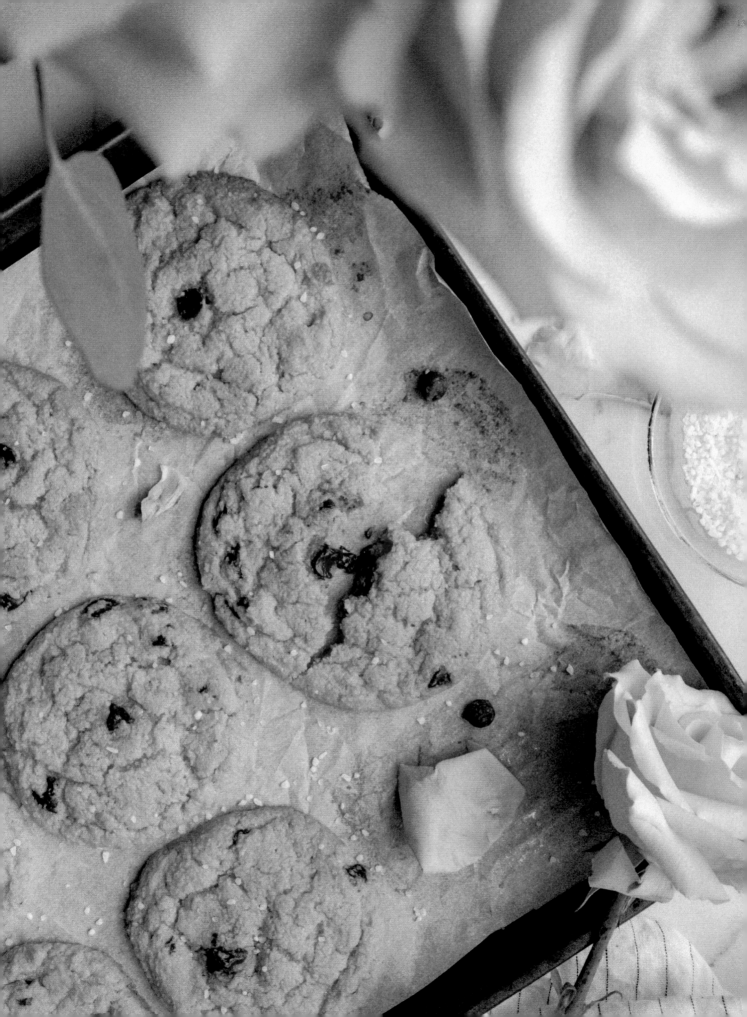

Classic Chewy Chocolate Chip

prep: *15 min*   **bake:** *10-12 min*   **cool:** *5-10 min*   **serves:** *12 cookies*

There is no question that a classic chocolate chip cookie is the most popular cookie of them all. This recipe was the first item I made when I started my bakery. I tested different combinations and perfected this beautiful bakery-style cookie by adding collagen to create that desired chewy texture! Now, my Chocolate Chip cookie is one of my number one sellers, and you will see why, once you have your first bite.

Dry ingredients

- 168g *(1½ cups)* almond flour
- 46g *(1/3 cup)* coconut flour
- 56g *(1/2 cup)* organic collagen *grass-fed*
- 152g *(3/4 cup)* sweetener
  monk fruit, erythritol, xylitol
- 1 teaspoon sea salt
- 1 teaspoon baking soda
- 110g *(1/2 cup)* chocolate chip
  the recipe is found on page 223
- flaky sea salt - *to garnish*

Wet ingredients

- 113g *(1/2 cup)* grass-fed butter *room temp*
  sub for palm shortening to make DF
- 1 free-run egg *room temp*
- 2 teaspoons blackstrap molasses
- 10mL *(2 teaspoons)* pure vanilla extract

Instructions

1. Mix all dry ingredients into a medium bowl; whisk until combined, and set aside.
2. Cream butter & sweetener in a stand mixer bowl with a beater blade/paddle attachment or an electric hand mixer. Beat until softened, 3-4 minutes. The butter should become lighter and almost double in volume.
3. Add the egg, vanilla, and molasses to the butter, and continue to cream for another 5 minutes.
4. Add all the dry ingredients to the butter mixture and beat again until incorporated.
5. Prepare a baking sheet with parchment paper, using a **medium-size 1.97-inch scoop**; scoop out cookies on a baking sheet, depending on the size of the scoop, 9 jumbo or 12 medium cookies.
6. Using the palm of your hand, slightly press down the cookie.
7. Place cookies in the fridge for 20min to allow them to chill.
8. **Preheat oven to 350°F/180°C.**
9. Bake smaller cookies for 9-10 minutes and 12-13 minutes for the jumbo.
10. Garnish with flaky sea salt, allow the cookies to cool completely on the trays & enjoy with a cup of coffee!
11. Store in an airtight container for five to six days and freeze for up to three months.

Note

- Make sure your butter is soft to the touch and at room temperature
- Let the egg sit out at room temperature for a few hours before using it
- The cookies will spread somewhat during baking, but you still need to pre-shape them. The more you pre-flatten them, the more they'll spread. The more they spread, the crispier they'll be, so if you like them cakier, don't flatten them too much!

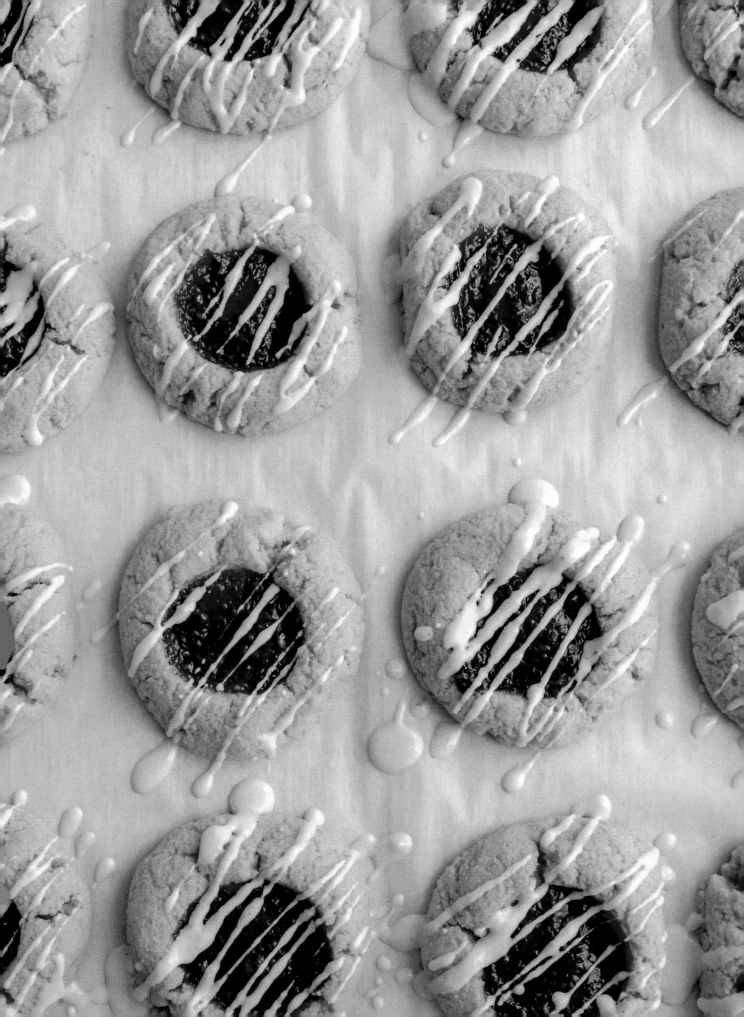

Raspberry Thumbprints

prep: *18 min*   **bake:** *10-12 min*   **cool:** *5-10 min*   **serves:** *12 cookies*

Thumbprint cookies have always been among my favourites, especially considering how easy it is to switch up the jams to make a completely different thumbprint cookie. One of my favourite flavour combinations is white chocolate and raspberry. The white chocolate drizzle is optional for this recipe, yet I believe it makes an ordinary thumbprint into a lovely masterpiece!

Dry ingredients

- 168g *(1½ cups)* almond flour
- 102g *(3/4 cup)* coconut flour
- 56g *(1/2 cup)* organic collagen *grass-fed*
- 152g *(3/4 cup)* sweetener
  monk fruit, erythritol, xylitol
- 1 teaspoon sea salt
- 1 teaspoon baking soda

Wet ingredients

- 113g *(1/2 cup)* grass-fed butter *room temp*
  sub for palm shortening to make DF
- 1 free-run egg *room temp*
- 10mL *(2 teaspoons)* pure vanilla extract
- 5mL *(1 teaspoon)* pure almond extract

Raspberry Jam

- 140g *(1/2 cup)* raspberry jam
  the recipe is found on page 193

White Chocolate

- 40g *(1/2 bar)* white chocolate bar
  the recipe is found on page 221

Instructions

1. Mix all dry ingredients into a medium bowl; whisk until combined, and set aside.
2. Cream butter & sweetener in a stand mixer bowl with a beater blade/paddle attachment or an electric hand mixer; beat until softened, 3-4 minutes; the butter should become lighter and almost double in volume.
3. Add the egg, vanilla, and molasses to the butter, and continue to cream for another 5 minutes.
4. Add all the dry ingredients to the butter mixture, and beat again until incorporated.
5. Prepare a baking sheet with parchment paper. Using a **medium-sized 1.97-inch scoop,** scoop out cookies on a baking sheet, depending on the size of the scoop, 9 jumbo or 12 medium cookies.
6. Using the palm of your hand, carefully roll the cookie dough to form a ball.
7. Using the back of a small **cookie/scoop size: 1.5 Tbsp/ 23 ml/ 0.8 oz),** press down to create a perfect round half whole.
8. Fill each cookie with 2 teaspoons of raspberry jam.
9. Place cookies in the fridge for 20min to allow them to chill.
10. **Preheat oven to 350°F/180°C.**
11. Bake smaller cookies for 9-10 minutes and 12-13 minutes for the jumbo.
12. As the cookies are cooling, prep the melted white chocolate.
13. In a small heatproof bowl, melt white in the microwave for 10-sec intervals, stirring between each interval, and repeat 3-5 times until completely melted.
14. Using a small scoop, drizzle the top of each cookie with white chocolate. Place in fridge to allow to set.
15. Store in an airtight container for three to four days and freeze for up to three months.

Note

- **If your thumbprints spread too much after baking, use a rubber spatula and carefully push around the edge of the cookie to reshape.**
- **Don't overfill with jam; it will overflow during baking, split & ruin the cookies.**

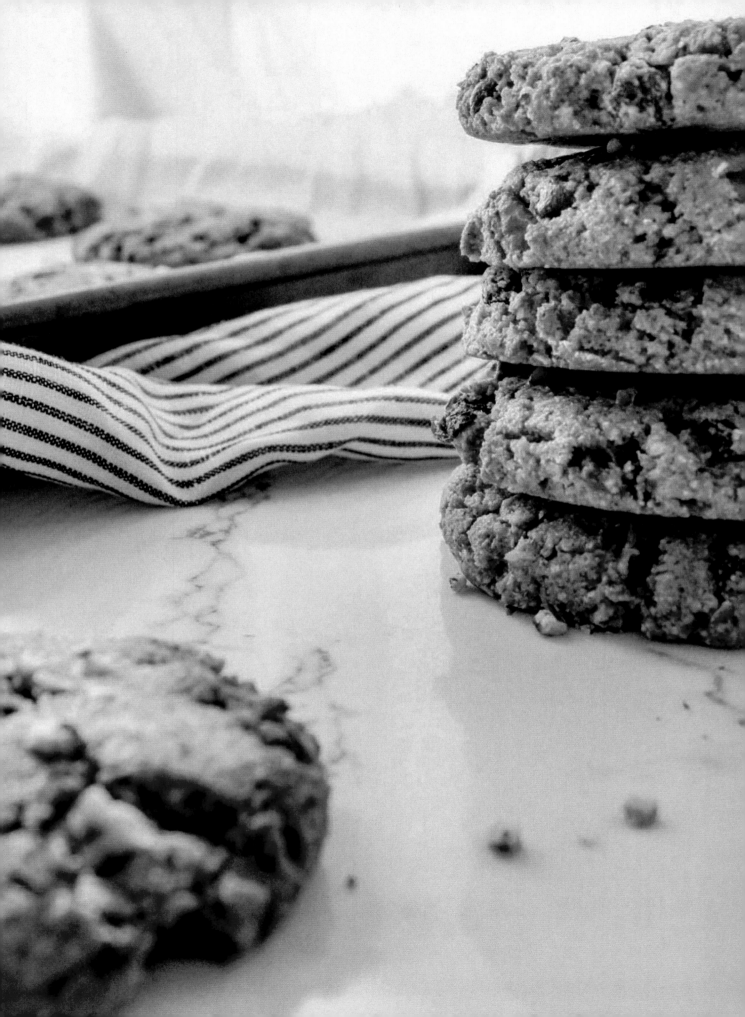

No-Oatmeal Breakfast Cookies

prep: *15 min* **bake:** *10-12 min* **cool:** *5-10 min* **serves:** *12 cookies*

These no-oatmeal, no-grain cookies simulate that beautiful breakfasty cookie so well! Have a few with some dairy-free nut milk, and you have a favourite morning ritual.

Dry ingredients
- 112g *(1 cup)* almond flour
- 46g *(1/3 cup)* coconut flour
- 42g *(1/2 cup)* coconut flakes *unsweetened*
- 14g *(2 tablespoons)* flax meal
- 55g *(1/2 cup)* pecans *chopped*
- 56g *(1/2 cup)* organic collagen *grass-fed*
- 110g *(1/2 cup)* chocolate chip
  the recipe is found on page 223
- 152g *(3/4 cup)* sweetener
  monk fruit, erythritol, xylitol
- 80g *(1/2 cup)* raisins *- optional if on paleo*
- 2 teaspoons cinnamon
- 1 teaspoon sea salt
- 1 teaspoon baking soda
- flaky sea salt *to garnish*

Wet ingredients
- 75g *(1/3 cup)* grass-fed butter *room temp*
  sub for palm shortening to make DF
- 75g *(1/4 cup)* almond butter
- 1 free-run egg *room temp*
- 2 teaspoons blackstrap molasses
- 10mL *(2 teaspoons)* pure vanilla extract

Instructions
1. **Preheat oven to 350°F/180°C. Prep** a cookie sheet with two small pieces of parchment paper side by side,
2. Toast coconut flakes for 4-5 minutes, and toast chopped pecans for 7 minutes; set aside.
3. Mix all dry ingredients into a medium bowl, including the toasted coconut and pecans; whisk until combined, and set aside.
4. Cream butter, almond butter & sweetener in a stand mixer bowl with a beater blade/paddle attachment or an electric hand mixer; beat until softened, 3-4 minutes; the butter should become lighter and almost double in volume.
5. Add the egg, vanilla, and molasses to the butter, and continue to cream for another 5 minutes.
6. Add all the dry ingredients to the butter mixture and beat again until incorporated.
7. Prepare a baking sheet with parchment paper. Using a **medium-size 1.97-inch scoop**, scoop out cookies on a baking sheet, depending on the size of the scoop, 9 jumbo or 12 medium cookies.
8. Using the palm of your hand, slightly press down the cookie.
9. Place cookies in the fridge for 20min to allow them to chill.
10. **Preheat oven to 350°F/180°C.**
11. Bake smaller cookies for 9-10 minutes and 12-13 minutes for the jumbo.
12. Garnish with flaky sea salt, allow the cookies to cool completely on the trays & enjoy with a cup of coffee!
13. Store in an airtight container for five to six days and freeze for up to three months.

Note

- **As noted in the recipe, the raisins add a great bite to the cookie; however, if you are on a keto diet, you can ditch them since they add up in carbs.**

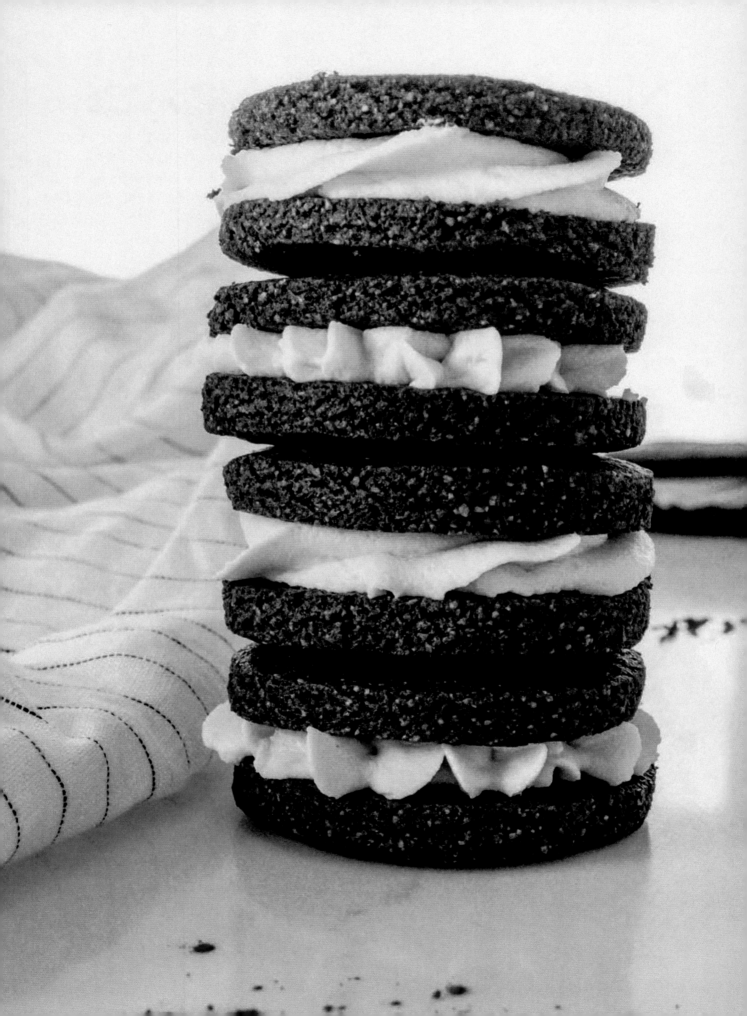

Homemade Oreos

prep: *12 min*   **bake:** *9-11 min*   **cool:** *5-10 min*   **serves:** *12 cookies*

It's true; those classic Oreo cookies have always been my favourite cookie! So it was a must to try to re-create these simple delights into a healthy version, and I absolutely adore them even more than the original ones.

Dry ingredients

- 140g *(1¼ cups)* almond flour
- 56g *(1/2 cup)* cocoa powder
- 18g *(2 tablespoons)* coconut flour
- 152g *(3/4 cup)* sweetener
  monk fruit, erythritol, xylitol
- 1 teaspoon sea salt
- 1 teaspoon baking soda
- 1/4 teaspoon espresso powder

Wet ingredients

- 75g *(1/3 cup)* grass-fed butter *room temp*
  sub for palm shortening to make DF
- 1 free-run egg *room temp*
- 5mL *(1 teaspoons)* pure vanilla extract

Filling/Icing ingredients

- 56g *(1/4 cup)* grass-fed butter *room temp*
  sub for palm shortening to make DF
- 14g *(1 tablespoon)* coconut oil *room temp*
- 120g *(1 cup)* powdered sweetener
  monk fruit, erythritol, xylitol
- 1/8 teaspoons sea salt
- 10mL *(2 teaspoons)* pure vanilla extract

Instructions

1. Mix all dry ingredients into a medium bowl; whisk until combined, and set aside.
2. Cream butter & sweetener in a stand mixer bowl with a beater blade/paddle attachment or an electric hand mixer; beat until softened, 3-4 minutes; the butter should become lighter and almost double in volume.
3. Add the egg, vanilla, and molasses to the butter, and continue to cream for another 5 minutes.
4. Add all the dry ingredients to the butter mixture, and beat again until incorporated.
5. Wrap Oreo dough with saran wrap and refrigerate for at least an hour.
6. **Preheat oven to 350°F/180°C** and line a baking tray with parchment paper.
7. Roll out the dough between two pieces of parchment paper until it is nice and thin. Cut out the rounds for the Oreos. They are roughly 1 3/4 inches in diameter; use a cookie cutter or the rim of a glass cup.
8. Transfer the cookies onto a prepared baking tray and place them in the freezer for 10-15 minutes before baking.
9. Bake for 8-12 minutes.
10. Allow cooling for 10 minutes before transferring to a cooling rack.
11. **Filling:** cream butter and coconut oil in a medium bowl with an electric mixer. Add the vanilla and a pinch of salt, and mix until fully incorporated. Add powdered sweetener and mix until fully incorporated and light and fluffy in texture.
12. Spread or pipe vanilla cream onto a cookie and sandwich between a second one. Refrigerate until set.
13. Store in an airtight container for five to six days and freeze for up to three months.

Note

- **Since these Oreos are already dark in colour, it's hard to tell if they are fully baked. It is important to add the baking time to get them to that nice and crisp Oreo texture. So just keep an eye out for them.**

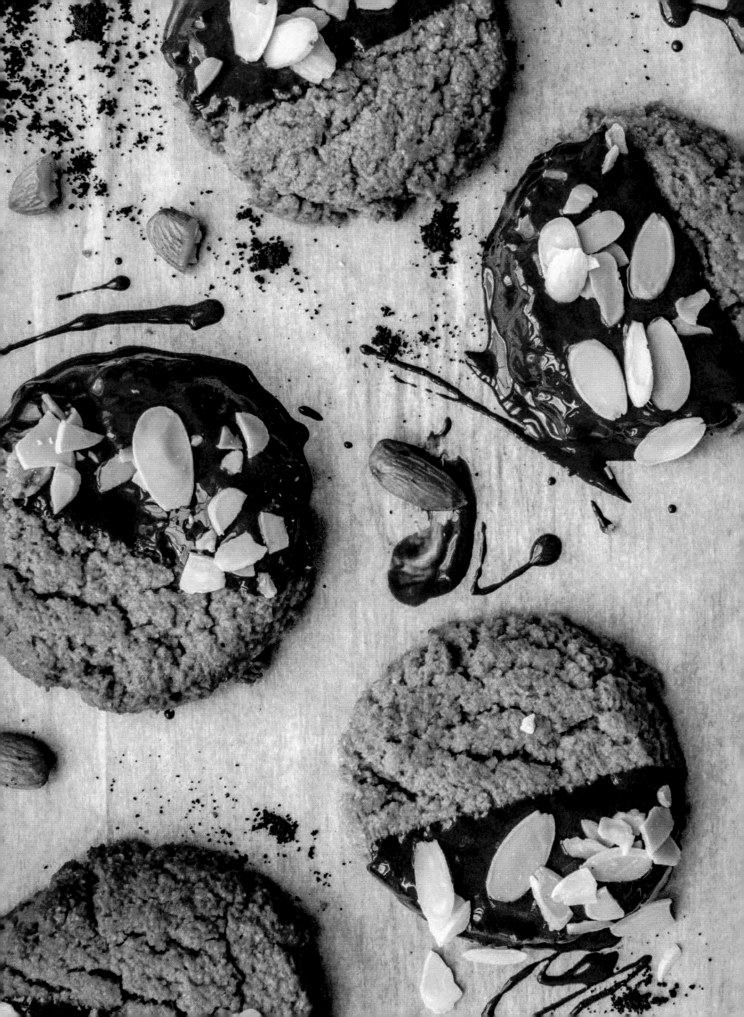

Espresso Almond Delights

prep: *12 min*   **bake:** *10-13 min*   **cool:** *5-10 min*   **serves:** *12 cookies*

Oh, these Espresso cookies are indeed delightful! And they give you a bright and bold boost of energy with the added caffeine from the espresso and dark chocolate. The hint of almond brings these cookies together by adding a lovely nutty aroma to your mouth.

Dry ingredients

- 168g *(1½ cups)* almond flour
- 68g *(1/2 cup)* coconut flour
- 56g *(1/2 cup)* organic collagen *grass-fed*
- 152g *(3/4 cup)* sweetener
  monk fruit, erythritol, xylitol
- 1 teaspoon sea salt
- 1 teaspoon baking soda

Wet ingredients

- 113g *(1/2 cup)* grass-fed butter *room temp*
  Sub for palm shortening to make DF
- 57g *(1/4 cup)* almond butter
  the recipe is found on page 229
- 1 free-run egg *room temp*
- 2 teaspoons blackstrap molasses
- 15g *(2oz)* double shot of espresso *organic*
- 10mL *(2 teaspoons)* pure vanilla extract
- 5mL *(1 teaspoon)* pure almond extract

Chocolate ganache/garnish

- 110g *(1/2 cup)* chocolate chips *melted*
  the recipe is found on page 223
- 14g *(1 tablespoon)* coconut oil *extra virgin*
- 46g *(1/2 cup)* almond slices *toasted/garnish*

Note

- **If you don't have an espresso machine, I recommend purchasing a high-quality instant espresso powder. Add 1tbsp of espresso powder, and dissolve it into 2oz of warm water.**

Instructions

1. **Preheat oven to 325°F/160°C** and line 1 baking sheet with parchment paper.
2. Bake almond slices on the baking sheet for 6min.
3. Mix all dry ingredients into a medium bowl; whisk until combined, and set aside.
4. Cream butter, almond butter & sweetener in a stand mixer bowl with a beater blade/paddle attachment or an electric hand mixer; beat until softened, 3-4 minutes; the butter should become lighter and almost double in volume.
5. Add the egg, espresso, vanilla, almond extract and molasses to the butter, and continue to cream for another 5 minutes.
6. Add all the dry ingredients to the butter mixture, and beat again until incorporated.
7. Prepare a baking sheet with parchment paper. Using a **medium-size 1.97-inch scoop,** scoop out cookies on a baking sheet, depending on the size of the scoop, 9 jumbo or 12 medium cookies.
8. Using the palm of your hand, slightly press down the cookie.
9. Place in the fridge for 20min to allow them to chill.
10. Bake smaller cookies for 9-10 minutes and 12-13 minutes for the jumbo.
11. Cool completely on the trays for about 20 minutes.
12. **Chocolate ganache:** In a small heatproof bowl, melt chocolate chips with coconut oil in the microwave for 10-sec intervals, stirring between intervals; repeat 3-5 times until completely melted.
13. Dunk half of the cookies in the chocolate ganache, and garnish the top with toasted sliced almonds.
14. Place in the fridge for 15 minutes to allow the chocolate to harden, & enjoy with a cup of coffee!
15. Store in an airtight container for one week in the fridge, and freeze for up to three months.

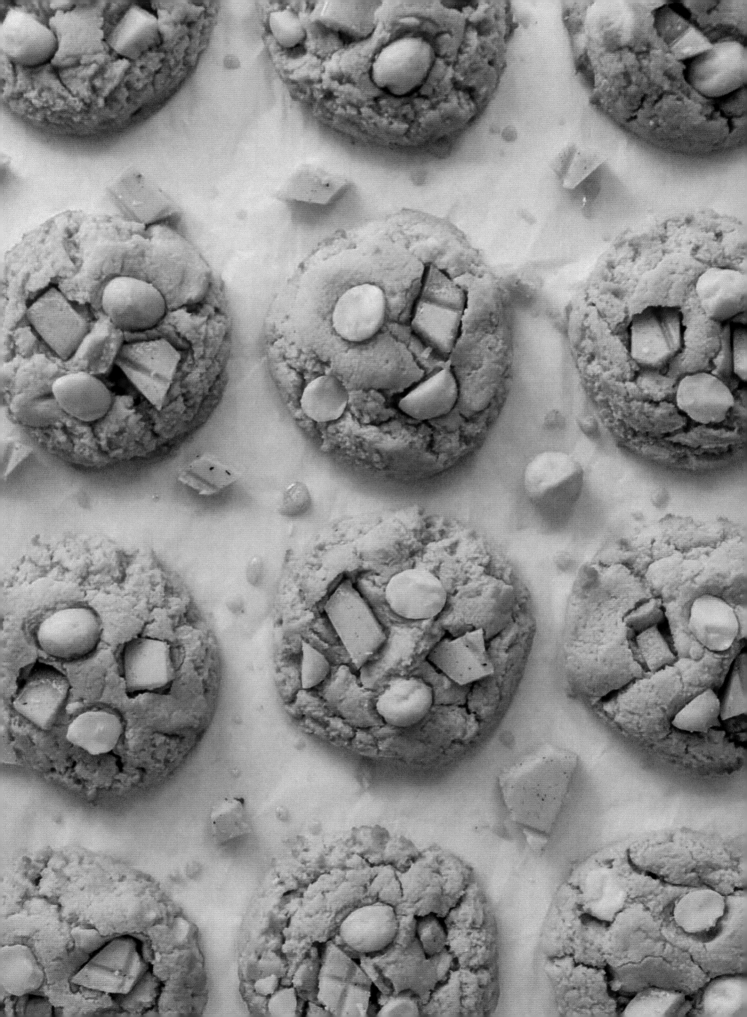

White Chocolate Macadamia

prep: *17 min*   **bake:** *10-13 min*   **cool:** *5-10 min*   **serves:** *12 cookies*

White chocolate macadamia cookies are my hubby's favourite! I wanted to make these cookies extra special and flavourful by adding toasted macadamia nut flour into the recipe. Let's be honest; you don't get the full macadamia experience when there are only three to four pieces on top!

Dry ingredients

- 112g *(1 cup)* almond flour
- 130g *(1 cup)* macadamia nuts *chop fine*
- 68g *(1/2 cup)* coconut flour
- 56g *(1/2 cup)* organic collagen *grass-fed*
- 40g *(1/2 bar)* white chocolate bar *chopped*
  The recipe is found on page 221
- 152g *(3/4 cup)* sweetener
  monk fruit, erythritol, xylitol
- 1 teaspoon sea salt
- 1 teaspoon baking soda

Wet ingredients

- 113g *(1/2 cup)* grass-fed butter *room temp*
  *Sub for palm shortening to make **DF***
- 1 free-run egg *room temp*
- 10mL *(2 teaspoons)* pure vanilla extract

Garnish

- 65g *(1/2 cup)* macadamia nuts
- 80g *(1/2 bar)* white chocolate bar *chopped*
  The recipe is found on page 221

Instructions

1. **Preheat oven to 325°F/160°C** and line 1 baking sheet with parchment paper.
2. Bake macadamia nuts on the baking sheet for 6-7min. Allow macadamia nuts to cool for 5 minutes.
3. Chop macadamia nuts into fine flour, similar to the same fineness of almond flour.
4. Mix all dry ingredients into a medium bowl; whisk until combined, and set aside.
5. Cream butter & sweetener in a stand mixer bowl with a beater blade/paddle attachment or an electric hand mixer. Beat until softened, 3-4 minutes; the butter should become lighter and almost double in volume.
6. Add the egg, vanilla, and molasses to the butter, and continue to cream for another 5 minutes.
7. Add all the dry ingredients to the butter mixture and beat again until incorporated.
8. Prepare a baking sheet with parchment paper. Using a **medium-size 1.97-inch scoop,** scoop out cookies on a baking sheet, depending on the size of the scoop, 9 jumbo or 12 medium cookies.
9. Using the palm of your hand, slightly press down the cookies and garnish the top with macadamia nuts.
10. Place cookies in the fridge for 20min to allow them to chill.
11. Preheat oven to 350°F/180°C. Bake smaller cookies for 9-10 minutes and 12-13 minutes for the jumbo.
12. **SEE NOTE:** Once cookies come out of the oven, garnish the top with the white chocolate chunks by pressing them into the cookie.
13. Allow the cookies to cool completely on the trays & enjoy with a cup of coffee!
14. Store in an airtight container for five to six days and freeze for up to three months.

Note

- **The white chocolate melts too quickly if baked on top of the cookies. That is why I recommend in Step 12 to add the chocolate after the cookies are baked.**
- **To truly bring out the flavour and aroma in any nut, it is best to toast the nut lightly first. That is why I roasted the macadamia nuts before making them into flour.**

White Chocolate Macadamia

prep: *17 min*   **bake:** *10-13 min*   **cool:** *5-10 min*   **serves:** *12 cookies*

White chocolate macadamia cookies are my hubby's favourite! I wanted to make these cookies extra special and flavourful by adding toasted macadamia nut flour into the recipe. Let's be honest; you don't get the full macadamia experience when there are only three to four pieces on top!

Dry ingredients

- 112g *(1 cup)* almond flour
- 130g *(1 cup)* macadamia nuts *chop fine*
- 68g *(1/2 cup)* coconut flour
- 56g *(1/2 cup)* organic collagen *grass-fed*
- 40g *(1/2 bar)* white chocolate bar *chopped*
  The recipe is found on page 221
- 152g *(3/4 cup)* sweetener
  monk fruit, erythritol, xylitol
- 1 teaspoon sea salt
- 1 teaspoon baking soda

Wet ingredients

- 113g *(1/2 cup)* grass-fed butter *room temp*
  *Sub for palm shortening to make **DF***
- 1 free-run egg *room temp*
- 10mL *(2 teaspoons)* pure vanilla extract

Garnish

- 65g *(1/2 cup)* macadamia nuts
- 80g *(1/2 bar)* white chocolate bar *chopped*
  The recipe is found on page 221

Note

- **The white chocolate melts too quickly if baked on top of the cookies. That is why I recommend in Step 12 to add the chocolate after the cookies are baked.**
- **To truly bring out the flavour and aroma in any nut, it is best to toast the nut lightly first. That is why I roasted the macadamia nuts before making them into flour.**

Instructions

- Preheat oven to 350°F/180°C.
- In a medium bowl, pour the entire bag of Chocolate Cupcake/cake Mix. (do not add the small bag of sweet powdered cocoa - leave for the buttercream frosting)
- Next, in a separate medium bowl, add all the wet ingredients. Whisk until well incorporated.
- Add the dry ingredients to the wet, and mix/whisk again until well incorporated.
- Using a rubber spatula, mix the batter until well incorporated.
- Line a cupcake tray with non-stick large parchment liners or a 6 -inch cake pan.
- Using a large cookie scoop, scoop out one level scoop into each cup.
- Bake the cupcakes for 25-30 minutes.
- Bake the cake for 45-60 minutes.
- Let cupcakes/cake completely cool to room temp on a cooling rack
- Chocolate Butter Cream: Using a stand mixer bowl (whisk attachment) or an electric hand mixer, whisk butter & vanilla on high until the buttercream becomes fully white & airy. Sift in the sweet powdered cocoa mix on top of the buttercream, and whisk again until well incorporated.
- Add buttercream into a piping bag with a piping tip. Starting at the edge of the cupcakes, swirl the buttercream into a mountain two and a half times to the top.
- When serving the cupcakes, ensure the frosting is at room temperature since it will harden when refrigerated.
- Store in the fridge in an airtight container for four to five days.
-

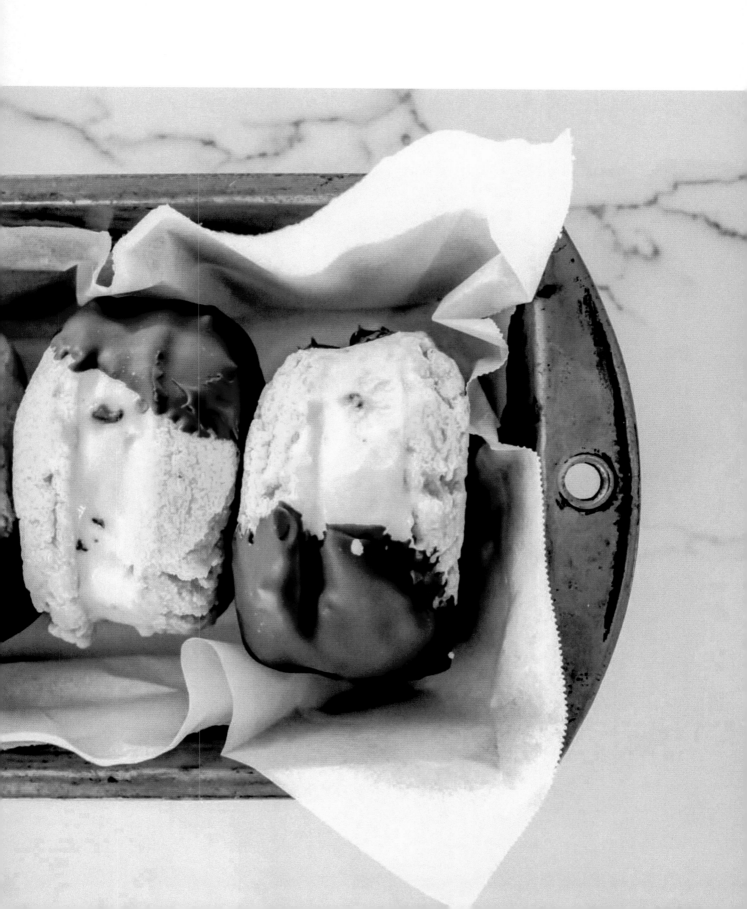

Ice-Cream Cookie Sandwiches

prep: *10 min*   **cool:** *5-10 min*   **serves:** *6 cookies sandwiches*

Who doesn't love ice-cream sandwiches? Especially when they are sandwiched between two delicious, freshly baked cookies! This recipe is so versatile that you can choose any cookie in this recipe book and just heap a scoop of delicious dairy-free ice cream inside!

Choose a cookie sandwich

- 1 dozen chewy chocolate chip cookies
  recipe found on page 31
- 1 dozen double chocolate chunk cookies
  recipe found on page 29
- 1 dozen peanut butter cookies
  recipe found on page 27
- 1 dozen espresso almond cookies
  recipe found on page 39

Choose an ice cream flavour

- 1 batch of Simply Vanilla Ice Cream DF
  recipe found on page 227
- 1 batch of Chocolate Ice Cream DF
  recipe found on page 225

Chocolate ganache

- 110g *(1/2 cup)* chocolate chips *melted*
  recipe found on page 223
- 14g *(1 tablespoon)* coconut oil *extra virgin*

Instructions

1. Have a batch of your choice of **Vanilla/Chocolate Ice Cream** pre-made in your freezer.
2. Choose what type of cookie you want to pair with your ice cream *(my favourite is the Classic Chewy Chocolate Chip cookie with the vanilla ice cream).*
3. Once cookies are baked and cooled completely, flip over half of the cookies so that bottom is facing upward.
4. Add three tablespoons of ice cream to each flipped cookie—sandwich it with the other cookie.
5. Place pre-made ice-cream cookie sandwiches back into the fridge & let sit.
6. **Chocolate ganache:** In a small heatproof bowl, melt chocolate chips with coconut oil in the microwave for 10-sec intervals, stirring between intervals; repeat 3-5 times until completely melted.
7. Dunk half of the cookies in the chocolate ganache, and garnish the top with toasted sliced almonds.
8. Place in the freezer for 15 minutes to allow the chocolate to harden, & enjoy!
9. Store leftovers in an air-tight container in the freezer for up to two-three months. Take out 10 minutes before serving.

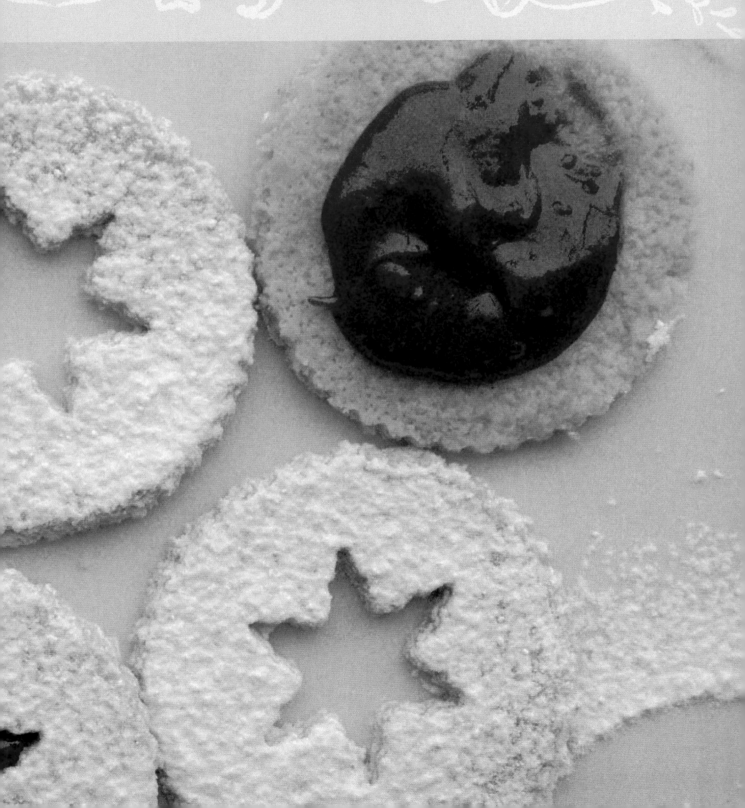

Christmas
COOKIES

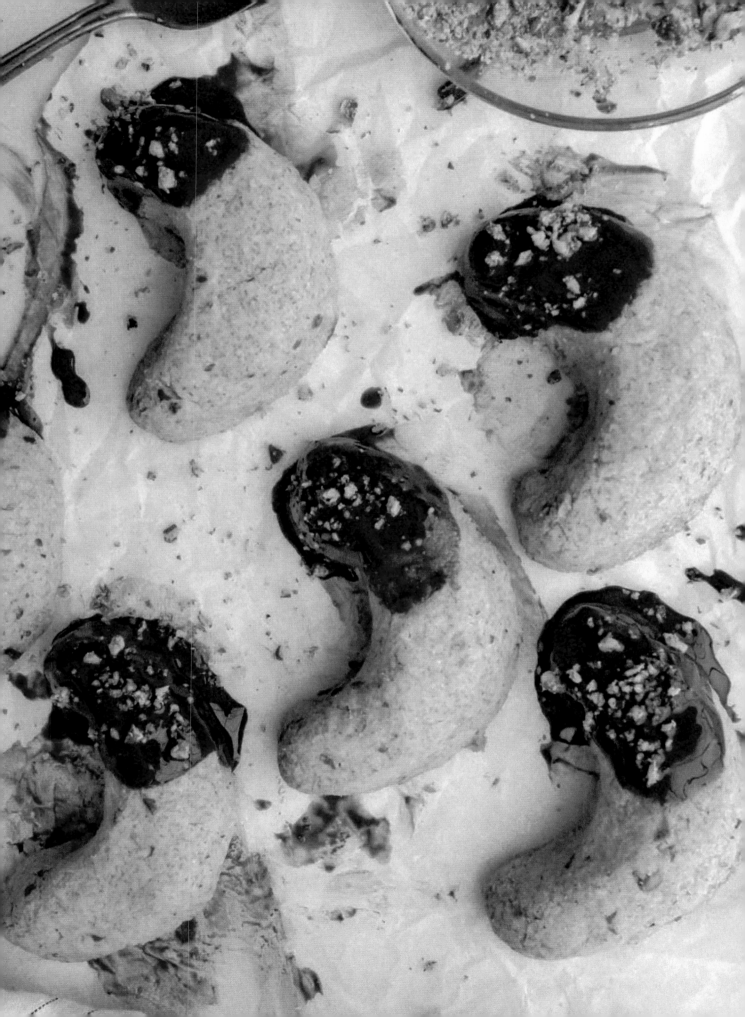

Shortbread Pecan Crescents

prep: *15 min*   **bake:** *10-12 min*   **cool:** *5-10 min*   **serves:** *12-15 cookies*

There isn't anything that reminds me more of Christmas baking than Shortbread. These cute pecan crescent cookies are a European tradition around Christmas time. They have such a warm, festive, nutty aroma while baking that everyone will be gathering in the kitchen while you're baking up a batch. I hope you enjoy these as much as I do.

Dry ingredients

- 90g *(1 cup)* pecans toasted *chopped fine*
- 140g *(1¼ cups)* almond flour
- 68g *(1/2 cup)* coconut flour
- 152g *(3/4 cup)* sweetener
  monk fruit, erythritol, xylitol
- 1 teaspoon sea salt
- 1 teaspoon baking soda

Wet ingredients

- 113g *(1/2 cup)* grass-fed butter *room temp*
  sub for palm shortening to make **DF**
- 10mL *(2 teaspoons)* pure vanilla extract
- 5mL *(1 teaspoon)* pure almond extract

Chocolate ganache/garnish

- 110g *(1/2 cup)* chocolate chips *melted*
  the recipe is found on page 223
- 14g *(1 tablespoon)* coconut oil *extra virgin*
- 23g *(1/ cup)* pecans toasted *chopped fine*
  to garnish

Instructions

1. **Preheat oven to 325°F/160°C.** You will need 1¼ cups *(115 g)* of finely chopped pecans *(some for garnish)*. Chop the pecans super fine. Line a baking sheet with parchment paper and place the chopped pecans on it— Bake for about 8 minutes.
2. In a medium bowl, measure out all your dry ingredients.
3. Beat the softened butter with a beater/paddle attachment in a stand mixer bowl or an electric hand mixer. Beat butter until creamed *(don't over-mix)*, about 2 to 3 minutes. Beat in the powdered sweetener, almond and vanilla extract.
4. Reduce speed to the lowest setting and gradually add the dry ingredients mixture in several additions. Mix until combined, being careful not to over-mix.
5. Place the cookie dough on a sheet of plastic wrap, and shape the dough into a log *(about 2 inches wide and 12 inches long)*. Roll the plastic wrap around the dough.
6. Pop the dough in the fridge for 30 minutes or until firm but not hard.
7. Once the dough is firm, unwrap dough; Using a round cookie cutter *(or the edge of a cup)*, cut the dough into half circles **"crescents"** until all cookies are cut out into desired shapes.
8. Reshape the dough using your hands to create a perfect moon shape crescent.
9. **Preheat the oven to 350°F/180°C** and line 1 baking sheet with parchment paper.
10. Place all the crescent cookies onto the baking sheet and refrigerate for an additional 15-20 minutes.
11. Bake cookies for 10-12 minutes. Cool the cookies for 30 min - they will be pretty soft.
12. **Chocolate Ganache:** In a small heatproof bowl, melt chocolate chips with coconut oil in the microwave for 10-sec intervals, stirring between intervals; repeat 3-5 times until completely melted.
13. Dip 1/2 of the crescent cookie into the melted chocolate, and place the cookie back on the parchment paper. Once all cookies are dipped in chocolate, you may dust some pecans on the melted chocolate and pop it back in the fridge for 5 min to allow the chocolate to harden up!

Note

- Toast all the pecans simultaneously, 1 1/4 cup (about *115g*) in total, so that you will have enough for the cookie dough and the garnish.

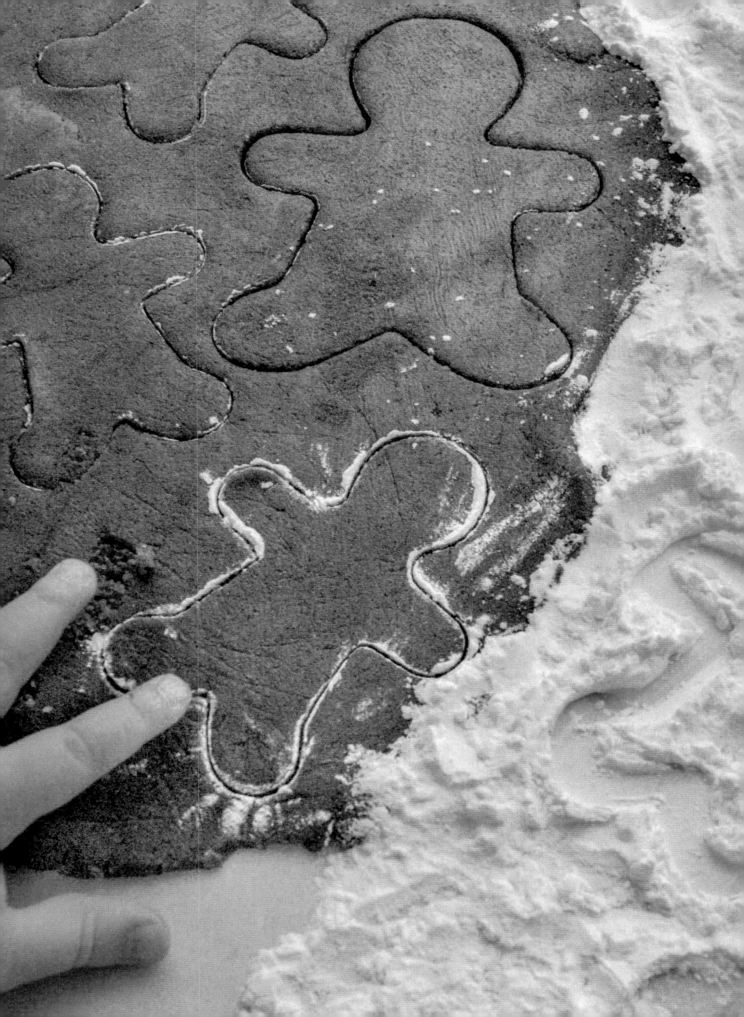

Gingerbread Cut-Outs

prep: *20 min*   **bake:** *10-17 min*   **cool:** *5-10 min*   **serves:** *12 cookies*

If you love a good kick, then you are just going to adore these fun, festive gingerbread cut-out cookies. You can decorate them as fancy or as light as you like. Either way, they are my family's favourite.

Dry ingredients

- 168g *(1 ½ cups)* almond flour
- 46g *(1/3 cup)* coconut flour
- 152g *(3/4 cup)* sweetener
  monk fruit, erythritol, xylitol
- 2 teaspoons ginger *powder*
- 2 teaspoons cinnamon
- 1/2 teaspoon allspice
- 1/2 teaspoon allspice
- 1 teaspoon baking soda
- 1/2 teaspoon sea salt

Wet ingredients

- 113g *(1/2 cup)* grass-fed butter *room temp*
  sub for palm shortening to make DF
- 1 free-run egg *room temp*
- 45g *(3 tablespoons)* blackstrap molasses
- 10mL *(2 teaspoons)* pure vanilla extract

Decorate/Icing

- 120g *(1 cup)* powdered sweetener
  monk fruit, erythritol, xylitol
- 30mL *(2 tablespoons)* coconut milk *high fat*

Note

- I have found that baking time varies wildly, depending on the cookies' thickness and length. So, keep an eye out for them, and note that if you like them crisp, you'll want to push the baking time as much as possible
- For the cute chocolate chip eyes, I recommend buying the chocolate chips as they look much better than making them.
- You may need to play with the consistency of the icing sugar, depending on what brand and type of powdered sweetener you use.

Instructions

1. Measure out all your dry ingredients in a med bowl, whisk until thoroughly combined, and set aside.
2. Cream butter in a large bowl with a beater/paddle attachment in a stand mixer bowl or an electric hand mixer for 1-2 minutes. Add in egg, molasses and vanilla and continue to cream. However, make sure not to overbeat. *(2-4 minutes)*
3. With your mixer on low, add half of your dry ingredients mixture - mixing until just incorporated. Mix in the rest. Wrap cookie dough with cling film *(saran wrap)* and refrigerate overnight *(best option)*. But if in a pickle, 3 hours will do.
4. **Preheat the oven to 350°F/180°C** and line a baking tray with parchment paper or a baking mat.
5. Roll out the dough between two pieces of parchment paper and cut out the shapes. The thickness will determine much of the texture: thinner cookies will be much crispier, while a thick dough *(particularly under-baked)* will yield a softer one. Place shaped cookies on the prepared baking tray and place in the freezer for 10 minutes before baking.
6. Bake for 10-17 minutes *(depending on the size of the cookies)* until fully golden.
7. Allow cooling for 10 minutes before transferring to a cooling rack. Allow cooling completely. They'll continue to harden up *(may take a few hours)*.
8. **Icing**: In a small bowl, mix powdered sweetener with the coconut milk until it creates a thick icing, and decorate cookies any way you desire. You can also melt chocolate chips and dip the cookies in chocolate ganache!
9. Store in an airtight container for five to six days and freeze for up to three months.

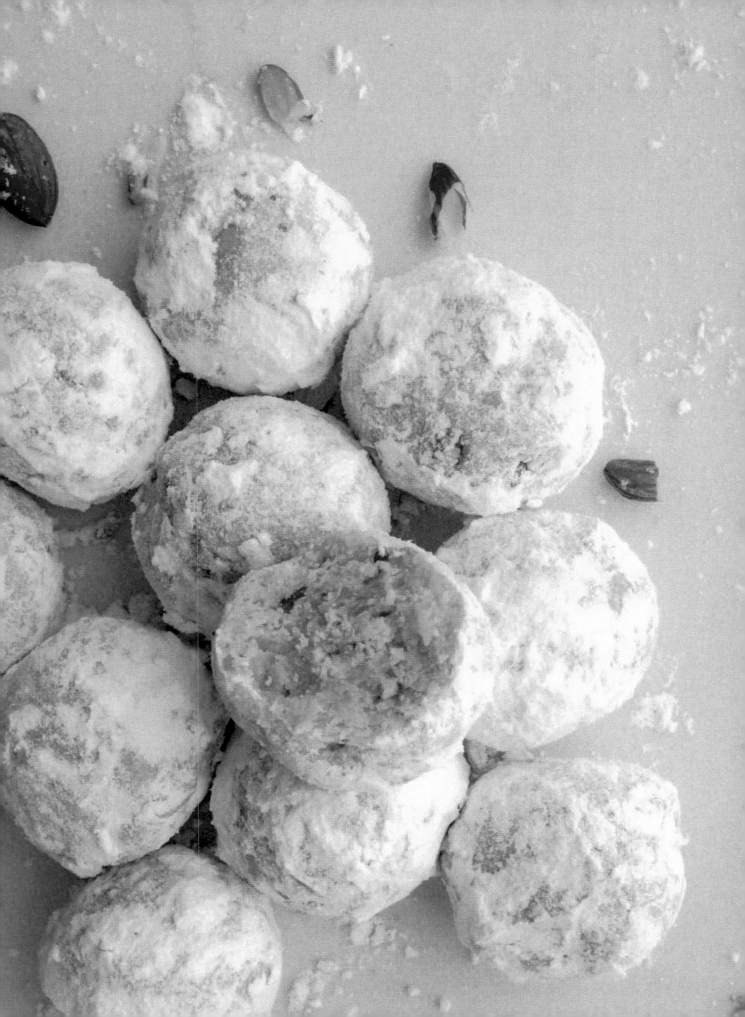

Toasted Almond Snowballs

prep: *8 min*   **bake:** *12-14 min*   **cool:** *5-10 min*   **serves:** *15-20 cookies*

For some reason, these simple little sweet snowball cookies have always been one of my warmest memories of Christmas baking. The combination of the nutty toasted almond flavour and the almond and vanilla extracts become like a beautiful Christmas carol in your mouth!

Dry ingredients

- 140g *(1 cup)* almonds toasted *chopped fine*
- 120g *(1 cup)* almond flour
- 68g *(1/2 cup)* coconut flour
- 120g *(1 cup)* powdered sweetener
  monk fruit, erythritol, xylitol
- 1 teaspoon sea salt

Wet ingredients

- 113g *(1/2 cup)* grass-fed butter *room temp*
  sub for palm shortening to make DF
- 10mL *(2 teaspoons)* pure vanilla extract
- 5mL *(1 teaspoon)* pure almond extract

Garnish/cover

- 120g *(1 cup)* powdered sweetener
  monk fruit, erythritol, xylitol

Instructions

1. **Preheat oven to 350°F/180°C** and line 1 baking sheet with parchment paper.
2. Measure out almond flour, and lightly toast for 4-5 minutes, then set it aside.
3. Chop raw whole almonds finely, place on a baking pan and bake for 6-7 minutes to allow the almonds to become more fragrant and flavourful.
4. In a medium bowl, add both dry and wet ingredients.
5. Mix the old-fashioned way *(by hand)* or with a beater/paddle attachment in a stand mixer bowl or an electric hand mixer. The dough will be on the crumbly/soft side.
6. **Using a small cookie dough scoop *(size: 1.5 Tbsp/ 23 ml/ 0.8 oz)*,** scoop out and place cookie almond dough on the baking sheet. Roll in the palms of your hand, and place in the fridge for 20 minutes or until firm but not hard.
7. Pop cookie dough snowballs in the preheated oven.
8. Bake snowball cookies for 12-14 minutes.
9. Once cookies are finished baking, let them cool for 30 min - they are delicate cookies.
10. Roll your cookie dough balls in the powdered sweetener until they are covered entirely.
11. Place all the rolled powdered cookies onto the baking sheet and back in the fridge to chill for an additional 15-20 minutes.
12. **Garnish:** Once they have cooled or before serving, roll the cookies in the powdered sweetener a second time. Be generous with the powdered sweetener; this is what makes these *"Snowball"* cookies!
13. Store in an airtight container for five to six days and freeze for up to three months.

Note

- **You can play around with the size of the scoop, yet I would recommend staying under 2 tablespoons per scoop.**

Cranberry Orange Linzers

prep: *20 min*   **bake:** *6-9 min*   **cool:** *5-10 min*   **serves:** *14-16 cookies*

When I was a little girl, my best friend's mom would always have the best Christmas baking. When she made linzers, I was so always so intrigued by their beautiful presentation!

Dry ingredients

- 168g *(1 ½ cups)* almond flour
- 46g *(1/3 cup)* coconut flour
- 152g *(3/4 cup)* sweetener
  monk fruit, erythritol, xylitol
- 1 tablespoon orange zest *fresh*
- 1 ½ teaspoons cinnamon
- 1/2 teaspoon sea salt

Wet ingredients

- 113g *(1/2 cup)* grass-fed butter *room temp*
  sub for palm shortening to make DF
- 1 teaspoon pure vanilla extract
- 1/2 teaspoon pure almond extract

Cranberry Jam

- 140g *(1/2 cup)* raspberry jam
  the recipe is found on page 193

Garnish/dust

- 30g *(1/4 cup)* powdered sweetener
  monk fruit, erythritol, xylitol

Instructions

1. In a medium bowl, measure/weigh out all your dry ingredients.
2. In a stand mixer bowl, beat the softened grass-fed butter with a beater/paddle attachment, or use an electric mixer. Beat butter until creamed *(don't over-mix)*, about 2 to 3 minutes. Beat in the powdered sweetener, orange zest and vanilla.
3. Reduce speed to the lowest setting and gradually add the dry ingredients mixture in several additions. Mix until just combined, being careful not to over-mix.
4. Divide the dough in half, shape it into disks, wrap securely in plastic wrap, and refrigerate for 1 hour or until firm but not hard! In a hurry? Pop the dough in the freezer for 20min; allow the dough to warm up on the counter until they are still firm but not soft.
5. **Preheat the oven to 350°F/180°C** and line 2 baking sheets with parchment paper.
6. On a lightly floured surface, roll out each piece of dough to 1/8-inch thickness. Cut out using a 3-inch cookie cutter and place on a prepared baking sheet, spacing them 1 inch apart. Using a one-inch cookie cutter, cut out the centres of the half of the cookie rounds, re-rolling the scraps.
7. Bake the bottoms and the tops *(the ones with the holes)* on separate cookie sheets!
8. Bake the bottom cookie dough sheet for 7-9 minutes. The tops bake faster; they only require about 6-8 minutes. Cool slightly on the cookie sheet, then transfer to a wire rack to cool completely.
9. Scoop 2 teaspoons of cranberry jelly in the centre of the bottom cookie *(without the small cut-out hole)*.
10. **Garnish:** When the tops have partially cooled, dust them generously with powdered sweetener.
11. Place tops on each bottom cookie, press gently to stick the cookies together and enjoy!
12. Store in an airtight container for five to six days and freeze for up to three months.

Note

- Linzers are so versatile; you can really put any jelly/jam filling inside you desire. Even a hazelnut chocolate ganache is wonderful - just be creative!

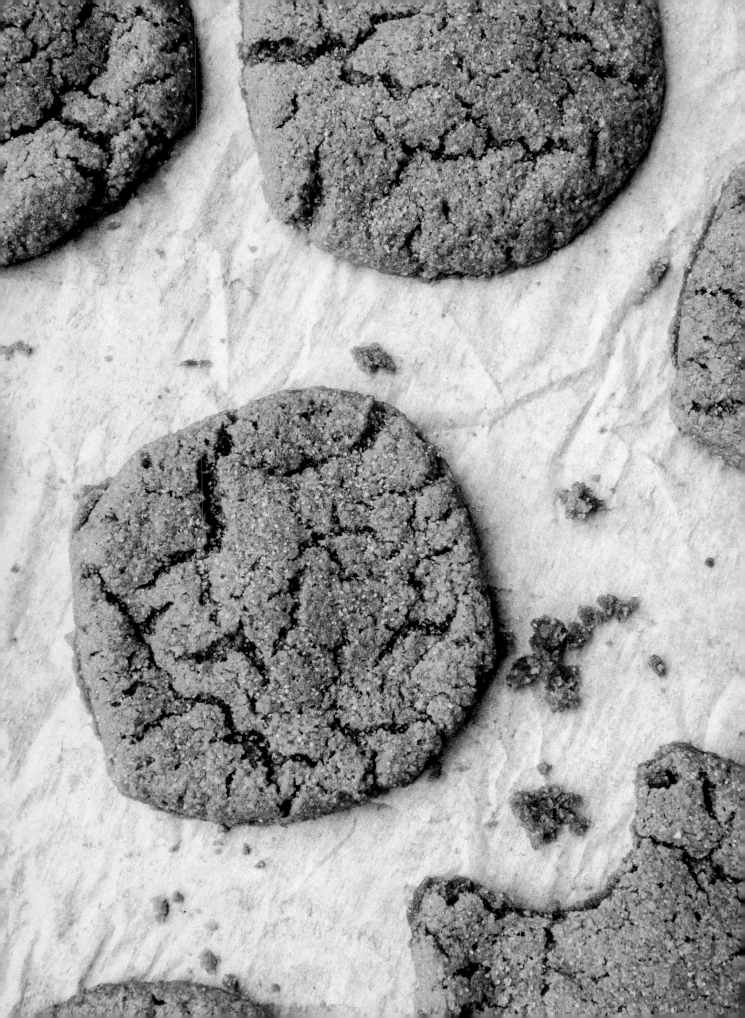

Soft & Chewy Gingersnaps

prep: *15 min*   **bake:** *10-12 min*   **cool:** *5-10 min*   **serves:** *12 cookies*

My bestseller during Christmas 2020 was my gingersnap cookies, and I would have to agree with my customers' flavour choice! If you love a bold and robust gingersnap, then do not hold back on the fresh ginger. The extra blackstrap molasses gives the gingersnaps the desired flavour and texture we love so much!

Dry ingredients

- 168g *(1½ cups)* almond flour
- 68g *(1/2 cup)* coconut flour
- 46g *(1/2 cup)* organic collagen *grass-fed*
- 152g *(3/4 cup)* sweetener
  monk fruit, erythritol, xylitol
- 1 tablespoon ginger *freshly grated*
- 1 teaspoon ginger powder
- 1 tablespoon cinnamon
- 1 teaspoon baking soda
- 1 teaspoon sea salt

Wet ingredients

- 113g *(1/2 cup)* grass-fed butter room temp
  sub for palm shortening to make DF
- 1 free-run egg *room temp*
- 60g *(1/4 cup)* blackstrap molasses
- 10mL *(2 teaspoons)* pure vanilla extract

Garnish/cover

- 100g *(1/2 cup)* sweetener
  monk fruit, erythritol, xylitol

Instructions

1. Mix all dry ingredients into a medium bowl; whisk until combined, and set aside.
2. Cream butter & sweetener in a stand mixer bowl with a beater/paddle attachment in a stand mixer bowl or an electric hand mixer. Beat until softened, 3-4 minutes; the butter should become lighter and almost double in volume.
3. Add the egg, vanilla, and molasses to the butter, and continue to cream for another 5 minutes.
4. Add all the dry ingredients to the butter mixture and beat until incorporated.
5. Prepare a baking sheet with parchment paper. Using a **medium-size 1.97-inch scoop,** scoop out cookies on the baking sheet, depending on the size of the scoop, 9 jumbo or 12 medium cookies.
6. **Garnish:** Using the palm of your hand, roll each cookie dough into a ball, and roll them in the granulated sweetener. Then lightly press down the cookie.
7. Place cookies in the fridge for 20min to allow them to chill.
8. **Preheat the oven to 350°F/180°C** and line a baking sheet with parchment paper.
9. Bake smaller cookies for 9-10 minutes and 12-13 minutes for the jumbo. Enjoy these gingersnap cookies with a cup of coffee!
10. Store in an airtight container for five to six days and freeze for up to three months.

Note

- **These cookies are on the spicier side - reduce ginger if sensitive to spice.**
- **This recipe works great for making snickerdoodles; just take out the ginger, and only add 5g *(1 teaspoon)* of blackstrap molasses.**

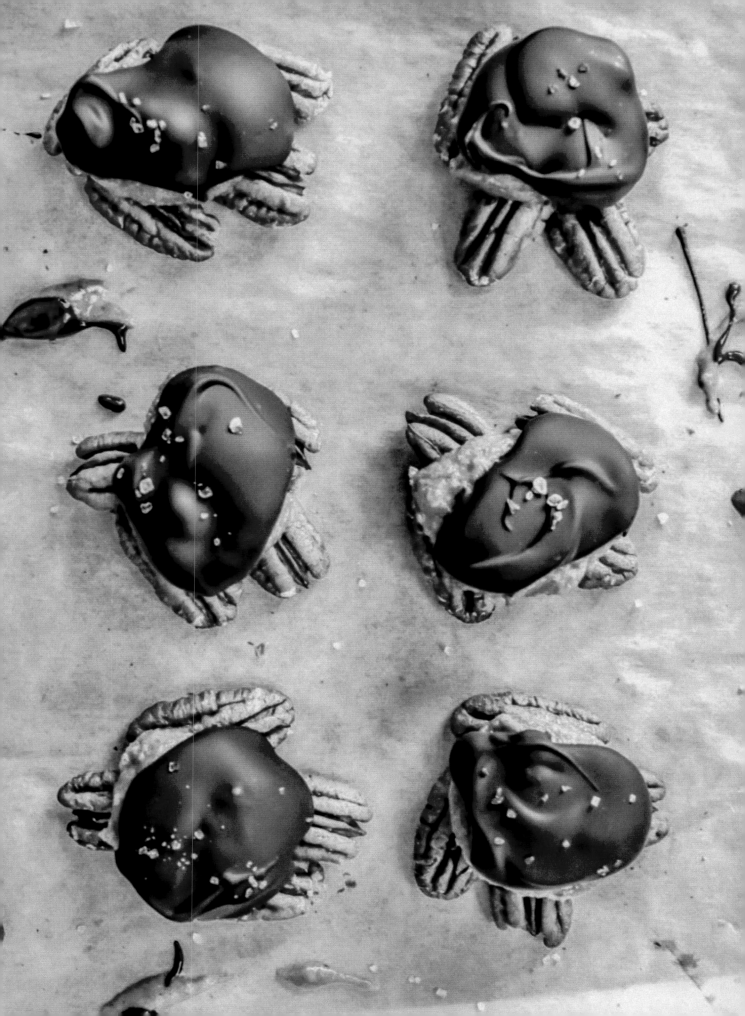

Turtles, Homemade!

prep: *10 min*   **bake:** *8 min*   **cool:** *5-10 min*   **serves:** *10-12 turtles*

I know turtles aren't considered a cookie; however, I had to add this recipe to my recipe book. These delicious little homemade turtles are just so lovely to serve at a Christmas gathering!

Ingredients

- 2 cups *(48 pieces)* pecans halves *toasted*
- 110g *(1/2 cup)* chocolate chips *melted*
  the recipe is found on page 214
- 14g *(1 tablespoon)* coconut oil *extra virgin*
- 1 cup caramel sauce
  the recipe is found on page 219

Assemble= 1 Turtle

- 4 pecans *toasted*
- 2 teaspoons melted chocolate
- 1 tablespoon caramel sauce
- 1 tablespoon melted chocolate
- garnish with flaky sea salt

Instructions

1. **Preheat oven to 325°F/160°C** and line a baking sheet with parchment paper.
2. Bake pecan halves on the baking sheet for 8min.
3. After the pecans are done, let them cool down. Arrange a cluster of 4 pecans on the baking sheet with the parchment paper, and make a total of 12 turtles.
4. In a small, heatproof bowl, place the chocolate chips and coconut oil.
5. Melt the chocolate and oil in the microwave, in 10-sec intervals, 3 to 5 times, stirring between each interval until the chocolate is melted.
6. Using a tablespoon, scoop out warmly melted chocolate *(about 2 teaspoons)* on top of each cluster of pecans. There will be chocolate leftover which will be used in **Step 9**.
7. Place the baking sheet in the fridge for 5 minutes to allow the chocolate to harden up, which will help the pecans stay together.
8. Once the chocolate has hardened, scoop a tablespoon of caramel on top of the hardened chocolate on each pecan cluster.
9. Using another tablespoon, scoop out the melted chocolate on top of the caramel on each turtle - one spoon for each turtle. *(reheat the chocolate in the microwave as instructed in **Step 5** if needed)*
10. Garnish with flaky sea salt.
11. Pop the baking sheet back into the fridge for an additional 20 minutes to allow the chocolate to harden.
12. Store in an airtight container in the fridge for six to eight days and freeze for up to 3 months.

Note

- **Prepping the caramel sauce ahead of time is best since it works better when the caramel is cold from the fridge. This allows everything else to harden together perfectly!**

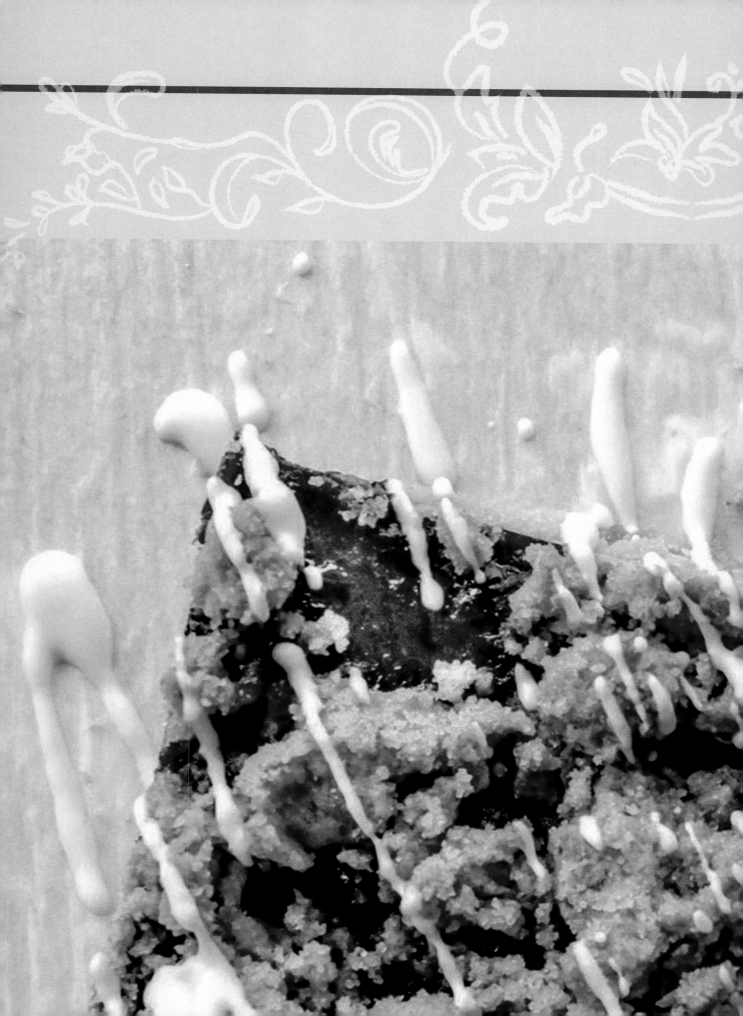

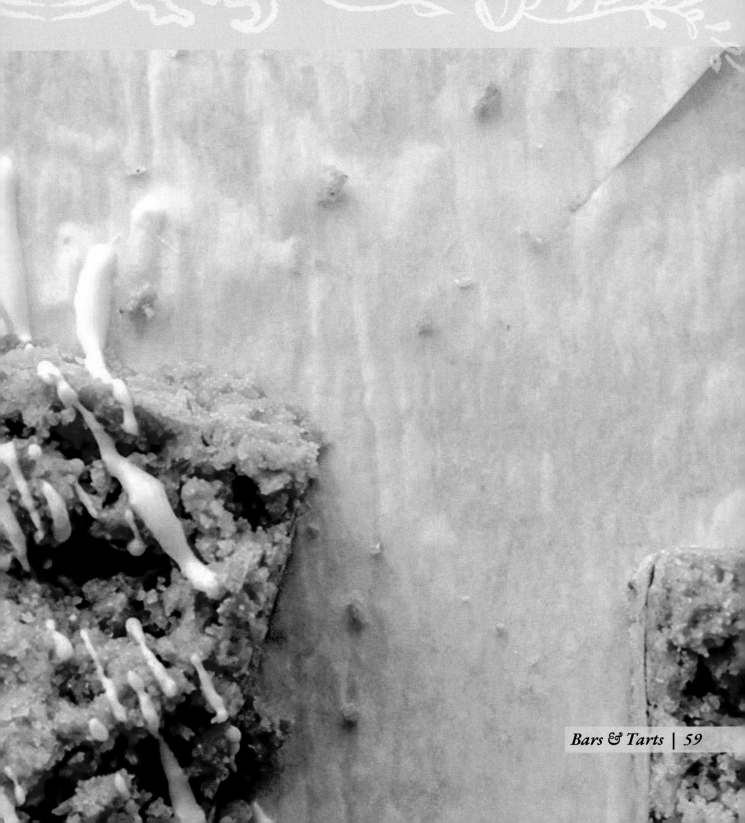

Chapter Two
BARS & TARTS

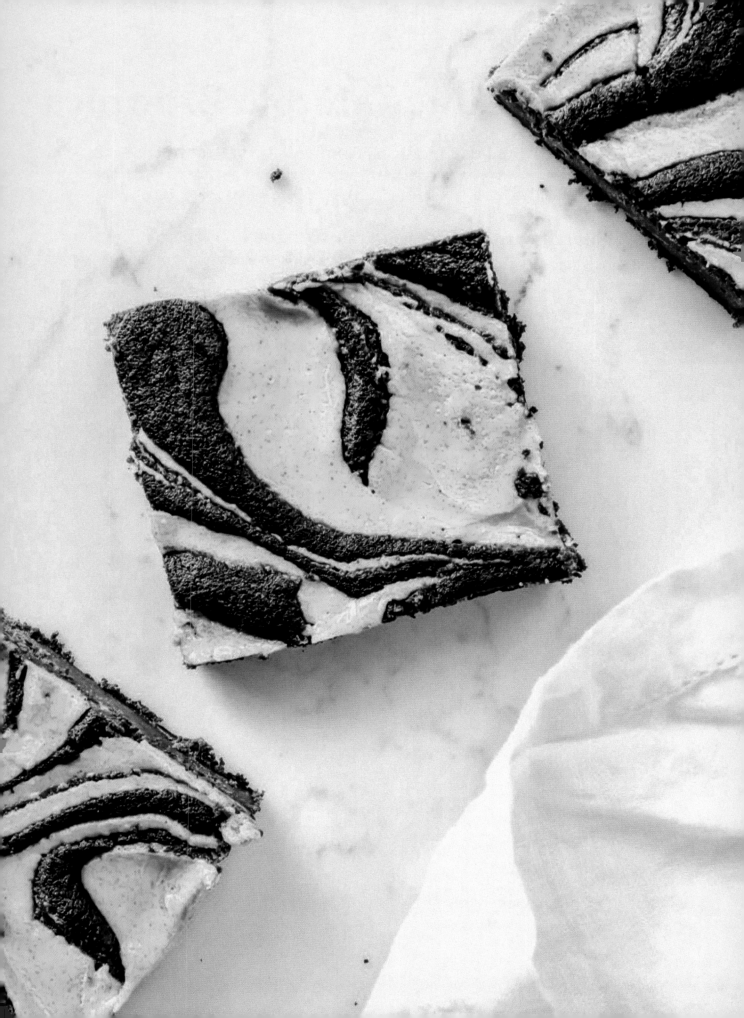

Peanut Butter Marble Brownies

prep: *12 min*   **bake:** *15-17 min*   **cool:** *5-10 min*   **serves:** *9 bars*

Oh, who doesn't love peanut butter in a fudge brownie? They are decadent and divine.

Wet ingredients

- 113g *(1/2 cup)* grass-fed butter *room temp*
  sub for palm shortening to make **DF**
- 80g *(1 full bar)* chocolate bar *melted*
  the recipe is found on page 223
- 57g *(1/4 cup)* peanut butter *natural*
- 4 free-run eggs *room temp*
- 2 teaspoons blackstrap molasses
- 10mL *(2 teaspoons)* pure vanilla extract

Dry ingredients

- 56g *(1/2 cup)* cocoa powder *sifted*
- 112g *(1 cup)* almond flour
- 34g *(1/4 cup)* coconut flour
- 28g *(1/4 cup)* organic collagen *grass-fed*
- 205g *(1 cup)* sweetener
  monk fruit, erythritol, xylitol
- 1 teaspoon sea salt

Top Marble ingredients

- 113g *(1/2 cup)* peanut butter *natural*

Instructions

1. Position a rack in the lower third of your oven and **preheat the oven to 350°F/180°C**. Line with parchment paper the bottom and sides of an 8x8-inch baking pan. Set aside. *(**Note:** The best baking pan is a lighter aluminum pan because it cooks consistently throughout)*
2. Add butter, chocolate chips and sweetener to a heatproof bowl. Melt over a water bath, constantly whisking *(or use the microwave, in 30sec intervals & stir in between until melted and mixed)*.
3. Remove from heat and allow the mixture to cool slightly. Add the peanut butter to allow the melted chocolate mixture to cool down even more.
4. Next, add one egg at a time, whisking well after each egg until completely incorporated. Add the molasses and vanilla - mix well.
5. In a medium bowl, sift the cocoa powder and add the remainder of the dry ingredients, whisking until thoroughly mixed. Then add the chocolate mixture on top and mix well.
6. Pour the brownie dough into the prepared pan.
7. **Marble:** Drizzle the peanut butter in 3-4 lines on top of the brownie mixture. Using a knife, swirl the peanut butter into the chocolate brownie for the marbled effect. *(make sure peanut butter is a runnier/oily consistency)*
8. Bake for 15-17 minutes. It's better to under-bake than to over-bake.
9. Take a look at the brownies around the 12-14min mark. Due to the high-fat content in the brownie, they will continue to cook while they cool. I let mine cool down for about 30min in the fridge.
10. Once the brownies are cooled, lift brownies using the edges of the parchment paper and cut them into the desired size.
11. Store in an airtight container in the fridge for six to eight days and freeze for up to 3 months.

Note

- **Baking time depends significantly on the oven and the type of baking pan. Darker/metal pans cook faster around the edges, yet ceramic pans take almost double the amount of time!**

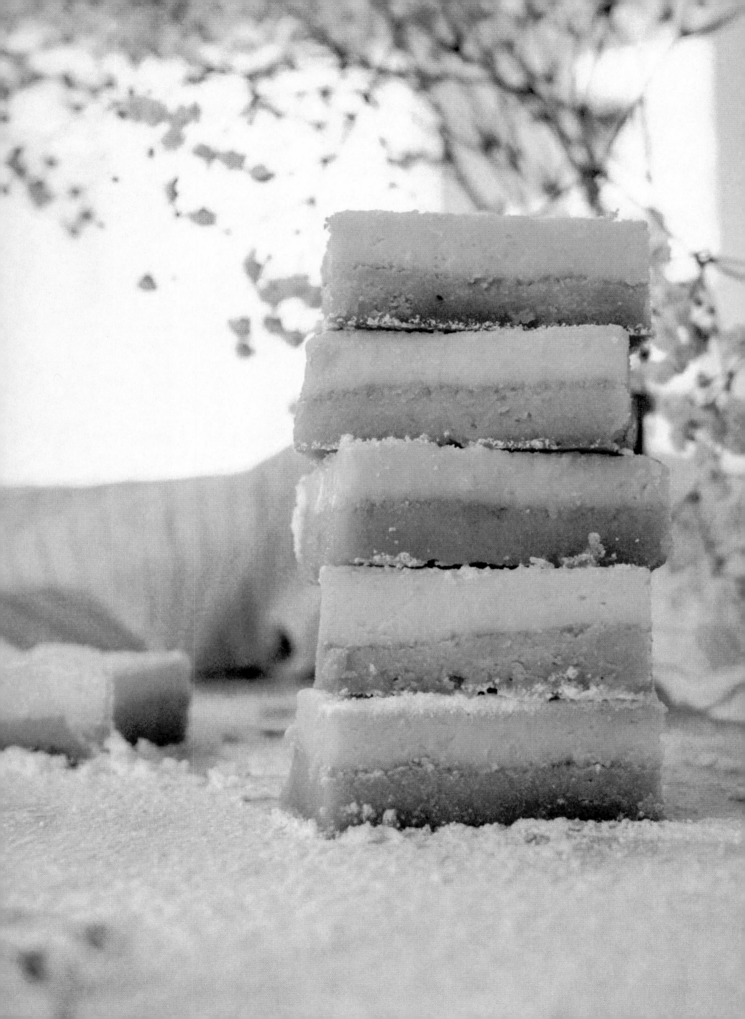

Custard Lemon Bars

prep: *12 min*   **bake:** *30-35 min*   **cool:** *1 hour*   **serves:** *9 bars*

These custard lemon bars are the perfect combination of something sweet, tart-like and slightly rich, yet so refreshing! You can also transform these custard bars into a tart. Both ways work wonderfully for this recipe. See page 67 for the instructions on making the tart crust and add custard lemon filling.

Crust ingredients

- 112g *(1 cup)* almond flour
- 34g *(1/4 cup)* coconut flour
- 20g *(1/4 cup)* shredded coconut *unsweetened*
- 28g *(1/4 cup)* organic collagen *grass-fed*
- 52g *(1/4 cup)* sweetener
  monk fruit, erythritol, xylitol
- 57g *(1/4 cup)* grass-fed butter *chilled*
  Sub for palm shortening to make DF
- 1 free-run egg *room temp*
- 1 teaspoon sea salt

Custard ingredients

- 75g *(1/3 cup)* grass-fed butter
- 70g *(1/3 cup)* coconut oil
- 4 free-run eggs *room temp*
- 80mL *(1/3 cup)* lemon juice
- 105g *(1/2 cup)* sweetener
  monk fruit, erythritol, xylitol
- 1 teaspoon pure vanilla extract
- 1-2 teaspoons pure lemon oil

Garnish

- 27g *(1/4 cup)* powdered sweetener
  monk fruit, erythritol, xylitol

Instructions

1. Position a rack in the lower third of your oven and **preheat the oven to 350°F/180°C.** Line with parchment paper the bottom and sides of an 8x8-inch baking pan.
2. In a bowl, whisk together all dry crust ingredients.
3. Add chilled butter *(cut into cubes)* & one egg. Using your hand, mix the crust dough the old-fashioned way, or use a stand mixer with a paddle/beater attachment. Mix/knead until it forms a ball.
4. Shape the dough into a circle and place it on your baking pan.
5. Push dough until a thin layer coats the entire pan.
6. Poke holes in the crust with a fork to allow a more even bake.
7. Bake for 12-15 minutes to par-cook the crust. As the crust is baking, start on the lemon custard.
8. **Custard:** In a small saucepan, combine all the custard ingredients **except the eggs.** Heat on medium-low until melted.
9. Add 1/4 cup of custard mixture from the saucepan into a small bowl. To temper the eggs, add one egg at a time and whisk together vigorously.
10. Once all eggs are added and tempered, pour the mixture into the saucepan. On low heat, whisk until it holds marks from the whisk and the first bubble appears on the surface, about 6 minutes.
11. Pour the custard onto the par-cooked crust and cook for an additional 15-17 minutes. Depending on the oven, you may have to par-cook for longer.
12. Once done baking, set it to cool for one full hour in the fridge to allow the custard to harden up.
13. **Garnish:** Cut lemon bars into 9 pieces, and garnish by dusting the top with powdered sweetener.
14. Store in an airtight container in the fridge for six to eight days and freeze for up to three months.

Note

- **When making the custard, make sure you continually whisk it so that the eggs don't curdle.**

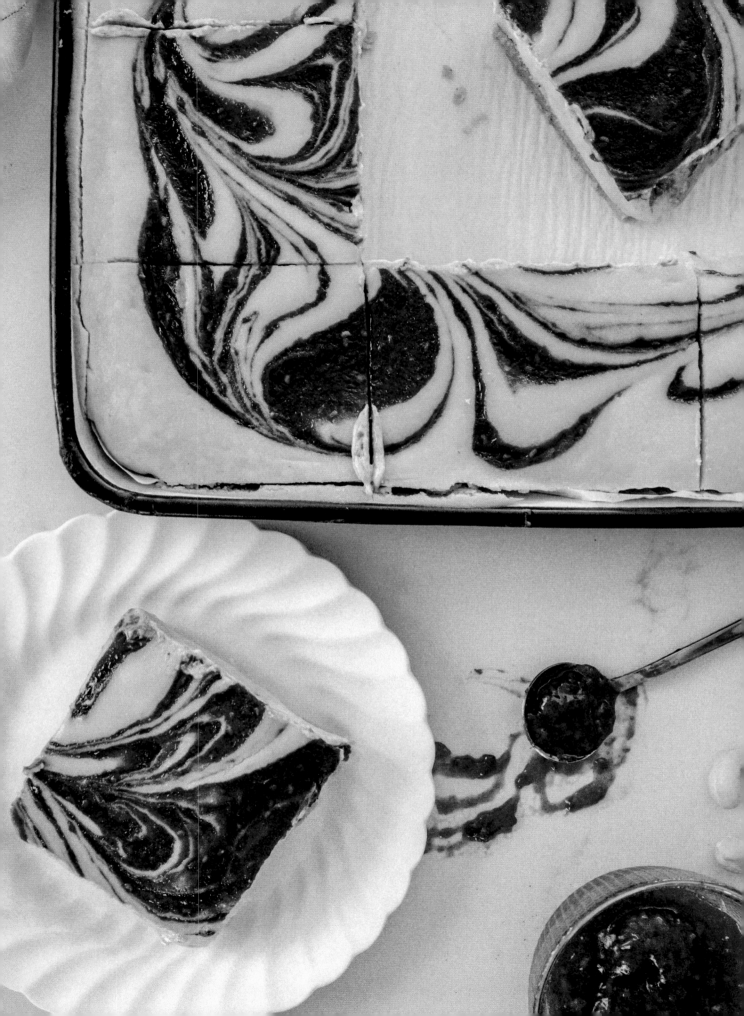

Raspberry Cheesecake Bars

prep: *12 min* **bake:** *35-40 min* **cool:** *1 hour* **serves:** *9 bars*

Cheesecake has always been one of those guilty pleasures of mine. When I found a way to replace the cream cheese with cashews, I was finally able to enjoy this delicious treat without the tummy pains. It's now a guilt-free pleasure!

Graham crust ingredients

- 112g *(1 cup)* almond flour
- 34g *(1/4 cup)* coconut flour
- 20g *(1/4 cup)* flaxseed *ground*
- 28g *(1/4 cup)* organic collagen *grass-fed*
- 53g *(1/4 cup)* sweetener
    monk fruit, erythritol, xylitol
- 57g *(1/4 cup)* grass-fed butter *chilled*
    Sub for palm shortening to make **DF**
- 1 free-run egg *room temp*
- 2 teaspoons cinnamon
- 1/2 teaspoon sea salt

Filling ingredients

- 280g *(2 cups)* raw cashews *soaked*
- 56g *(1/4 cup)* coconut oil *melted*
- 157g *(3/4 cup)* sweetener
    monk fruit, erythritol, xylitol
- 3 free-run eggs *room temp*
- 2 tablespoons lemon juice
- 1 teaspoon pure vanilla extract
- 1/2 teaspoon sea salt

Raspberry jam

- 140g *(1/2 cup)* raspberry jam
    The recipe is found on page **193**

Instructions

1. Position a rack in the lower third of your oven and **preheat to 350°F/180°C**. Line with parchment paper the bottom and sides of an 8x8-inch baking pan.
2. **Graham crust:** Mix almond flour, coconut flour, ground flaxseeds, collagen, sweetener, cinnamon and sea salt into a bowl and whisk together.
3. Add chilled cubes of butter & one egg. Using your hand, mix the crust dough the old-fashioned way, or use a stand mixer with a paddle/beater attachment. Mix/knead until it forms a ball.
4. Shape the dough into a circle in the baking pan, and flatten it into your prepared parchment pan.
5. Push dough in the pan until a thin layer coats the entire pan.
6. Poke holes in the crust with a fork to allow a more even bake.
7. Bake for 12-15 minutes to par-cook the crust.
8. As the crust is baking, start on the cashew cheesecake filling. **NOTE:** Ensure you soak the cashews for at least 4-8 hours.
9. **Filling:** In a high-speed blender, combine all the filling ingredients. Blend on high speed until creamy & smooth.
10. Pour cashew cheesecake filling onto the par-cooked crust.
11. **Jam:** Drizzle/pour the raspberry jam on the cashew filling in 3-4 lines. Use a butter knife to swirl the jam portion into the cheesecake portion to create the marbled look. *(jam pours best when warm)*
12. Bake for an additional 17-20 minutes. Depending on the oven, you may have to cook for longer.
13. Cool for one full hour in the fridge to harden up.
14. Cut cheesecake into 9 bars, and enjoy!
15. Store in an airtight container in the fridge for six to eight days and freeze for up to three months.

Note

- **Soaking the cashews is a must for this recipe. If you are tight for time, try soaking the cashews in hot water for an hour. Soak overnight in the fridge for best results.**

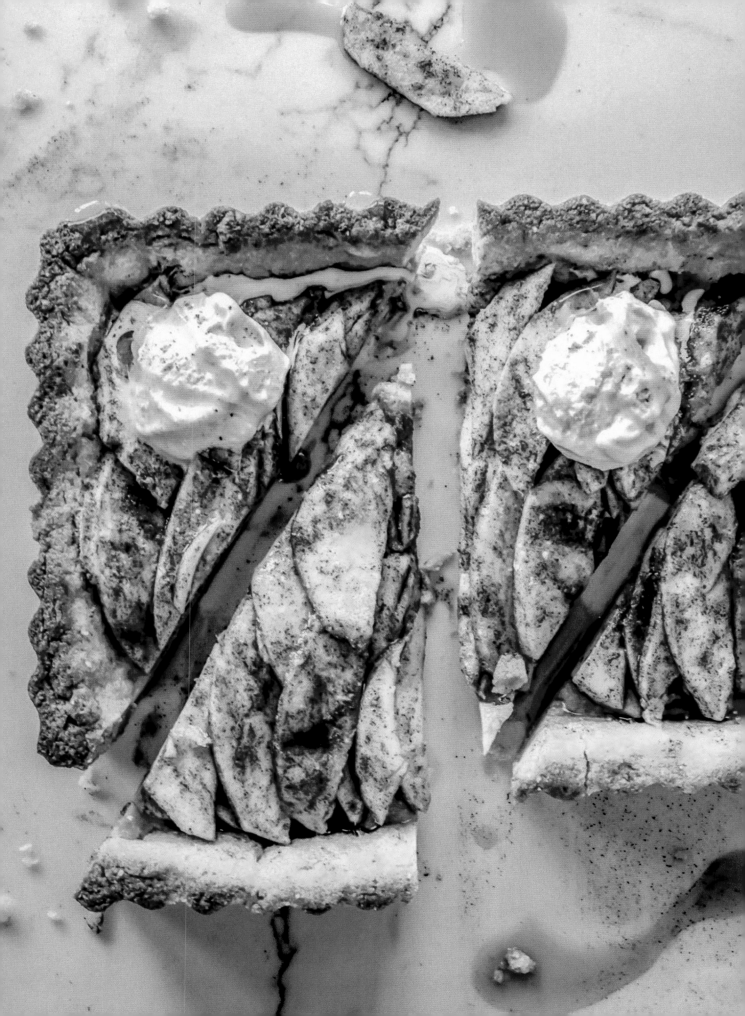

Spiced Brown Butter Apple Tart

prep: *25 min*   **bake:** *40-45 min*   **cool:** *15-20 min*   **serves:** *8 slices*

Serve this mouth-watering warm recipe three ways, slice it into bars, serve as a lovely tart, or even add crumble on top of the apple filling (see page 71 for crumble topping) and enjoy it as an apple crumble pie.

Crust ingredients

- 112g *(1 cup)* almond flour
- 46g *(1/3 cup)* coconut flour
- 11g *(1 tablespoon)* psyllium husk powder
- 52g *(1/4 cup)* sweetener
  monk fruit, erythritol, xylitol
- 57g *(1/4 cup)* grass-fed butter *chilled*
  sub for palm shortening to make DF
- 1 free-run egg *room temp*
- 15mL *(1 tablespoon)* apple cider vinegar
- 1 teaspoon baking soda
- 1 teaspoon sea salt

Filling ingredients:

- 57g *(1/4 cup)* grass-fed butter *browned*
- 105g *(1/2 cup)* sweetener
  monk fruit, erythritol, xylitol
- 3 medium organic apples *peeled*
- 2 teaspoons cinnamon
- 1 teaspoon allspice
- 15mL *(1 tablespoon)* lemon juice
- 1 teaspoon pure vanilla extract
- 1 teaspoon sea salt

Garnish

- 1 scoop Vanilla Ice Cream
  the recipe is found on page 227

Instructions

1. **Preheat oven to 350°F/180°C.**
2. **Crust:** Mix almond flour, coconut flour, psyllium husk powder, sweetener, baking soda and sea salt into a bowl, and whisk together.
3. Add chilled cubes of butter, one egg and apple cider vinegar. Using your hand, mix the crust dough the old-fashioned way, or use a stand mixer with a paddle/beater attachment. Mix/knead until it forms a ball.
4. Grease a 8 x 6 tart pan or an 8" pie baking pan.
5. Place dough in greased pan and flatten it until a thin layer coats the entire pan and creates an edge crust.
6. Poke holes in the crust with a fork to allow a more even bake.
7. Bake for 12-15 minutes at 350°F/180°C to par-cook.
8. **Filling:** Brown the butter: In a small saucepan on medium heat, allow the butter to come to a foaming stage, reduce heat slightly and stir until butter goes from a yellow hue to a golden hue.
9. Add sweetener. Allow the browned buttery sugar sauce to cool for 10 minutes off the heat.
10. While the browned butter is cooling, peel and slice the apples into thin slices in a medium bowl.
11. Place apples in a large bowl. Add cinnamon, vanilla extract, lemon juice and sea salt. Toss to combine until all the apple slices are evenly coated.
12. Fill the bottom of the crust with apple slices. Drizzle the melted browned butter on top of the apple slices filling. Pour any extra liquids left from the apple slices into the saucepan with the brown butter.
13. Bake for 30 to 35 minutes or until the apples are tender and the pie is golden brown on top.
14. **Garnish:** Slice and serve the tart with a big scoop of vanilla ice cream!
15. Store in an airtight container in the fridge for six to eight days and freeze for up to three months.

Note

- **The tart/pie crust may bake too quickly; place tin foil around the edges of the crust, so it does not brown too fast.**

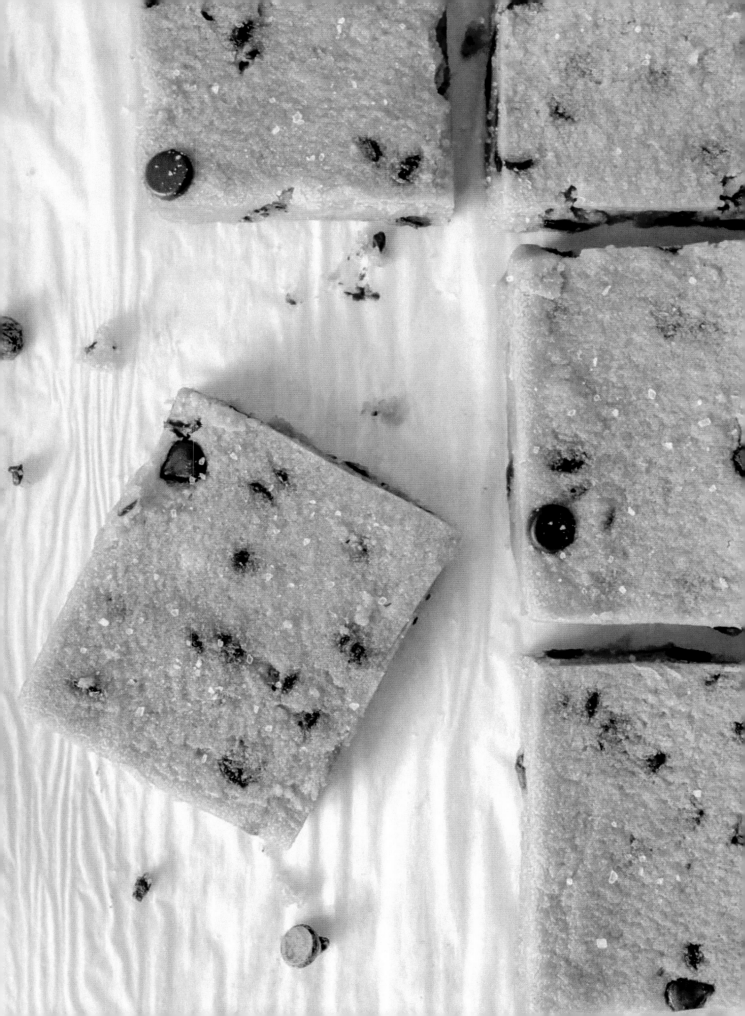

Salted Brown Butter Blondies

prep: *12 min*   **bake:** *15-17 min*   **cool:** *5-10 min*   **serves:** *9 bars*

Adding the simple step of browning your butter will enhance the depth, richness and nuttiness of any baked good. Brown butter is pretty amazing, but remember, don't burn the BUTTA!

Dry ingredients
- 168g *(1½ cups)* almond flour
- 46g *(1/3 cup)* coconut flour
- 110g *(1/2 cup)* chocolate chips
  the recipe is found on page 223
- 28g *(1/4 cup)* organic collagen *grass-fed*
- 152g *(3/4 cup)* sweetener
  monk fruit, erythritol, xylitol
- 1 teaspoon sea salt

Wet ingredients
- 170g *(3/4 cup)* grass-fed butter *room temp*
- 4 free-run eggs *room temp*
- 2 teaspoons blackstrap molasses
- 10mL *(2 teaspoons)* pure vanilla extract

Garnish
- flaky sea salt to garnish

Instructions

1. Position a rack in the lower third of your oven and **preheat to 350°F/180°C.** Line with parchment paper the bottom and sides of an 8x8-inch baking pan.
2. In a medium to large saucepan, melt the butter on medium heat.
3. The butter will become very foamy *(this is good, but make sure it's not too hot, so the butter does not burn).* With a rubber spatula, stir the butter constantly for about 2 minutes until it passes from a yellow-golden hue to a golden blond and finally to a lovely light brown.
4. Set the brown butter aside to cool down for 10 minutes.
5. Add all the dry ingredients to a medium bowl, and whisk until thoroughly mixed.
6. Add butter on top of the dry ingredients. Then add one egg at a time, whisking well after each until completely incorporated. Mix in the molasses and vanilla.
7. Pour the blondie mixture into the prepared baking pan. Use an offset spatula to level out the top.
8. Bake for 16-18 minutes. It's better to under-bake than over-bake.
9. Take a look at the blondies at around the 14-15min mark and remove them if they look ready. Due to the high-fat content, they will continue to cook while cool. I let mine cool for about 30min in the fridge.
10. Once blondies are cooled, lift them using the edges of the parchment paper and cut them into the desired size.
11. **Garnish:** Sprinkle flaky sea salt on top.
12. Store in an airtight container for five to six days and freeze for up to three months.

Note

- **In this recipe you can only use butter to make the brown butter. However, you can skip this browning step and use palm shortening to make it dairy-free.**

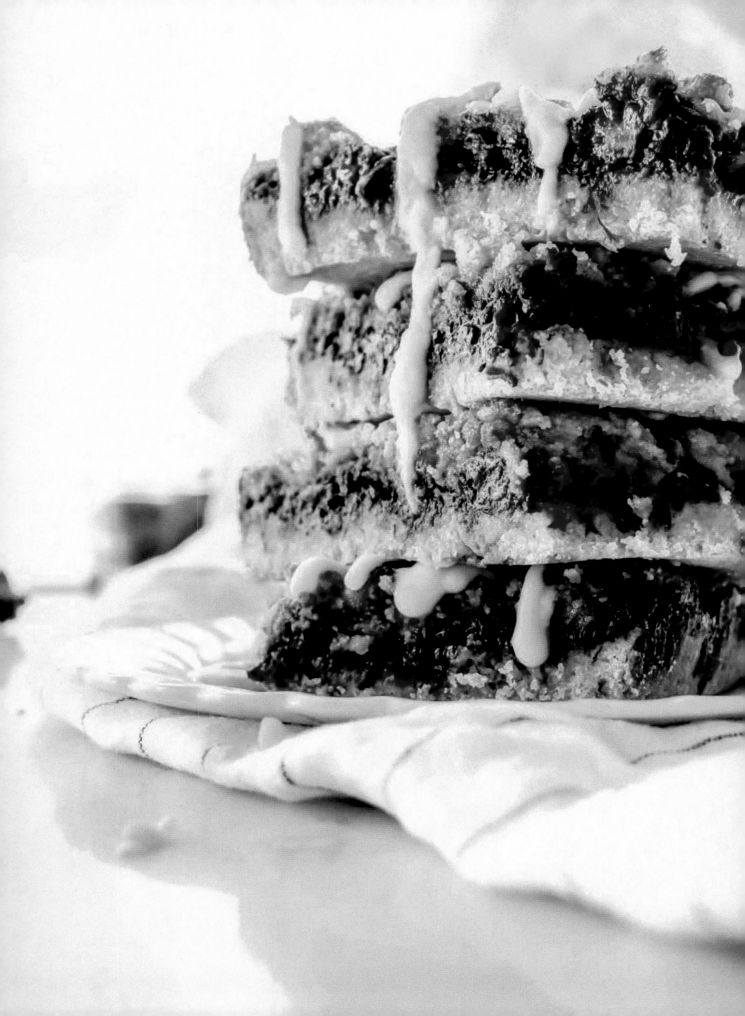

Berry Crumble Bars

prep: *15 min*   **bake:** *30-35 min*   **cool:** *15-20 min*   **serves:** *9 bars*

Berry crumble bars are our favourite dessert. This recipe is highly versatile - you can add any flavour jam/jelly your heart desires (apple butter is my top 3 combos), and they always taste incredible.

Crust ingredients

- 112g *(1 cup)* almond flour
- 46g *(1/3 cup)* coconut flour
- 28g *(1/4 cup)* organic collagen *grass-fed*
- 52g *(1/4 cup)* sweetener
    monk fruit, erythritol, xylitol
- 57g *(1/4 cup)* grass-fed butter *chilled*
    sub for palm shortening to make DF
- 1 egg *room temp*
- 1 teaspoon sea salt

Fillings

- 280g *(1 cup)* berry jams *recipe on page 193*
    OR
- 290g *(1 cup)* apple butter *recipe on page 195*

Crumble ingredients:

- 57g *(1/4 cup)* grass-fed butter *room temp*
- 94g *(3/4 cup)* almond flour
- 30g *(1/4 cup)* coconut flour
- 52g *(1/4 cup)* sweetener
    monk fruit, erythritol, xylitol
- 1 teaspoon cinnamon
- 1 teaspoon pure vanilla extract

Garnish/drizzle

- 27g *(1/4 cup)* powdered sweetener
    monk fruit, erythritol, xylitol
- 15mL *(1 tablespoon)* lemon juice

Instructions

1. Position a rack in the lower third of your oven and **preheat to 350°F/180°C.** Line with parchment paper the bottom and sides of an 8x8-inch baking pan.
2. Add all dry crust ingredients into a bowl & whisk together.
3. Add chilled cubes of butter & one egg. Using your hand, mix the crust dough the old-fashioned way, or use a stand mixer. Mix/knead until it forms a ball.
4. Flatten the dough and place it onto your prepared parchment pan. Stretch the dough until a thin layer coats the entire pan.
5. Poke holes in the crust with a fork to allow a more even bake.
6. Bake for 12-15 minutes at 350°F/180°C to par-cook the crust. As the crust is baking, start on the crumble, and have the jam pre-made.
7. **Crumble:** Place all the crumble ingredients into a bowl and, using your hands, mix the crumble until it is well incorporated.
8. **Filling:** Spread the jam of choice onto the par-cooked crust, then evenly sprinkle the crumble on top of the jam and bake for an additional 15-17 minutes. Depending on the oven, you may have to par-cook for longer.
9. Once the crumble bars are done, set them to cool for 15 min. Then cut it into 9 pieces.
10. **Garnish/drizzle:** Mix powdered sweetener and lemon juice to garnish by drizzling the top with icing.
11. Store in an airtight container for three to four days and freeze for up to three months.

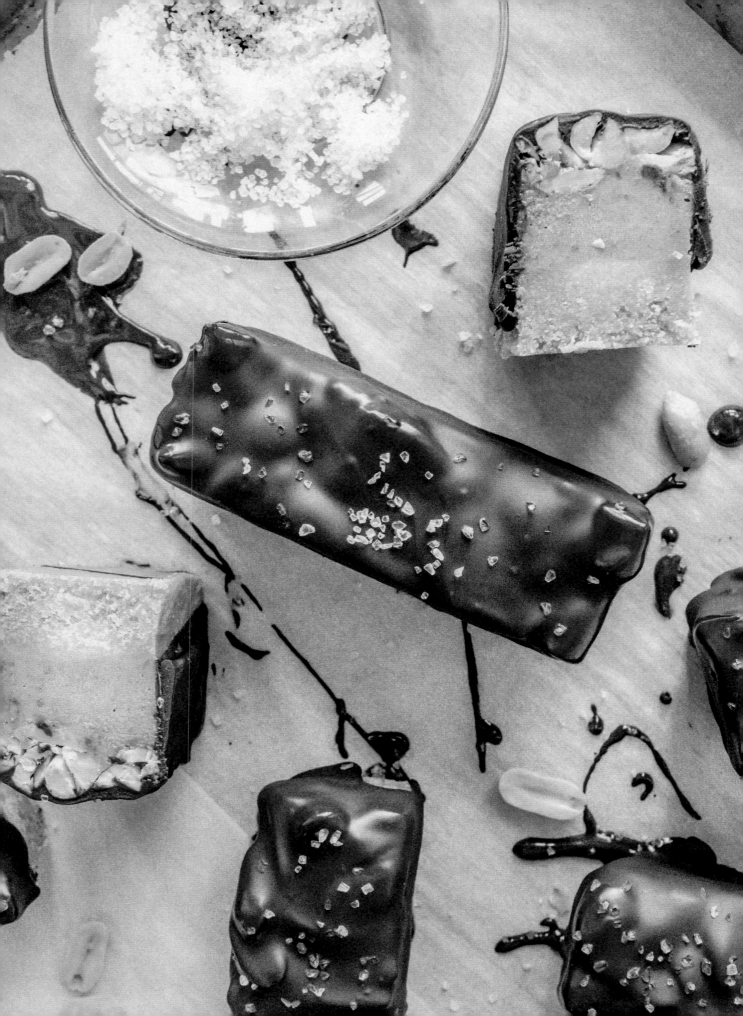

Homemade Raw Snickers Bars

prep: *20 min*   **cool:** *2 hours*   **serves:** *6 jumbo bars / 8 medium bars*

My husband marvels at this recipe. Every time I make it, he exclaims that "They taste even better than the real snicker bars!" So of course I had to add this recipe to my collection, even though there is no baking required.

Nougat/crust layer

- 140g *(1 1/4 cups)* almond flour
- 34g *(1/4 cup)* coconut flour
- 120g *(1/2 cup)* caramel sauce
  - *the recipe is found on page 219*
- 1 teaspoon sea salt

Caramel peanut butter layer

- 250g *(1 cup)* caramel sauce
  - *the recipe is found on page 219*
- 113g *(1/2 cup)* peanut butter *natural*
- 1 teaspoon sea salt

Peanut layer

- 145g *(1 cup)* dry roasted peanuts *salted*

Chocolate ganache layer

- 220g *(1 cup)* chocolate chips
  - *the recipe is found on page 223*
- 1 tablespoon coconut oil

Garnish

- flakey sea salt *to garnish*

Instructions

1. Prep caramel sauce ahead of time. I recommend doing it the day before since this recipe works much better with a cold caramel sauce.
2. **Nougat layer:** In a medium bowl, mix all the nougat ingredients until it forms a thick, crust-like dough.
3. Line with parchment paper an 8x4 inch loaf pan. Make sure the parchment paper is bigger than the loaf pan, so you can easily remove the snicker bars by lifting the parchment paper in step 9.
4. Press the nougat crust evenly in the bottom of the loaf pan.
5. **Caramel peanut butter layer:** Add caramel peanut butter ingredients in another small/medium bowl. Mix until well incorporated and evenly distributed over the nougat layer.
6. **Peanut layer:** Sprinkle the peanuts on the caramel peanut butter layer and slightly press the peanuts into the caramel.
7. Pop the loaf pan in the freezer for about an hour.
8. **Ganache layer:** Prep the chocolate layer by melting the chocolate chips in a heat-proof bowl in the microwave in 10-sec intervals *(mix after every 10 sec until melted completely)*, or place the bowl over the simmering water in a saucepan.
9. Once the snicker bars are chilled & solid, lift them out using parchment paper's edges. Cut the slab directly down the centre and cut each side into 3 slices, just over 1 inch, leaving you with 6 jumbo candy bars.
10. Prep a baking sheet with parchment paper. Roll snicker bars in melted chocolate using a fork, scoop out and place the bars onto the baking sheet.
11. **Garnish:** Before the chocolate ganache has hardened, sprinkle it with flaky sea salt and place them in the fridge to harden up.
12. Store in an airtight container in the fridge for up to two weeks and freeze for three months.

Note

- **As I noted in the recipe, the caramel should be made a day in advance since the cashews work best when soaked for 6+ hours or even overnight.**

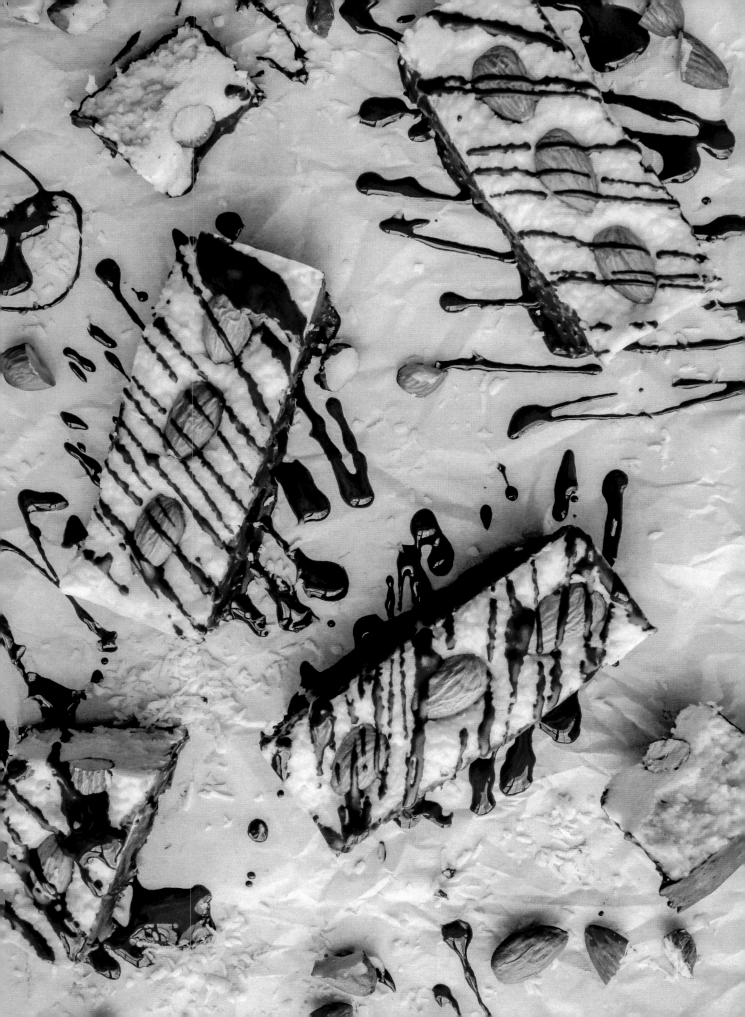

Raw Almond Joy Bars

prep: *20 min*   **cool:** *2 hours*   **serves:** *6 candy bars*

These Almond Joy Candy Bars are so easy to make and beyond delicious! If you are a coconut & chocolate lover, then I know you will LOVE these candy bars.

Coconut base

- 170g *(2 cups)* coconut flakes *unsweetened*
- 80g *(3/4 cup)* powdered sweetener
  monk fruit, erythritol, xylitol
- 118g *(1/2 cup)* coconut oil *melted*
- 1 teaspoon pure vanilla extract
- 1/8 teaspoon almond extract *optional*
- 1/2 teaspoon sea salt

Almond layer

- 80g *(1/2 cup)* raw almonds

Chocolate ganache layer

- 165g *(3/4 cup)* chocolate chips
  the recipe found on page 223
- 14mL *(1 tablespoon)* coconut oil

Instructions

1. **Coconut base:** Mix all coconut base ingredients in a medium bowl until a thick, paste-like dough is formed. *(make sure coconut oil is melted)*
2. Line an 8x4-inch loaf pan with parchment paper. Make sure the parchment paper is bigger than the loaf pan so you can easily remove the almond joy bars by lifting the parchment paper out of the pan in **Step 8**.
3. Press the coconut base evenly on the bottom of the loaf pan.
4. Using a knife, slice lightly down the center. Then cut three even slices per side, making six bars in total.
5. **Almond layer:** Add three almonds in a row on each bar.
6. Pop the loaf pan in the freezer for about an hour.
7. **Ganache layer:** Prep the chocolate layer by melting the chocolate chips in a heat-proof bowl, in the microwave in 10-sec intervals *(mixing at every interval),* or over a simmering double broiler with a heat-proof bowl.
8. Once the almond joy bars are chilled & solid, lift them out using the parchment paper's edges. Cut them entirely through where you made the marks in **Step 4,** making six jumbo bars *(about 3/4 inch wide),*
9. Prep a baking sheet with parchment paper.
10. Dunk the bottoms of the bars in melted chocolate using a fork, scoop out and place the bars onto the baking sheet.
11. Drizzle the bars with chocolate ganache and flaky sea salt and place them in the fridge or freezer to harden up.
12. Store in an airtight container in the fridge for up to three weeks and freeze for three months.

Note

- **If you want an extra coconut flavour, try adding 1 teaspoon of coconut extract to bring out the flavour.**

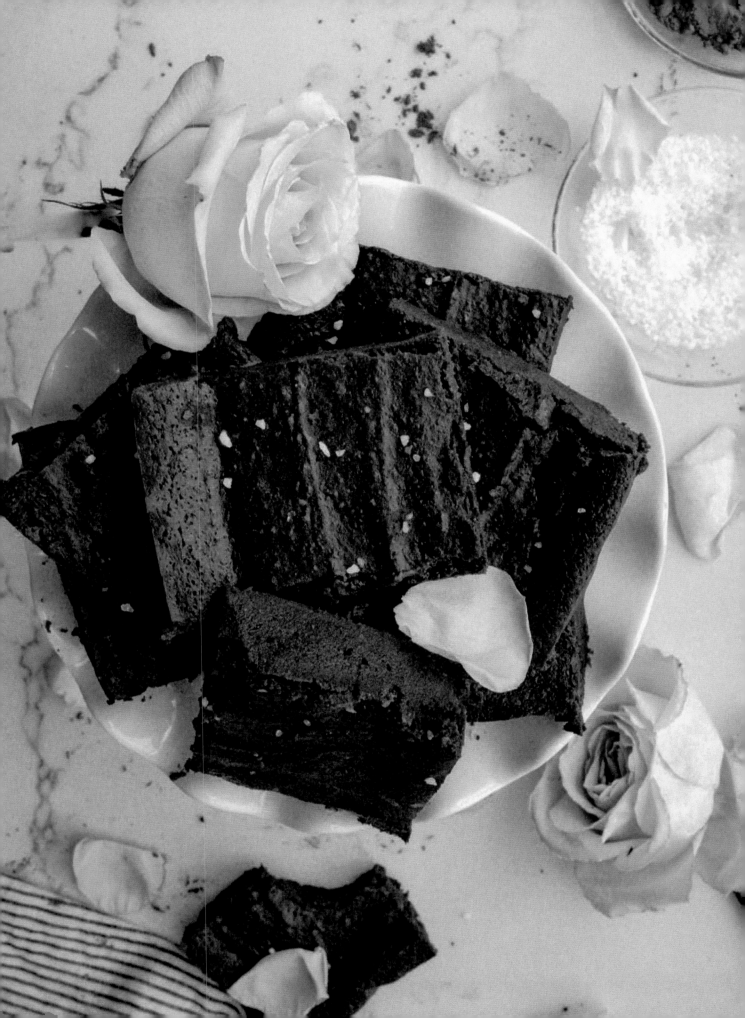

Gooey Fudge Brownies

prep: *12 min*   **bake:** *15-17 min*   **cool:** *5-10 min*   **serves:** *9 bars*

My Gooey Fudge Brownies are another one of my top sellers; they are always one of the first items sold out! These are for the dark chocolate lovers who adore a rich, thick, decadent brownie. Make sure you make this recipe! The extra added collagen and chocolate make these brownies gooey and oh so gooey.

Dry ingredients

- 56g *(1/2 cup)* cocoa powder *sifted*
- 112g *(1 cup)* almond flour
- 34g *(1/4 cup)* coconut flour
- 56g *(1/2 cup)* organic collagen *grass-fed*
- 205g *(1 cup)* sweetener
  monk fruit, erythritol, xylitol
- 1 teaspoon sea salt
- flaky sea salt *to garnish*

Wet ingredients

- 170g *(3/4 cup)* grass-fed butter *room temp*
  sub for palm shortening to make **DF**
- 110g *(1/2 cup)* chocolate chips *melted*
  the recipe is found on page 223
- 4 free-run eggs *room temp*
- 10mL *(2 teaspoons)* pure vanilla extract

Garnish

- flaky sea salt to garnish

Instructions

1. Position a rack in the lower third of your oven and **preheat to 350°F/180°C.** Line with parchment paper the bottom and sides of an 8x8-inch baking pan. (*The best baking pan is a lighter aluminum pan because it cooks consistently throughout.*) Set aside.
2. Add butter, chocolate chips, sweetener and vanilla extract to a heatproof bowl. Melt over a water bath, constantly whisking (*or use the microwave, in 30sec intervals & stir in between*).
3. Remove from heat and allow the mixture to cool slightly.
4. Add one egg at a time, whisking well after each egg is completely incorporated.
5. In a medium bowl, sift the cocoa powder, and add the remainder of the dry ingredients whisking until thoroughly mixed. Add in the melted chocolate mixture and mix well.
6. Pour the brownie mixture into the prepared pan, and then, using an offset spatula, even out the top if needed.
7. Bake for 15-17 minutes. It's better to under-bake than to over-bake.
8. **NOTE:** Take a look at the brownies at around the 12-14min time mark. Due to the high-fat content in the brownie, they will continue to cook while they cool. I let mine cool for about 30min in the fridge.
9. Once the brownies are cooled, lift them using the edges of the parchment paper and cut them into the desired size.
10. **Garnish:** Sprinkle with flaky sea salt.
11. Store in an airtight container for up to five days. and freeze for up to three months.

Note

- **The baking time depends significantly on the oven & baking pan. Darker/metal pans cook faster around the edges, yet ceramic pans take almost double the amount of time!**

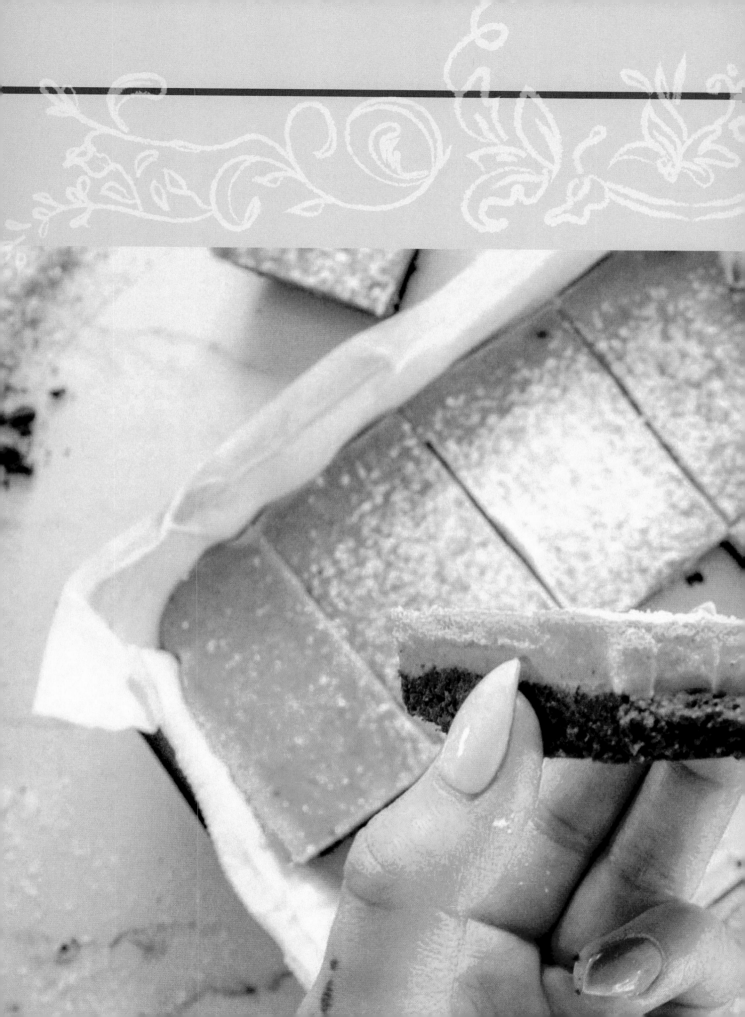

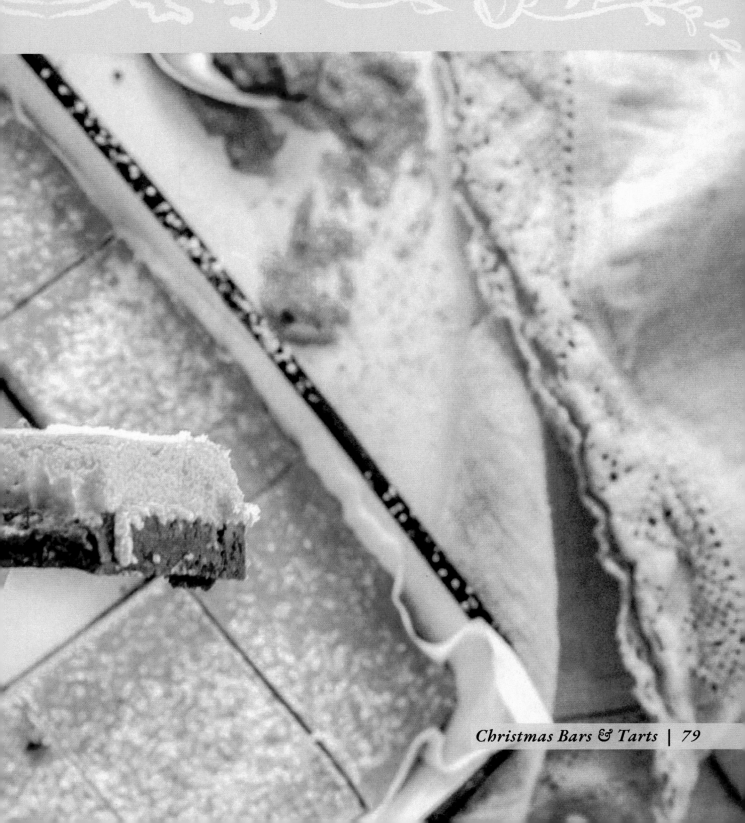

Christmas
BARS & TARTS

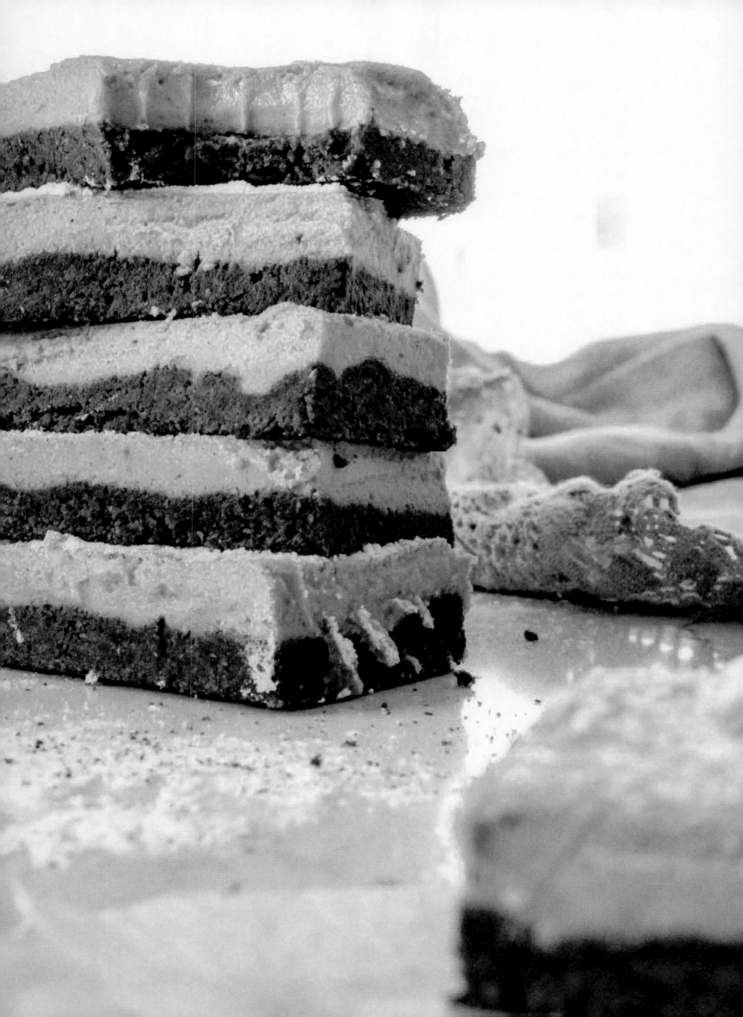

Pumpkin Eggnog Custard Bars

prep: *12 min*   **bake:** *30-35 min*   **cool:** *20-30 min*   **serves:** *9 bars*

Eggnog & spiced pumpkin - can it get any more festive than that? Like the Lemon Custard Bars on page 63, this pumpkin eggnog bars recipe may also be transformed into a tart! See page 67 for the instructions on making the tart crust and add custard pumpkin filling.

Crust ingredients
- 112g *(1 cup)* almond flour
- 34g *(1/4 cup)* coconut flour
- 28g *(1/4 cup)* cocoa powder
- 52g *(1/4 cup)* sweetener
     monk fruit, erythritol, xylitol
- 57g *(1/4 cup)* grass-fed butter *chilled*
     sub for palm shortening to make **DF**
- 1 free-run egg *room temp*
- 1/2 teaspoon sea salt

Custard ingredients
- 75g *(1/3 cup)* grass-fed butter
     sub for palm shortening to make **DF**
- 56g *(1/4 cup)* pumpkin purée *unsweetened*
- 80g *(1/3 cup)* coconut oil
- 80mL *(1/3 cup)* coconut milk *full fat*
- 105g *(1/2 cup)* sweetener
     monk fruit, erythritol, xylitol
- 4 free-run eggs *room temp*
- 2 teaspoons rum extract
- 2 teaspoons pure vanilla extract
- 2 teaspoons nutmeg *fresh or powder*
- 1/2 teaspoon pumpkin spice
- 1/2 teaspoon sea salt

Garnish
- 27g *(1/4 cup)* powdered sweetener
     monk fruit, erythritol, xylitol

Note

- **If you don't like the eggnog flavour, ditch the rum extract and nutmeg, and you will have yourself pumpkin custard bars!**

Instructions
1. Position a rack in the lower third of your oven and **preheat to 350°F/180°C.** Line with parchment paper the bottom and sides of an 8x8-inch baking pan.
2. **Crust:** Measure almond flour, coconut flour, cocoa powder, sweetener and sea salt into a bowl and whisk well.
3. Add chilled cubes of butter & one egg. Using your hand, mix the crust dough the old-fashioned way, or use a stand mixer with a paddle/beater attachment. Mix/knead until it forms a ball.
4. Place the dough onto the prepared pan and flatten until a thin layer coats the entire pan.
5. Poke holes in the crust to allow a more even bake.
6. Bake for 12-15 minutes at 350°F/180°C to par-cook the crust. As the crust is baking, start on the lemon custard.
7. **Custard:** In a small saucepan, combine all the custard ingredients **except the eggs.** Heat on medium-low heat until melted.
8. Add 1/4 cup of the saucepan melted custard content into a small bowl; temper the eggs by adding one egg at a time and whisking them together vigorously.
9. Once all eggs are tempered, pour the egg mixture into the saucepan. On low heat, whisk until it holds marks from the whisk and the first bubble appears on the surface, about 6 minutes. *If eggs curdle, don't worry; blend in a high-speed blender for 2-3 minutes.*
10. Pour the custard onto the crust and cook for an additional 15-17 minutes. Depending on the oven, you may have to par-cook a bit longer.
11. Cool for one full hour in the fridge to allow the custard to harden up.
12. **Garnish:** Cut eggnog bars into 9 pieces, and garnish by dusting the top with powdered sweetener.
13. Store in an airtight container for three to four days and freeze for up to three months.

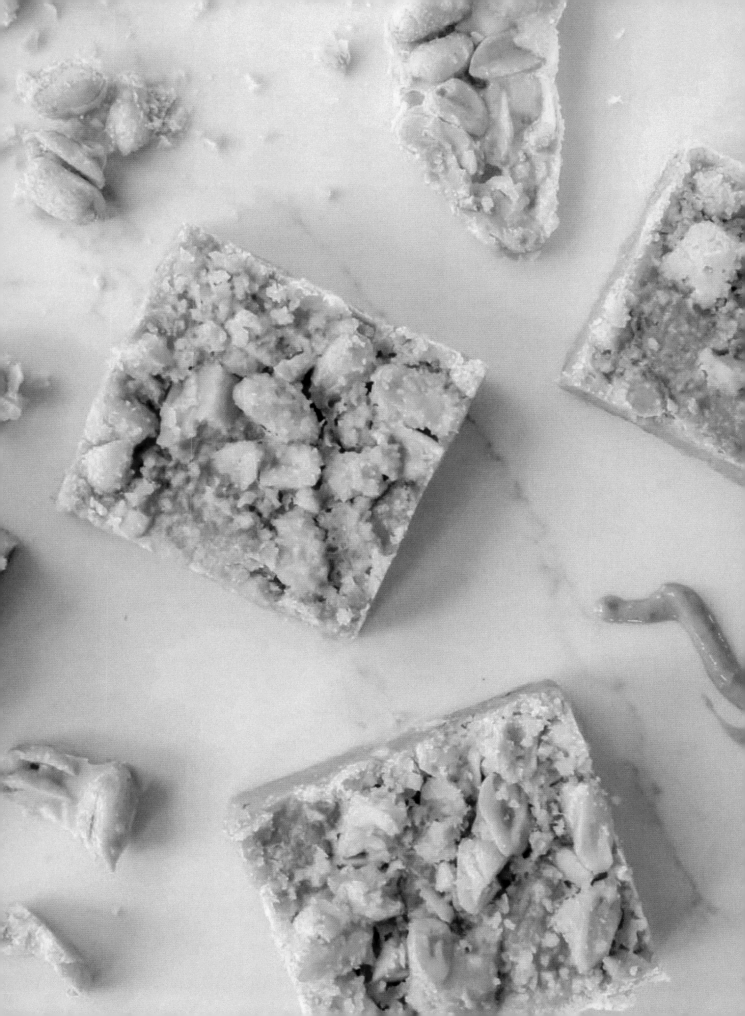

Peanut Brittle Blondies

prep: *12 min*   **bake:** *15-17 min*   **cool:** *5-10 min*   **serves:** *9 bars*

Adding the simple step of browning your butter will enhance the depth, richness and nuttiness of any baked good.
Brown butter is pretty impressive, but remember, don't burn the BUTTA!

Dry ingredients

- 168g *(1½ cups)* almond flour
- 46g *(1/3 cup)* coconut flour
- 28g *(1/4 cup)* organic collagen *grass-fed*
- 152g *(3/4 cup)* sweetener
    monk fruit, erythritol, xylitol
- 1 teaspoon sea salt

Wet ingredients

- 113g *(1/2 cup)* grass-fed butter *browned*
- 113g *(1/2 cup)* peanut butter *natural*
- 2 teaspoons blackstrap molasses
- 4 free-run eggs *room temp*
- 10mL *(2 teaspoons)* pure vanilla extract

Peanut brittle ingredients

- 145g *(1 cup)* dry roasted peanuts *salted*
- 57g *(1/4 cup)* grass-fed butter *melted*
- 105g *(1/2 cup)* sweetener
    monk fruit, erythritol, xylitol
- 5mL *(1 teaspoon)* pure vanilla extract

Instructions

1. **Peanut brittle:** In a small saucepan on medium heat, add butter, sweetener, and vanilla.
2. Cook the mixture to a golden caramel. Do not under-cook the caramel, as it will be highly brittle & grainy. It should be a deep brown colour.
3. Pour the brittle caramel mixture over the dry roasted peanuts and leave it to cool completely in the fridge for around 40-50 minutes.
4. **Preheat oven to 350°F/180°C.**
5. Line with parchment paper the bottom and sides of an 8x8-inch baking pan.
6. In a medium saucepan, melt butter on medium heat until it becomes liquified.
7. Set melted butter aside to cool down for 10 minutes.
8. Add all the dry ingredients to a medium bowl, whisking until thoroughly mixed.
9. Add the melted butter to the dry ingredients, then add one egg at a time, whisking well after each added egg until completely incorporated. Then mix in peanut butter, molasses and vanilla.
10. Pour the mixture into the prepared pan. Then add the peanut butter on top. Use an offset spatula to spread and level out the top.
11. Break the cooled peanut and caramel brittle into small pieces and sprinkle it over the top of the blondies.
12. Bake for 16-18 minutes. It's better to under-bake than over-bake.
13. Take a look at the blondies around 14-15min. Remove from the oven if they look ready. Due to the high-fat content, they will continue to cook while cool. I let mine cool for about 30min in the fridge.
14. Once the blondies are cooled, lift them using the edges of the parchment paper. Cut into the desired size.
15. Store in an airtight container for one week and freeze for up to three months.

Note

- **You can only use butter to make the brown butter. However, you can skip the browning step and use palm shortening to make it dairy-free.**

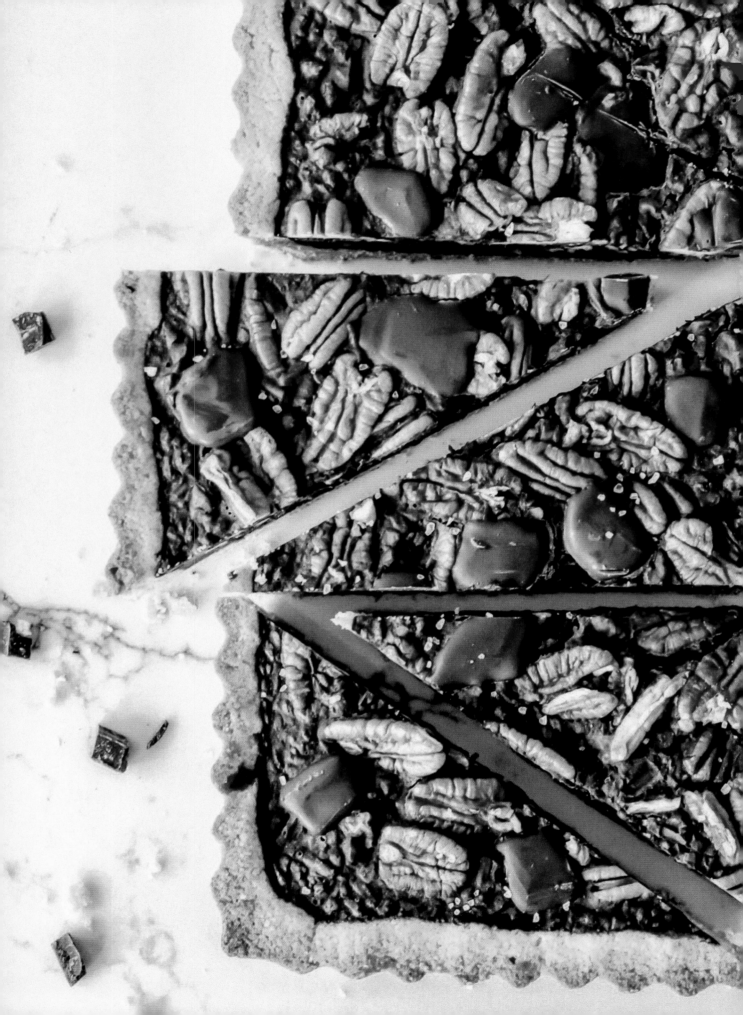

Pecan Chocolate Tart

prep: *25 min* **bake:** *40-45 min* **cool:** *15-20 min* **serves:** 8 slices

Serve this pecan chocolate gooey tart warm with a nice big scoop of vanilla ice cream (recipe on page 210)!

Crust ingredients
- 112g *(1 cup)* almond flour
- 46g *(1/3 cup)* coconut flour
- 11g *(1 tablespoon)* psyllium husk powder
- 52g *(1/4 cup)* sweetener
    - *monk fruit, erythritol, xylitol*
- 57g *(1/4 cup)* grass-fed butter *chilled*
- 1 free-run egg *room temp*
- 15mL *(1 tablespoon)* apple cider vinegar
- 1 teaspoon baking soda
- 1 teaspoon sea salt

Filling ingredients:
113g *(1/2 cup)* grass-fed butter *browned*
- 110g *(1/2 cup)* chocolate chips
    - *the recipe is found on page 223*
- 152g *(1/2 cup)* sweetener
    - *monk fruit, erythritol, xylitol*
- 4 free-run eggs *room temp*
- 62g *(1/2 cup)* pecan halves
- 57mL *(1/2 cup)* coconut milk *full fat*
- 25g *(1/4 cup)* cocoa powder
- 62g *(1/2 cup)* pecan halves
- 1 teaspoon pure vanilla extract
- 1 teaspoon sea salt

Garnish
- 62g *(1/2 cup)* pecan halves
- 85g *(1 full)* chocolate bar
    - *the recipe is found on page 223*

Note

- **The tart/pie crust may bake too quickly; place tin foil around the edges of the crust, so it does not brown too fast.**

Instructions
1. **Preheat oven to 350°F/180°C.**
2. **Crust:** Mix almond flour, coconut flour, psyllium husk powder, sweetener, baking soda and sea salt into a bowl, and whisk together.
3. Add chilled cubes of butter, one egg and apple cider vinegar. Using your hand, mix the crust dough the old-fashioned way, or use a stand mixer with a paddle/beater attachment. Mix/knead until it forms a ball.
4. Grease an 8x6-inch tart pan or an 8-inch pie baking pan.
5. Place dough onto the greased pan and push the dough into the pan until a thin layer coats the entire pan and creates an edge crust.
6. Poke holes in the crust with a fork to allow a more even bake.
7. Bake for 12-15 minutes at 350°F/180°C to par-cook.
8. **NOTE:** When the tart crust is finished par-cooking, bake 1 cup *(125g)* of pecans halves for 7 minutes for the filling and the garnish.
9. **Filling:** Brown the butter in a small saucepan on medium heat. Allow the butter to come to a foaming stage, reduce heat slightly and stir until butter goes from a yellow hue to a golden/light brown hue.
10. Add chocolate chips and sweetener to the butter and mix until the chocolate chips are melted.
11. In a medium bowl, whisk together eggs, full-fat coconut milk/cream, sifted cocoa powder, toasted pecan pieces, vanilla extract and sea salt.
12. Transfer the creamy pecan mixture to the cooled chocolate-butter mixture; Stir together until thoroughly combined and smooth!
13. With a spatula, pour the entire mixture into the pre-baked pie crust.
14. **Garnish:** Top the pie/tart with the pecan halves.
15. Bake the tart for 25 minutes.
16. Once the tart is out of the oven, cool for 20 minutes, chop up the Chocolate Bar and slightly press the chucks on top of the pecan pie.
17. Let pie cool for 2 hours before slicing in and enjoying.
18. Store in an airtight container for three to four days and freeze for up to three months.

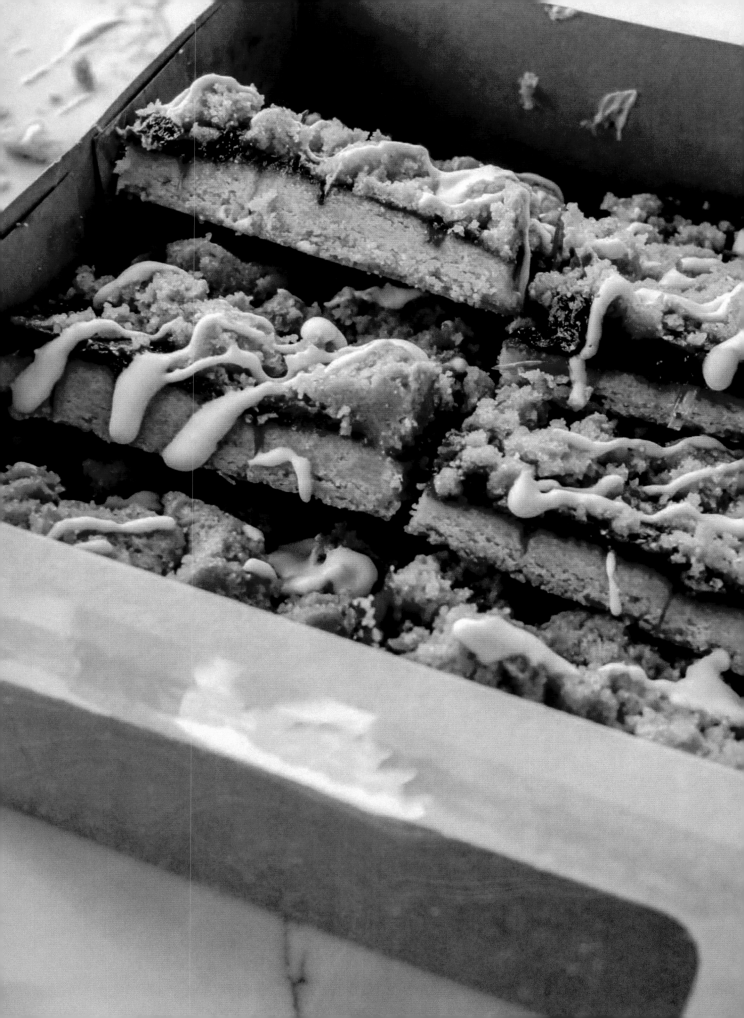

Cranberry Orange Streusel Bars

prep: *15 min*   **bake:** *30-35 min*   **cool:** *15-20 min*   **serves:** *9 bars*

Have an unforgettable Christmas gathering with these lovely festive Cranberry Orange Streusel Bars!

Crust ingredients

- 112g *(1 cup)* almond flour
- 46g *(1/3 cup)* coconut flour
- 28g *(1/4 cup)* organic collagen *grass-fed*
- 52g *(1/4 cup)* sweetener
  monk fruit, erythritol, xylitol
- 57g *(1/4 cup)* grass-fed butter *chilled*
  sub for palm shortening to make DF
- 1 free-run egg *room temp*
- 1 teaspoon sea salt

Fillings

- 280g *(1 cup)* cranberry jam
  the recipe is found on page 193

Crumble ingredients:

- 57g *(1/4 cup)* grass-fed butter *room temp*
  sub for palm shortening to make DF
- 94g *(3/4 cup)* almond flour
- 30g *(1/4 cup)* coconut flour
- 52g *(1/4 cup)* sweetener
  monk fruit, erythritol, xylitol
- 1 teaspoon cinnamon
- 1 zest of a large orange
- 1 teaspoon pure vanilla extract

Garnish/drizzle

- 27g *(1/4 cup)* powdered sweetener
  monk fruit, erythritol, xylitol
- 15mL *(1 tablespoon)* lemon juice

Instructions

1. Pre-make your jam *(the recipe is found on page 193)*
2. Position a rack in the lower third of your oven and **preheat to 350°F/180°C.** Line with parchment paper the bottom and sides of an 8x8-inch baking pan.
3. **Crust:** Mix almond flour, coconut flour, collagen, sweetener and sea salt into a bowl and whisk together.
4. Add chilled cubes of butter and one egg. Using your hand, mix the crust dough the old-fashioned way, or use a stand mixer. Mix/knead until it forms a ball.
5. Place dough onto the prepared pan and push the dough into the pan until a thin layer coats the entire pan.
6. Poke holes in the crust with a fork to allow a more even bake.
7. Bake for 12-15 minutes to par-cook the crust. As the crust is baking, start on the crumble, and have the jam pre-made.
8. **Crumble:** Place all crumble ingredients into a bowl, and mix using your hands until it is well incorporated.
9. **Filling:** Spread the jam of choice onto baked crust, sprinkle the crumble on top of the jam and bake for an additional 15-17 minutes. Depending on the oven, you may have to par-cook for longer.
10. Once the crumble bars are done, set them to cool for 15 min, then cut them into 9 pieces.
11. **Garnish:** Mix powdered sweetener and lemon juice & garnish by drizzling the top with icing.
12. Store in an airtight container for four to five days and freeze for up to three months.

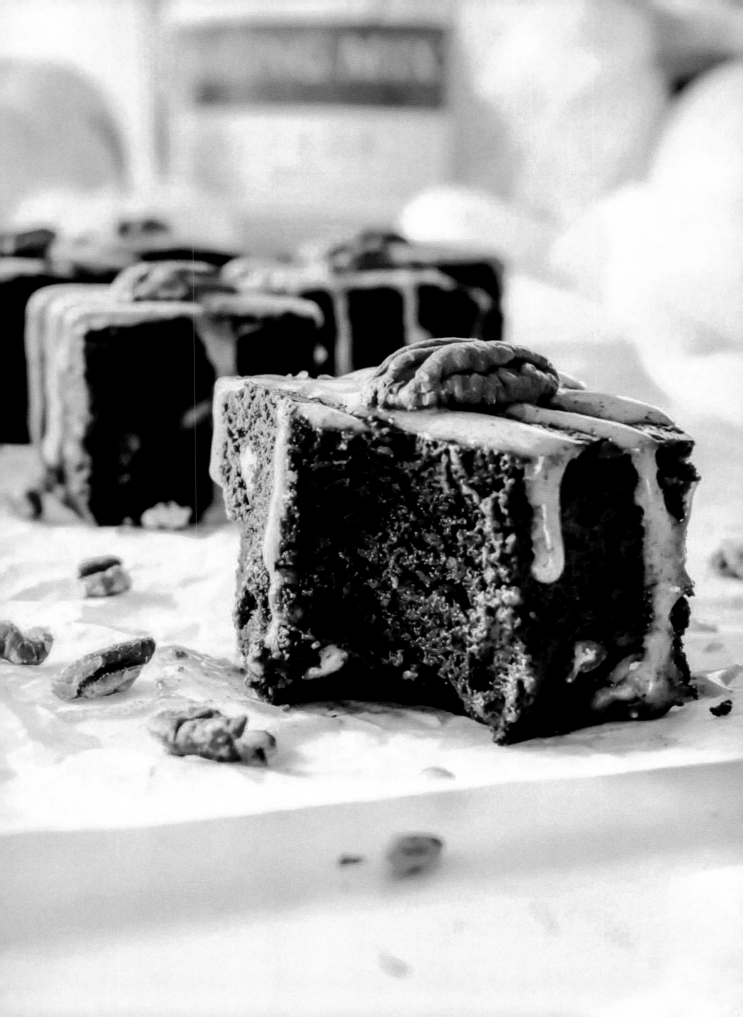

Pumpkin Turtle Brownies

prep: *12 min*   **bake:** *15-17 min*   **cool:** *5-10 min*   **serves:** *9 bars*

Brownies, with a pumpkin spiced turtle surprise, scream Christmas time. They require a bit of extra work if you are going to make the homemade caramel sauce, yet it's so worth it!

Dry ingredients

- 112g *(1 cup)* almond flour
- 65g *(1/2 cup)* pecan halves *toasted & chopped*
- 205g *(1 cup)* sweetener
  monk fruit, erythritol, xylitol
- 56g *(1/2 cup)* cocoa powder sifted
- 34g *(1/4 cup)* coconut flour
- 56g *(1/2 cup)* organic collagen *grass-fed*
- 205g *(1 cup)* sweetener
- 1 teaspoon pumpkin spice
- 1 teaspoon sea salt

Wet ingredients

- 113g *(1/2 cup)* grass-fed butter *room temp*
  sub for palm shortening to make DF
- 110g *(1/2 cup)* chocolate chips *melted*
  the recipe is found on page 214
- 56g *(1/4 cup)* pumpkin purée *unsweetened*
- 4 eggs *room temp*
- 10mL *(2 teaspoons)* pure vanilla extract

Garnish

- 120g *(1/2 cup)* caramel sauce
  the recipe is found on page 219
- 32g *(1/4 cup)* pecan halves *toasted*

Instructions

1. **Preheat to 350°F/180°C.** Line a baking sheet with parchment paper and bake pecan halves for 7 minutes for the garnish and dry ingredients, and set aside.
2. Prep an 8x8-inch baking pan with parchment paper to cover the bottom and sides of the pan. Set aside.
3. Add butter, chocolate chips and sweetener to a heatproof bowl. Melt over a water bath, constantly whisking *(or use the microwave, in 30sec increments & stir every 30 seconds)*.
4. Remove from heat and allow the mixture to cool slightly.
5. Add pumpkin purée and one egg at a time to the chocolate mixture, whisking well after each egg is completely incorporated, and add vanilla extract.
6. Chop half of the pecans to add them to the brownie mixture.
7. In a medium bowl, add chopped pecans, sift the cocoa powder, and add the remainder of the dry ingredient, whisking until thoroughly mixed.
8. Add the chocolate mixture to the dry ingredients to create the brownie dough. Stir together until thoroughly combined.
9. Pour the brownie mixture into the prepared pan, and then using an off-set spatula, even out the top if needed.
10. Bake for 15-17 minutes. It's better to under-bake than over-bake.
11. **NOTE:** Take a look at the brownies around the 12-14min mark. Due to the high-fat content in the brownie, they will continue to cook while they cool. I let mine cool for about 30min in the fridge. Remove from the oven if ready.
12. Once the brownies are cooled, Lift brownies using the edges of the parchment paper and cut them into the desired size.
13. **Garnish:** Drizzle with warmed-up caramel sauce, and add pecan on top of the caramel.
14. Store in an airtight container for three to four days and freeze for up to three months.

Note

- **The baking time depends significantly on the oven & baking pan. Darker/metal pans cook faster around the edges, yet ceramic pans take almost double the amount of time!**

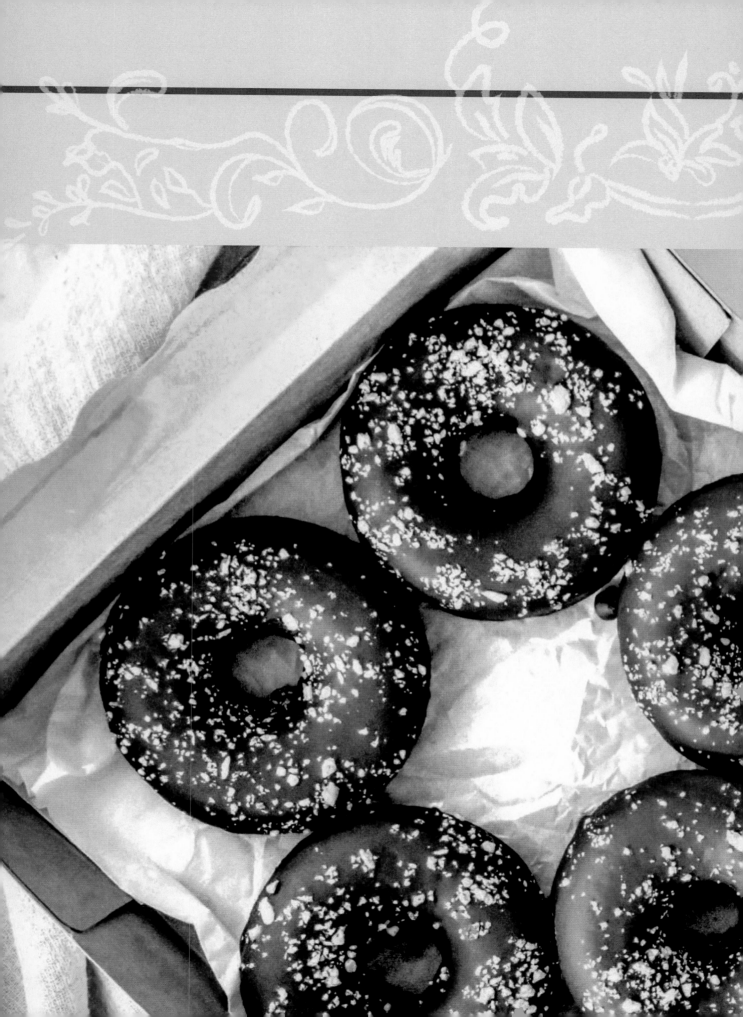

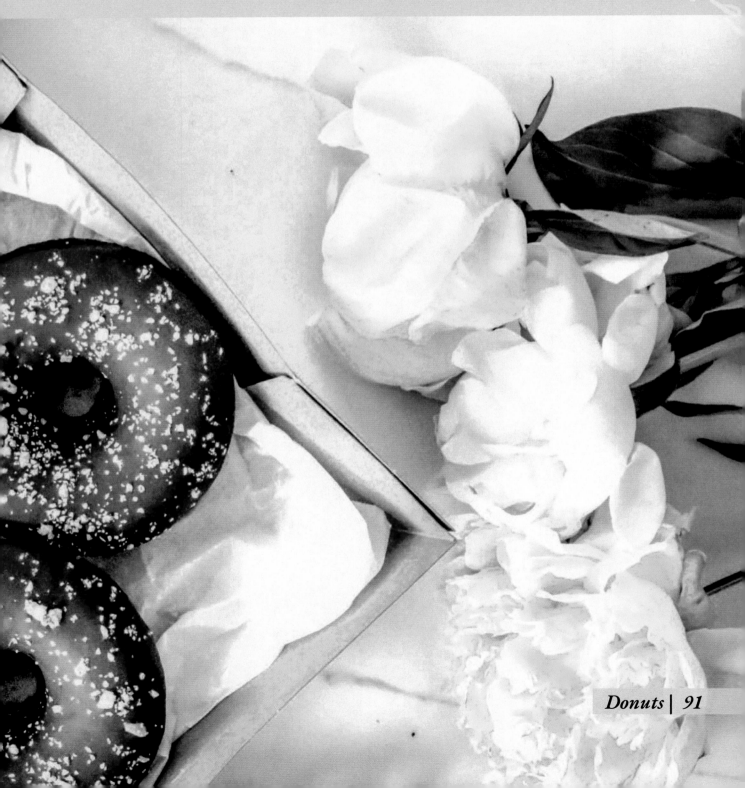

Chapter Three
DONUTS

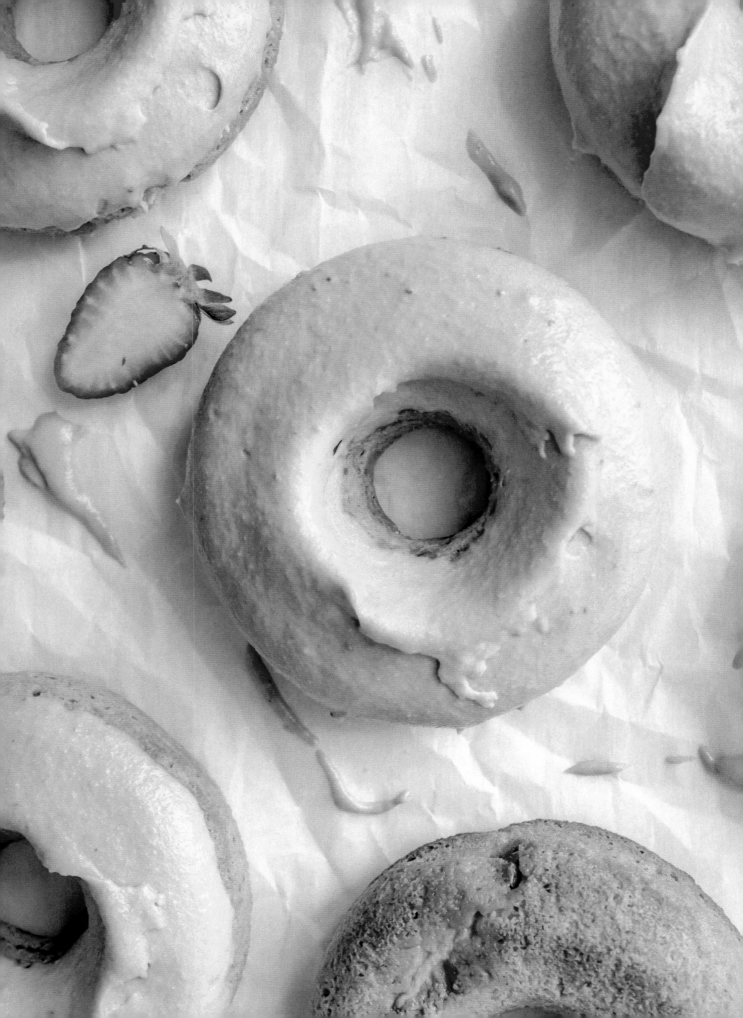

Strawberry Cream Donuts

prep: *20 min*   **bake:** *17-20 min*   **cool:** *15-20 min*   **serves:** *9 large donuts*

I honestly was never a huge fan of donuts until I created my own donut recipes! These donuts are far from the traditional dry or bready ones - they are moist, fluffy and absolutely to die for!

Dry ingredients:

- 84g *(3/4 cup)* almond flour
- 46g *(1/3 cup)* coconut flour
- 125g *(1 cup)* chopped strawberries *fresh*
- 33g *(3 tablespoons)* psyllium husk powder
- 56g *(1/2 cup)* organic collagen *grass-fed*
- 152g *(3/4 cup)* sweetener

  monk fruit, erythritol, xylitol
- 1 teaspoon baking soda
- 1 teaspoon baking powder
- 2 teaspoons instant yeast
- 1 teaspoon sea salt

Wet ingredients:

- 4 free-run eggs *room temp*
- 15mL *(1 tablespoon)* apple cider vinegar
- 118mL *(1/2 cup)* avocado oil
- 118mL *(1/2 cup)* coconut milk *full fat*
- 15mL *(1 tablespoon)* honey *activates yeast*
- 15mL *(1 tablespoon)* apple cider vinegar
- 1 teaspoon pure vanilla extract

Strawberry cream glaze:

- 120g *(1 cup)* powdered sweetener
- 140g *(1/2 cup)* strawberry jam

  the recipes is found on page 193
- 57mL *(1/4 cup)* coconut milk *full fat*
- 1/8 teaspoon sea salt

Instructions

1. **Preheat oven to 350°F/180°C.**
2. Mix all dry ingredients in a bowl. Add the chopped strawberries.
3. **NOTE:** *Make sure strawberries are finely chopped into small pieces.* Whisk together with the dry ingredients, and set aside.
4. Add all the wet ingredients to a stand mixer or regular bowl. Whisk until well incorporated.
5. Add the dry ingredients to the wet, and mix/whisk again until well incorporated.
6. Using a rubber spatula, scrape donut dough around the bowl, and use a large cookie scoop to transfer the dough into a piping bag *(you can also use a big ziplock bag)*.
7. Grease a silicone donut baking pan with coconut or avocado oil to ensure it does not stick.
8. Cut the bottom of the piping bag & squeeze out the dough just enough to fill halfway up to the rim of the donut pan.
9. Bake for 17-20 minutes at 350°F/180°C.
10. As the donuts are baking, you can prepare the strawberry cream glaze.
11. **Strawberry cream glaze:** In a small bowl, add all glaze ingredients *(make sure coconut milk is well mixed)*. Whisk all together until it's a creamy smooth consistency.
12. Once the donuts are out of the oven, wait about 10 minutes before flipping them over on a cooling rack. Let donuts cool for an additional 20 minutes in the fridge.
13. Dunk donuts into the strawberry cream glaze. Carefully twist in a circular motion and transfer the donuts to a cookie sheet lined with parchment paper to allow them to sit before serving. Enjoy!
14. Refrigerate and store in an airtight container for one week, or freeze for three months.
15. Serve them cold, or take them out of the fridge 20min before eating.

Note

- **Make sure you chop/slice strawberries small enough to fit through the hole in the piping bag.**

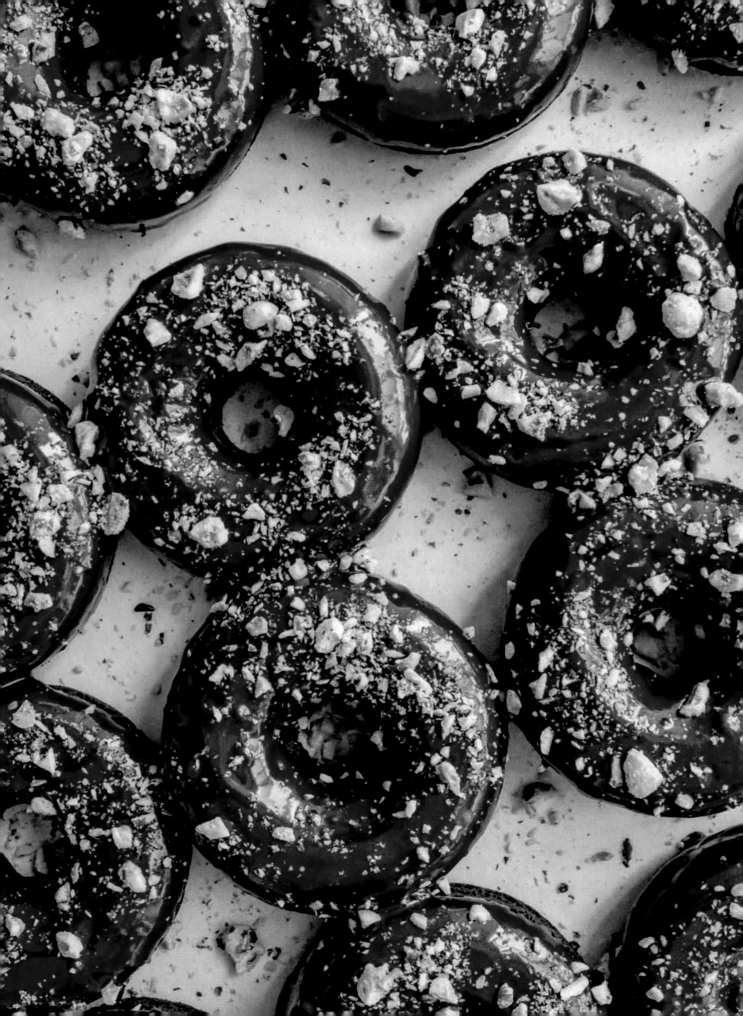

Decadent Hazelnut Donuts

prep: *20 min*   **bake:** *17-20 min*   **cool:** *15-20 min*   **serves:** *9 large donuts*

Chocolate and hazelnuts have always been one of my favourite combos, and incorporating those two exquisite flavours into a donut is just brilliant!

Dry ingredients:

- 112g *(1 cup)* hazelnut flour *toasted*
- 34g *(1/4 cup)* coconut flour
- 56g *(1/2 cup)* cacao powder
- 22g *(2 tablespoons)* psyllium husk powder
- 56g *(1/2 cup)* organic collagen *grass-fed*
- 152g *(3/4 cup)* sweetener
    monk fruit, erythritol, xylitol
- 1 teaspoon baking soda
- 1 teaspoon baking powder
- 2 teaspoons instant yeast
- 1 teaspoon sea salt

Wet ingredients:

- 4 free-run eggs *room temp*
- 177mL *(3/4 cup)* avocado oil
- 118mL *(1/2 cup)* coconut milk *full fat*
- 15mL *(1 tablespoon)* apple cider vinegar
- 15mL *(1 tablespoon)* honey *activates yeast*
- 1 teaspoon pure vanilla extract

Chocolate ganache glaze:

- 220g *(1 cup)* chocolate chips
    the recipe is found on page 223
- 15mL *(1 tablespoon)* coconut oil *melted*
- 135g *(1 cup)* whole hazelnuts *toasted*

Instructions

1. **Preheat oven to 350°F/180°C.**
2. Measure hazelnut flour and toast for 6 minutes on a baking sheet, and set aside. For the garnish, bake the whole hazelnuts for 12 minutes.
3. Once hazelnut flour has cooled down, measure out all dry ingredients in a medium bowl. Whisk together and set aside.
4. Next, in a separate medium bowl, add all the wet ingredients. Whisk until well incorporated.
5. Add the dry ingredients to the wet, and mix/whisk again until well incorporated.
6. Using a rubber spatula, scrape donut dough around the bowl, and use a large cookie scoop to transfer the dough into a piping bag *(you can also use a big ziplock bag)*.
7. Grease a silicone donut baking pan with coconut or avocado oil to ensure it does not stick.
8. Cut the bottom of the piping bag & squeeze out the dough just enough to fill halfway up to the rim of the donut pan.
9. Bake for 17-20 minutes at 350°F/180°C.
10. Once the donuts are out of the oven, wait about 10 minutes before flipping them over on a cooling rack. Let donuts cool for an additional 20 minutes in the fridge.
11. **Chocolate ganache glaze:** In a small, heat-proof bowl, melt chocolate chips over a water bath *(constantly whisking)* or use the microwave in 30sec increments, stirring every time.
12. Dunk donuts into the chocolate ganache. Carefully twist in a circular motion and transfer the donuts to a cookie sheet lined with parchment paper.
13. Sprinkle with chopped toasted hazelnuts and pop them into the fridge for 15-20minutes to allow the ganache to harden up.
14. Refrigerate and store in an airtight container for one week, or freeze for three months.
15. Serve them cold, or take them out of the fridge 20min before eating.

Note

- **The first step is critical for adding that lovely aroma and flavour of hazelnuts to the donuts.**

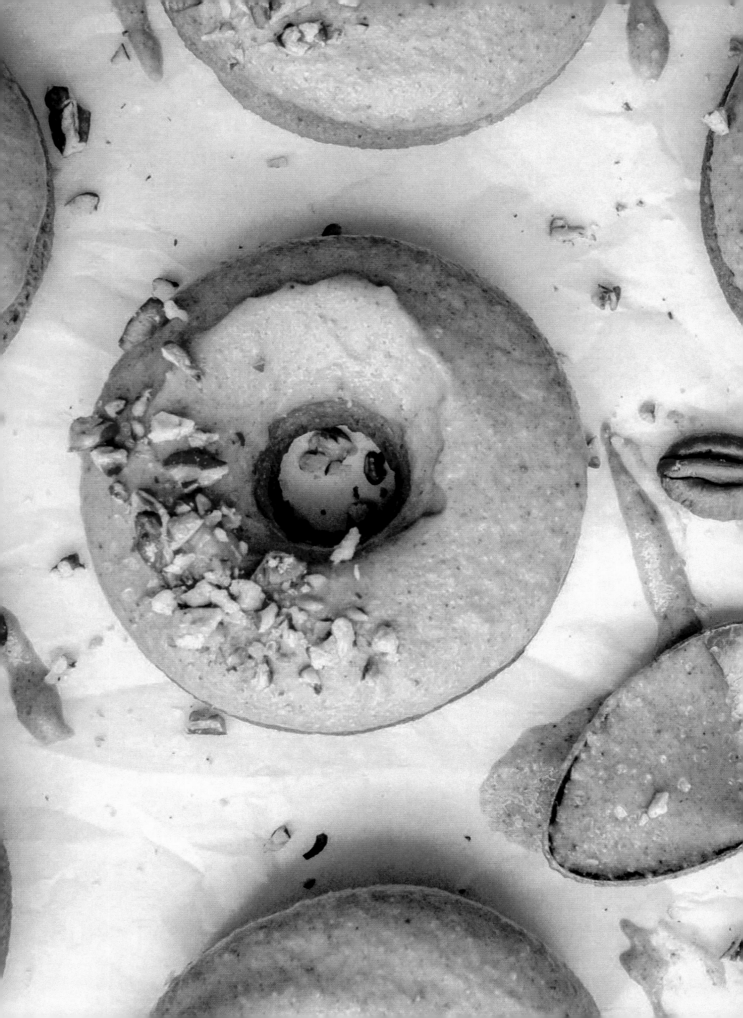

Salted Caramel Donuts

prep: *20 min*   **bake:** *17-20 min*   **cool:** *15-20 min*   **serves:** *9 large donuts*

There is no doubt that my raw caramel sauce has been one of my favourite ingredients to incorporate into so many of my Bakerlita recipes. Glazing your donuts in this sauce is next level AMAZING!

Dry ingredients:

- 84g *(3/4 cup)* almond flour
- 46g *(1/3 cup)* coconut flour
- 33g *(3 tablespoons)* psyllium husk powder
- 56g *(1/2 cup)* organic collagen *grass-fed*
- 152g *(3/4 cup)* sweetener
    monk fruit, erythritol, xylitol
- 1 teaspoon baking soda
- 1 teaspoon baking powder
- 2 teaspoons instant yeast
- 1 teaspoon sea salt

Wet ingredients:

- 4 free-run eggs *room temp*
- 118mL *(1/2 cup)* avocado oil
- 118mL *(1/2 cup)* coconut milk *full fat*
- 15mL *(1 tablespoon)* honey *activates yeast*
- 15mL *(1 tablespoon)* apple cider vinegar
- 1 teaspoon pure vanilla extract
- 1 teaspoon caramel extract

Caramel glaze:

- 240g *(1 cup)* salted caramel sauce
    the recipe is found on page 219
- 55g *(1/2 cup)* pecans *toasted & chopped*

Instructions

1. **Preheat oven to 350°F/180°C.**
2. In a medium bowl, measure out all dry ingredients. Whisk together and set aside.
3. Next, in a separate medium bowl, add all the wet ingredients. Whisk until well incorporated.
4. Add the dry ingredients to the wet, and mix/whisk again until well incorporated.
5. Using a rubber spatula, scrape donut dough around the bowl, and use a large cookie scoop to transfer the dough into a piping bag *(you can also use a big ziplock bag)*.
6. Grease a silicone donut baking pan with coconut or avocado oil to ensure it does not stick.
7. Cut the bottom of the piping bag & squeeze out the dough just enough to fill halfway up to the rim of the donut pan.
8. Bake for 17-20 minutes at 350°F/180°C.
9. Once the donuts are out of the oven, wait about 10 minutes before flipping them over on a cooling rack. Let donuts cool for an additional 20 minutes in the fridge.
10. For the garnish, bake the pecans for 5-6 minutes. Chop and set them aside.
11. **Caramel glaze:** In a small bowl, add caramel sauce. It is best to make the caramel sauce the day before. This allows the cashews extra time to soak, which yields an extra creamy caramel.
12. Dunk donuts into the caramel cream glaze, carefully twisting in a circular motion. Transfer the donuts to a cookie sheet lined with parchment paper and allow them to sit before serving. Enjoy!
13. Refrigerate and store in an airtight container for one week, or freeze for three months.
14. Serve them cold, or take them out of the fridge 20min before eating.

Note

- **The caramel sauce is the highlight of this recipe. Be sure to make it ahead of time to ensure the best creamy consistency.**

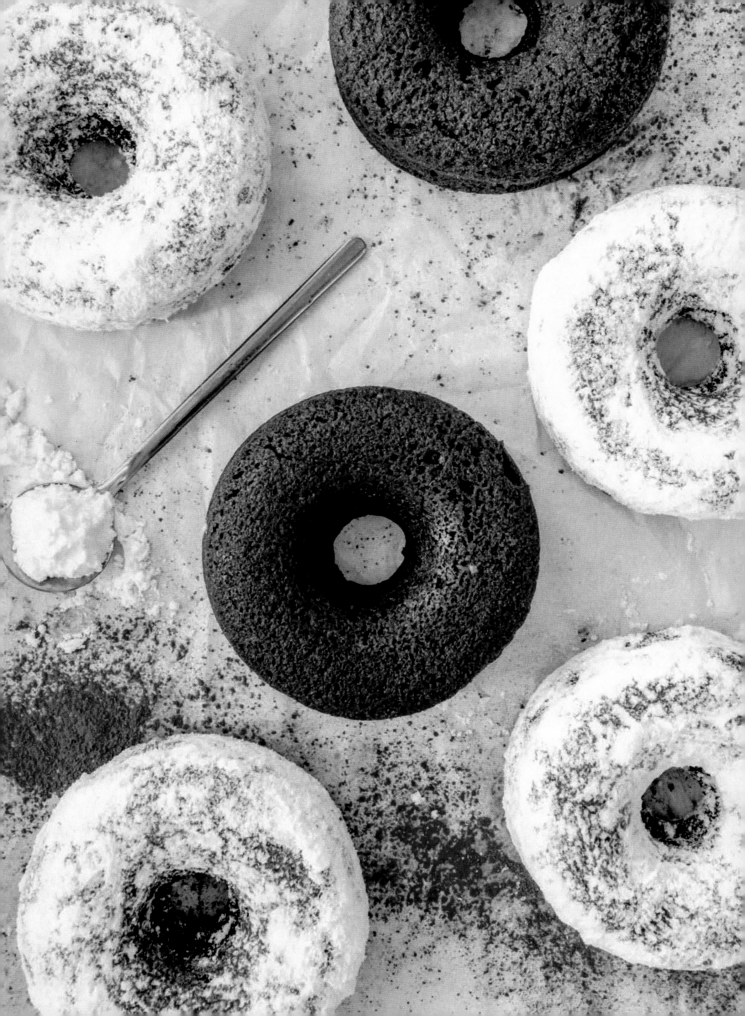

Powdered Sugar Donuts

prep: *20 min*   **bake:** *17-20 min*   **cool:** *15-20 min*   **serves:** *9 large donuts*

These are so simple to make and they are are the prefect satisfaction for your sweet chocolate cravings - all in one glorious donut!

Dry ingredients:

- 84g *(3/4 cup)* almond flour
- 34g *(1/4 cup)* coconut flour
- 56g *(1/2 cup)* cacao powder
- 22g *(2 tablespoons)* psyllium husk powder
- 56g *(1/2 cup)* organic collagen *grass-fed*
- 152g *(3/4 cup)* sweetener

    monk fruit, erythritol, xylitol

- 1 teaspoon baking soda
- 1 teaspoon baking powder
- 2 teaspoons instant yeast
- 1 teaspoon sea salt

Wet ingredients:

- 220g (1/2 cup) chocolate chips *melted*

    recipe is found on page 223

- 4 free-run eggs *room temp*
- 118mL *(1/2 cup)* avocado oil
- 118mL *(1/2 cup)* coconut milk *full fat*
- 15mL *(1 tablespoon)* apple cider vinegar
- 15mL *(1 tablespoon)* honey *activates yeast*
- 1 teaspoon pure vanilla extract

Powder garnish:

- 120g *(1 cup)* powdered sweetener

    monk fruit, erythritol, xylitol

Note

- **You may also make these with a vanilla base donut. Look on page 96, just omit the caramel extract.**

Instructions

1. **Preheat oven to 350°F/180°C.**
2. In a small, heat-proof bowl, melt chocolate chips over a water bath *(constantly whisking)* or use the microwave in 30sec increments, stirring every time.
3. Add all the wet ingredients in a medium bowl, including the melted chocolate chips. Whisk until well incorporated.
4. Next, in a separate medium bowl, add all the dry ingredients. Whisk until well incorporated.
5. Add the dry ingredients to the wet, and mix/whisk again until well incorporated.
6. Using a rubber spatula, scrape donut dough around the bowl, and use a large cookie scoop to transfer the dough into a piping bag *(you can also use a big ziplock bag)*.
7. Grease a silicone donut baking pan with coconut or avocado oil to ensure it does not stick.
8. Cut the bottom of the piping bag & squeeze out the dough just enough to fill halfway up to the rim of the donut pan.
9. Bake for 17-20 minutes at 350°F/180°C.
10. Once the donuts are out of the oven, wait about 10 minutes before flipping them over on a cooling rack.
11. **Powder garnish:** In a small bowl, add powder sweetener.
12. Dunk the donut's top and bottom into the powdered sweetener while still slightly warm to ensure the sweetener sticks to the donut.
13. Carefully twist in a circular motion and transfer the donuts to a cookie sheet lined with parchment paper & allowing them to cool a bit longer.
14. Dunk the donuts in the powdered sweetener one last time before serving. Enjoy!
15. Refrigerate and store in an airtight container for one week, or freeze for three months.
16. Serve them cold, or take them out of the fridge 20min before eating.

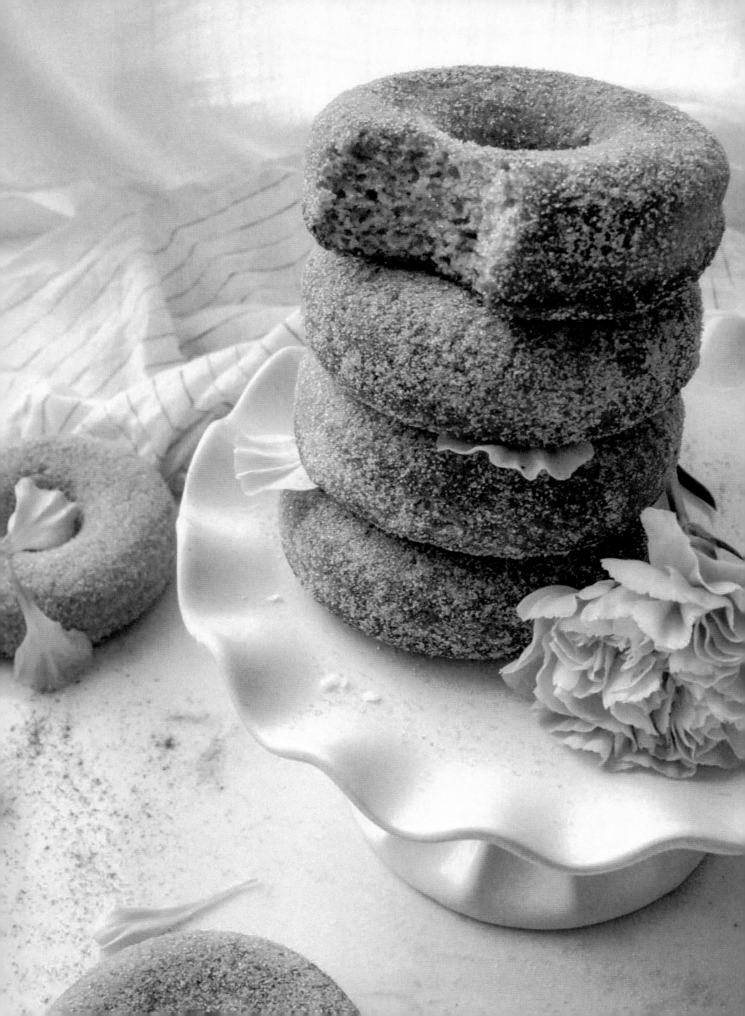

Cinnamon Sugar Donuts

prep: *20 min*   **bake:** *17-20 min*   **cool:** *15-20 min*   **serves:** *9 large donuts*

Honestly, these donuts are my favourite. These Cinnamon Sugar Donuts taste like something you would find at a specialty donut shop. You would never guess that they are entirely gluten, sugar, dairy and guilt FREE!

Dry ingredients:
- 84g *(3/4 cup)* almond flour
- 46g *(1/3 cup)* coconut flour
- 33g *(3 tablespoons)* psyllium husk powder
- 56g *(1/2 cup)* organic collagen *grass-fed*
- 152g *(3/4 cup)* sweetener
  monk fruit, erythritol, xylitol
- 1 tablespoon cinnamon
- 1 teaspoon baking soda
- 1 teaspoon baking powder
- 2 teaspoons instant yeast
- 1 teaspoon sea salt

Wet ingredients:
- 4 free-run eggs *room temp*
- 118mL *(1/2 cup)* avocado oil
- 118mL *(1/2 cup)* coconut milk *full fat*
- 15mL *(1 tablespoon)* apple cider vinegar
- 15mL *(1 tablespoon)* honey *activates yeast*
- 1 teaspoon pure vanilla extract

Sugar garnish:
- 152g *(3/4 cup)* sweetener
  monk fruit, erythritol, xylitol

Instructions

1. **Preheat oven to 350°F/180°C.**
2. In a medium bowl, measure out all dry ingredients. Whisk together and set aside.
3. Next, in a separate medium bowl, add all the wet ingredients. Whisk until well incorporated.
4. Add the dry ingredients to the wet, and mix/whisk again until well incorporated.
5. Using a rubber spatula, scrape donut dough around the bowl, and use a large cookie scoop to transfer the dough into a piping bag *(you can also use a big ziplock bag)*.
6. Grease a silicone donut baking pan with coconut or avocado oil to ensure it does not stick.
7. Cut the bottom of the piping bag & squeeze out the dough just enough to fill halfway up to the rim of the donut pan.
8. Bake for 17-20 minutes at 350°F/180°C.
9. Once the donuts are out of the oven, wait about 10 minutes before flipping them over on a cooling rack.
10. **Sugar garnish:** In a small bowl, add sweetener *(see note)*.
11. Dunk the donut's top and bottom into the sweetener while still slightly warm to ensure the sweetener sticks to the donut.
12. Carefully twist in a circular motion and transfer the donuts to a cookie sheet with parchment paper to allow them to cool a bit longer.
13. Dunk the donuts in the sweetener one last time before serving. Enjoy!
14. Refrigerate and store in an airtight container for one week, or freeze for three months.
15. Serve them cold, or take them out of the fridge 20min before eating.

Note

- **I love to use Lakanto's Golden monk fruit Sweetener; it gives these donuts such a gorgeous golden hue, with a more caramelly flavour.**

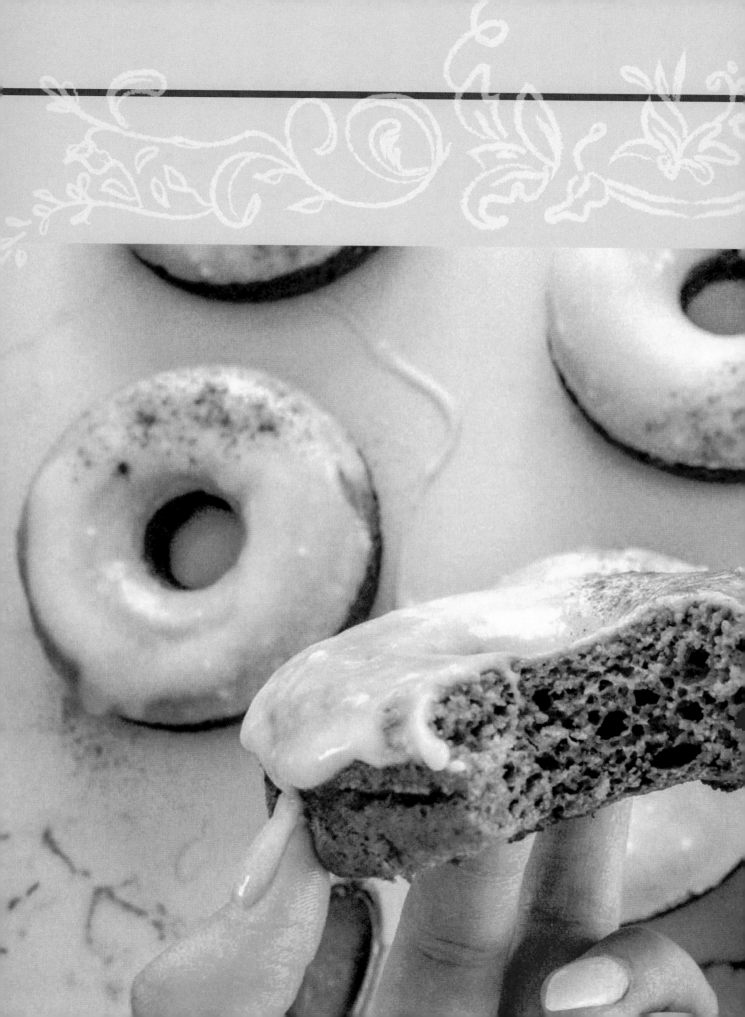

Christmas
DONUTS

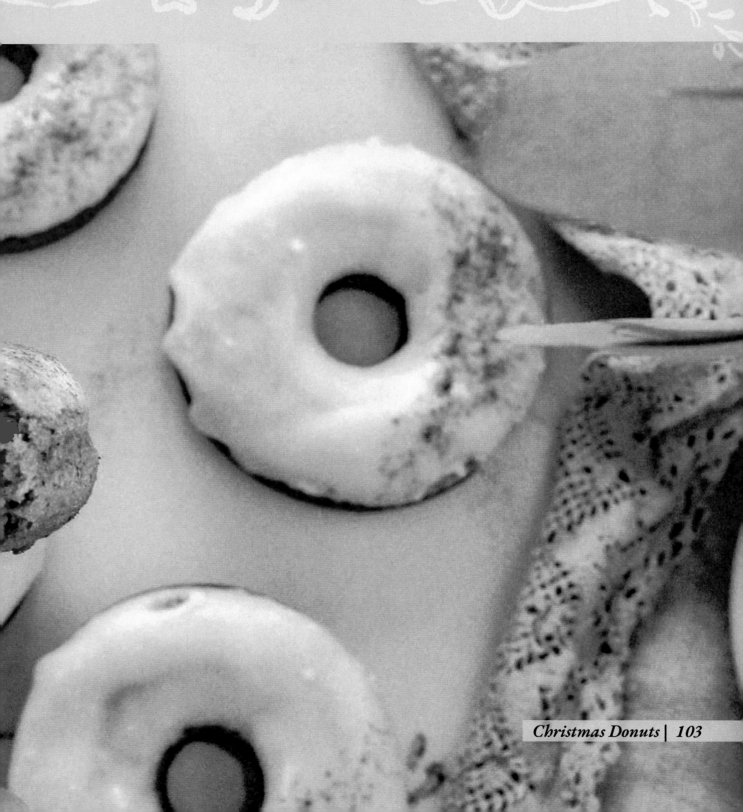

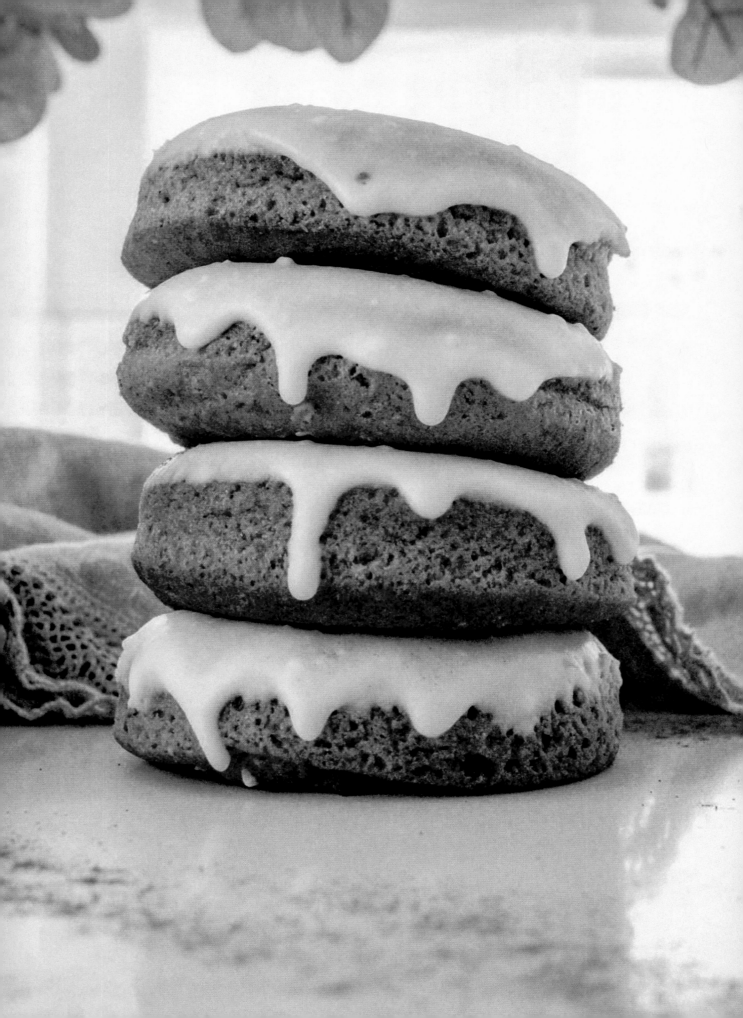

Pumpkin Pie Donuts

prep: *20 min* **bake:** *17-20 min* **cool:** *15-20 min* **serves:** *9 large donuts*

Pumpkin pie always makes its mark around the holiday season. These moist, fluffy, pumpkin pie spice donuts are such a perfect way to welcome the festive fun into your home.

Dry ingredients:
- 112g *(1 cup)* almond flour
- 46g *(1/3 cup)* coconut flour
- 33g *(3 tablespoons)* psyllium husk powder
- 56g *(1/2 cup)* organic collagen *grass-fed*
- 152g *(3/4 cup)* sweetener
  monk fruit, erythritol, xylitol
- 1 tablespoon pumpkin spice
- 1 teaspoon baking soda
- 1 teaspoon baking powder
- 2 teaspoons instant yeast
- 1 teaspoon sea salt

Wet ingredients:
- 120mL *(1/2 cup)* pumpkin purée *unsweet.*
- 4 free-run eggs *room temp*
- 118mL *(1/2 cup)* avocado oil
- 118mL *(1/2 cup)* coconut milk *full fat*
- 15mL *(1 tablespoon)* honey *activates yeast*
- 15mL *(1 tablespoon)* apple cider vinegar
- 1 teaspoon pure vanilla extract

Glaze:
- 57mL *(1/4 cup)* coconut milk *full fat*
- 120g *(1 cup)* powdered sweetener
  monk fruit, erythritol, xylitol

Instructions
1. **Preheat oven to 350°F/180°C.**
2. In a medium bowl, measure out all dry ingredients. Whisk together and set aside.
3. Next, in a separate medium bowl, add all the wet ingredients. Whisk until well incorporated.
4. Add the dry ingredients to the wet, and mix/whisk again until well incorporated.
5. Using a rubber spatula, scrape donut dough around the bowl, and use a large cookie scoop to transfer the dough into a piping bag *(you can also use a big ziplock bag).*
6. Grease a silicone donut baking pan with coconut or avocado oil to ensure it does not stick.
7. Cut the bottom of the piping bag & squeeze out the dough just enough to fill halfway up to the rim of the donut pan.
8. Bake for 17-20 minutes at 350°F/180°C.
9. Once the donuts are out of the oven, wait about 10 minutes before flipping them over on a cooling rack. Let donuts cool for an additional 20 minutes in the fridge.
10. **Glaze:** Mix the powdered sweetener and coconut milk in a small bowl.
11. Dunk the top of the donut into the glaze, carefully twisting it in a circular motion. Transfer the donuts to a cookie sheet lined with parchment paper and allow them to sit before serving. Enjoy!
12. Refrigerate and store in an airtight container for one week, or freeze for three months.
13. Serve them cold, or take them out of the fridge 20min before eating.

Note

- If you don't have pumpkin spice, use 1 teaspoon cinnamon, 1/2 teaspoon ginger, 1/8 teaspoon cloves and 1/8 teaspoon nutmeg.

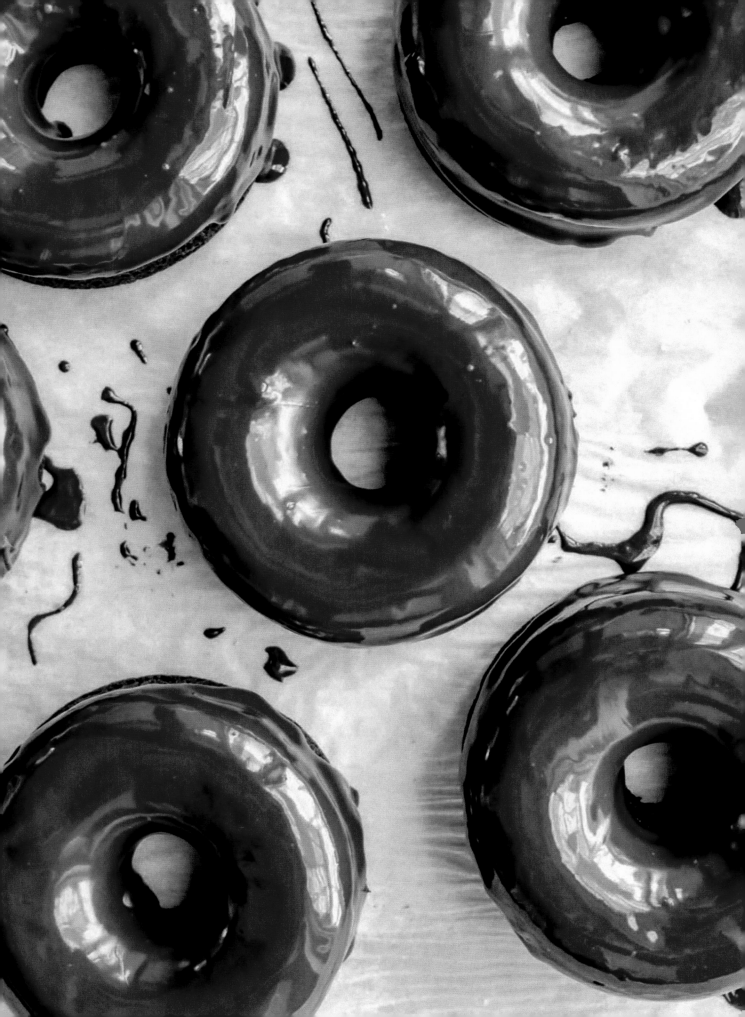

Dark Chocolate Mint Donuts

prep: *20 min* **bake:** *17-20 min* **cool:** *15-20 min* **serves:** *9 large donuts*

These are so simple to make and they perfectly satisfy those sweet chocolate cravings!

Dry ingredients:
- 84g *(3/4 cup)* almond flour
- 34g *(1/4 cup)* coconut flour
- 56g *(1/2 cup)* cacao powder
- 22g *(2 tablespoons)* psyllium husk powder
- 56g *(1/2 cup)* organic collagen *grass-fed*
- 152g *(3/4 cup)* sweetener
  monk fruit, erythritol, xylitol
- 1 teaspoon baking soda
- 1 teaspoon baking powder
- 2 teaspoons instant yeast
- 1 teaspoon sea salt

Wet ingredients:
- 110g *(1/2 cup)* chocolate chips *melted*
  the recipe is found on page 223
- 4 free-run eggs *room temp*
- 113mL *(1/2 cup)* avocado oil
- 113mL *(1/2 cup)* coconut milk *full fat*
- 15mL *(1 tablespoon)* honey *activates yeast*
- 15mL *(1 tablespoon)* apple cider vinegar
- 1 teaspoon pure peppermint oil
- 1 teaspoon pure vanilla extract

Chocolate ganache glaze:
- 220g *(1 cup)* chocolate chips *melted*
- 15mL *(1 tablespoon)* coconut oil

Instructions

1. **Preheat oven to 350°F/180°C.**
2. In a medium bowl, measure out all dry ingredients. Whisk together and set aside.
3. Next, in a separate medium bowl, add all the wet ingredients. Whisk until well incorporated.
4. Add the dry ingredients to the wet, and mix/whisk again until well incorporated.
5. Using a rubber spatula, scrape donut dough around the bowl, and use a large cookie scoop to transfer the dough into a piping bag *(you can also use a big ziplock bag)*.
6. Grease a silicone donut baking pan with coconut or avocado oil to ensure it does not stick.
7. Cut the bottom of the piping bag & squeeze out the dough just enough to fill halfway up to the rim of the donut pan.
8. Bake for 17-20 minutes at 350°F/180°C.
9. Once the donuts are out of the oven, wait about 10 minutes before flipping them over on a cooling rack. Let donuts cool for an additional 20 minutes in the fridge.
10. **Chocolate ganache glaze:** In a small, heat-proof bowl, melt chocolate chips over a water bath *(constantly whisking)* or use the microwave in 30sec increments, stirring every time.
11. Dunk donuts into the chocolate ganache glaze, carefully twisting in a circular motion. Transfer the donuts to a cookie sheet lined with parchment paper and allow them to sit before serving. Enjoy!
12. Refrigerate and store in an airtight container for one week, or freeze for three months.
13. Serve them cold, or take them out of the fridge 20min before eating.

Note

- You can also make these donuts with a vanilla base. Check out page 97 and follow the instructions, just omit the caramel extract.

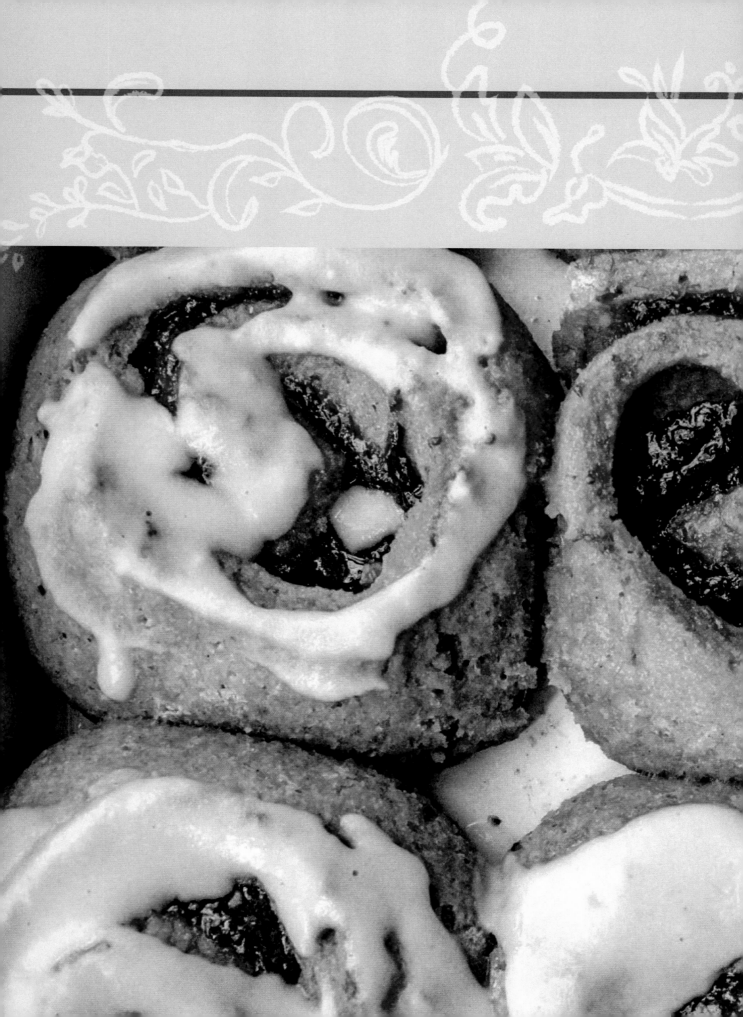

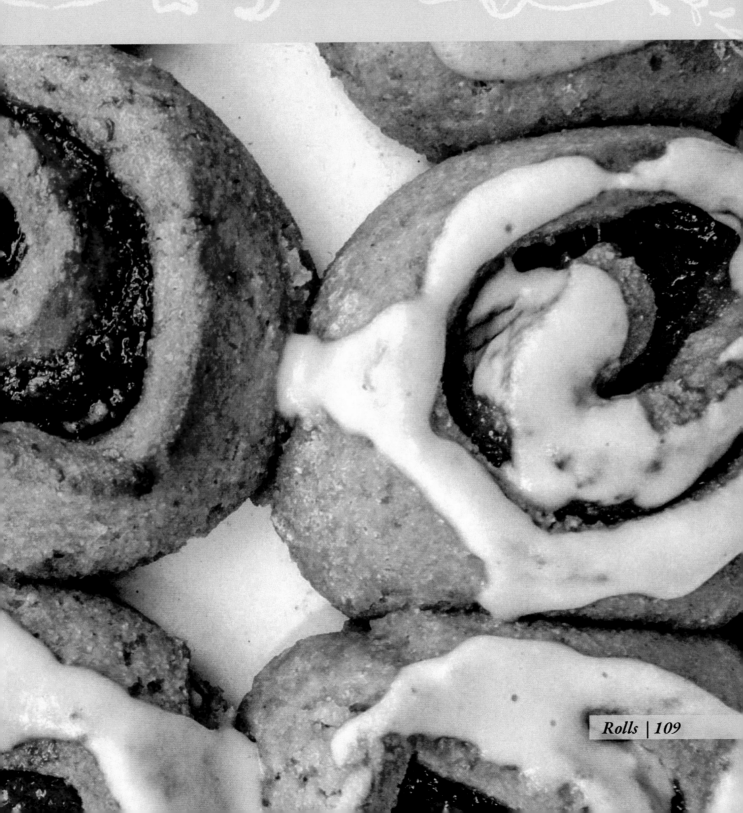

Chapter Four
ROLLS

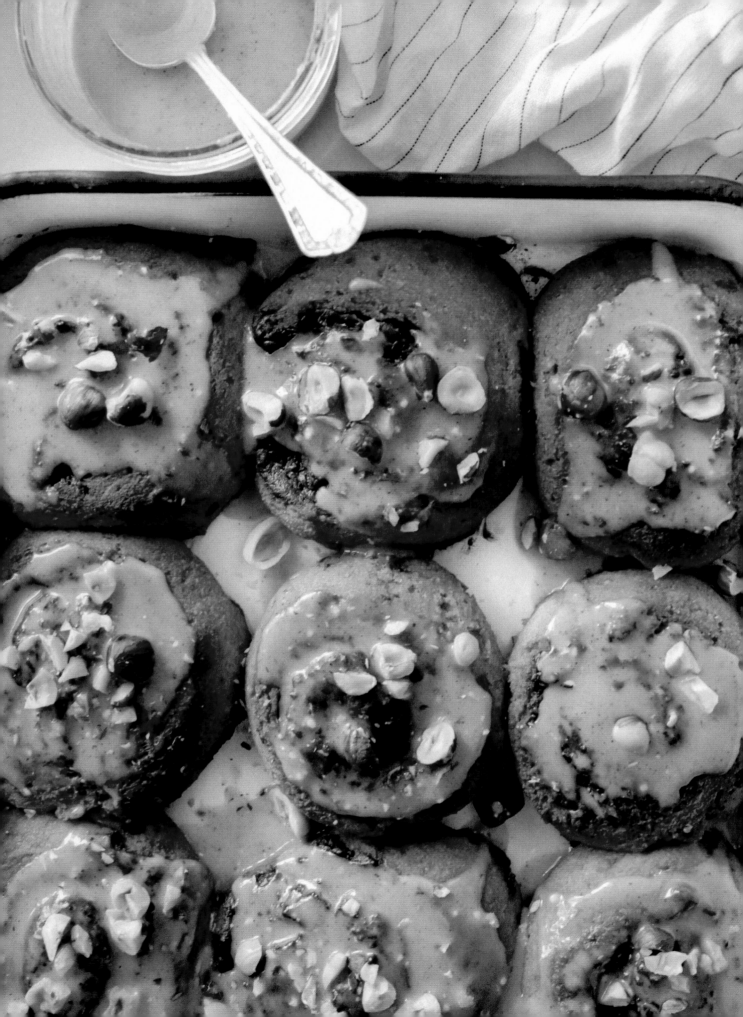

Hazelnut Chocolate Rolls

prep: *25 min*   **bake:** *25-30 min*   **cool:** *15-20 min*   **serves:** *6-8 rolls*

Dry ingredients:

- 168g *(1 1/2 cups)* hazelnut flour *toasted*
- 46g *(1/3 cup)* coconut flour
- 33g *(3 tablespoons)* psyllium husk powder
- 56g *(1/2 cup)* organic collagen *grass-fed*
- 152g *(3/4 cup)* sweetener
  monk fruit, erythritol, xylitol
- 1 teaspoon baking soda
- 1 teaspoon baking powder
- 2 teaspoons instant yeast
- 1 teaspoon sea salt

Wet ingredients:

- 3 free-run eggs *room temp*
- *118mL (1/2 cup)* coconut milk *full fat*
- 15mL *(1 tablespoon)* honey *activates yeast*
- 30mL *(2 tablespoons)* apple cider vinegar
- 1 teaspoon pure vanilla extract

Filling:

- 110g *(1/2 cup)* chocolate chips *melted*
  the recipe is found on page 223
- 152g *(3/4 cup)* sweetener
  monk fruit, erythritol, xylitol
- 57g *(1/4 cup)* hazelnut butter

Garnish topping:

- 120g *(1 cup)* powdered sweetener
- 120g *(1/2 cup)* hazelnut butter
  make homemade on page 229
- 75mL *(3 tablespoons)* nut milk
- 65g *(1/2 cup)* hazelnuts *toasted & chopped*

Instructions

1. **Preheat oven to 350°F/180°C.** Prep an 8x8 inch pan with parchment paper & toast hazelnut flour for 5-6 minutes. Toast whole hazelnuts for 10 minutes.
2. In a medium bowl, measure all dry ingredients. Whisk together well and set aside.
3. Measure all wet ingredients in a separate medium bowl. Whisk together until fully incorporated. Pour the wet ingredients on the dry ingredients; Using a rubber spatula, mix well until completely integrated.
4. Place a piece of saran wrap to cover the bowl, and place the dough in the fridge for about 15 minutes to firm up.
5. **Filling:** In a small bowl, melt chocolate chips over a water bath *(constantly whisking)* or using a microwave in 10sec increments & stirring in between until melted. Mix the hazelnut butter and sweetener into the melted chocolate.
6. Place a large piece of saran wrap onto the surface of your countertop.
7. Place the chilled dough onto the saran wrap surface. Take another piece of saran wrap, place it on top of the dough and press down.
8. Using a rolling pin, roll the dough out into a 16x8-inch rectangle
9. Spread the chocolate hazelnut filling evenly over the whole surface of the dough.
10. Roll the dough and fold the saran wrap under it until it rolls into a big log roll.
11. Cut the roll in half using a sharp knife, then cut each half into 3-4 pieces, leaving you with 6-8 even rolls. Place rolls in buttered baking pans.
12. Bake for 25-35 minutes or until lightly golden brown on top.
13. **Garnish topping:** Add the powdered sweetener, hazelnut butter, and nut milk in a small bowl. Whisk/stir until silky smooth. Add more or less milk if needed.
14. Once baked, let the rolls cool down for about 20 min. Once cooled, drizzle the glaze, and sprinkle with toasted chopped hazelnuts. Enjoy!
15. Store in the fridge in an airtight container for four to five days or freeze for up to three months.

Note

- **Chilling the dough before rolling it out makes it much easier to roll tightly.**

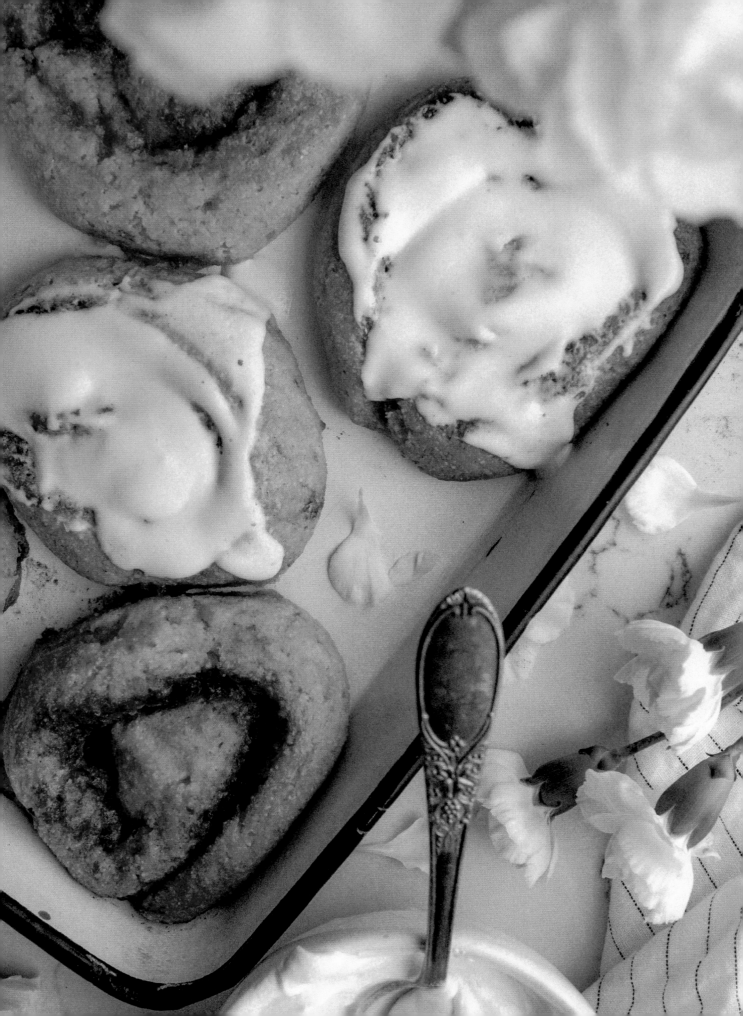

Classic Cinnamon Rolls

prep: *25 min*   **bake:** *25-30 min*   **cool:** *15-20 min*   **serves:** *6-8 rolls*

Dry ingredients:

- 168g *(1 1/2 cups)* almond flour
- 46g *(1/3 cup)* coconut flour
- 33g *(3 tablespoons)* psyllium husk powder
- 56g *(1/2 cup)* organic collagen *grass-fed*
- 152g *(3/4 cup)* sweetener
  - *monk fruit, erythritol, xylitol*
- 1 teaspoon baking soda
- 1 teaspoon baking powder
- 2 teaspoons instant yeast
- 1 teaspoon sea salt

Wet ingredients:

- 3 eggs *room temp*
- 118mL *(1/2 cup)* coconut milk *full fat*
- 15mL *(1 tablespoon)* honey *activates yeast*
- 30mL *(2 tablespoons)* apple cider vinegar
- 1 teaspoon pure vanilla extract

Filling:

- 57g *(1/4 cup)* grass-fed butter *softened*
  - *sub for palm shortening to make DF*
- 105g *(1/2 cup)* sweetener
  - *monk fruit, erythritol, xylitol*
- 16g *(2 tablespoons)* cinnamon

Cream Cheese Glaze:

- 120g *(1 cup)* powdered sweetener
- 120g *(1/2 cup)* cashew cream cheese
  - *the recipe is found on page 235*
- 75mL *(3 tablespoons)* nut milk

Instructions

1. **Preheat oven to 350°F/180°C.** Prep an 8x8-inch pan with parchment paper.
2. In a medium bowl, measure all dry ingredients. Whisk together well and set aside.
3. Measure all wet ingredients in a separate medium bowl. Whisk together until fully incorporated. Pour the wet ingredients on the dry ingredients; Using a rubber spatula, mix well until completely integrated.
4. Place a piece of saran wrap to cover the bowl, and place the dough in the fridge for about 15 minutes to firm up.
5. In a small bowl, mix the sweetener and the cinnamon. Set aside *(for the filling)*
6. Place a large piece of saran wrap on your countertop.
7. Place the chilled dough on the saran-wrapped surface. Take another piece of saran wrap, place it on top of the dough and press down.
8. Using a rolling pin, roll the dough out into a 16x8-inch rectangle.
9. **Filling:** Spread the softened grass-fed butter all over the surface of the dough and sprinkle the cinnamon-sweetener mixture evenly over the whole surface of the dough.
10. Roll the dough and fold the saran wrap under it until it rolls into a big log roll.
11. Cut the roll in half using a sharp knife, then cut each half into 3-4 pieces, leaving you with 6-8 even rolls. Place rolls in buttered baking pans.
12. Bake the rolls for 25-35 minutes or until lightly golden brown on top.
13. **Cream cheese glaze:** Add all the glaze ingredients into a small bowl. Whisk/stir until silky smooth. Add more or less milk if needed.
14. Let rolls cool down for 20 min. Once cinnamon rolls are cooled, it's time to drizzle the glaze all over your rolls. Enjoy!
15. Store in the fridge in an airtight container for four to five days or freeze for up to three months.

Note

- **Chilling the dough before rolling it out makes it much easier to roll tightly.**

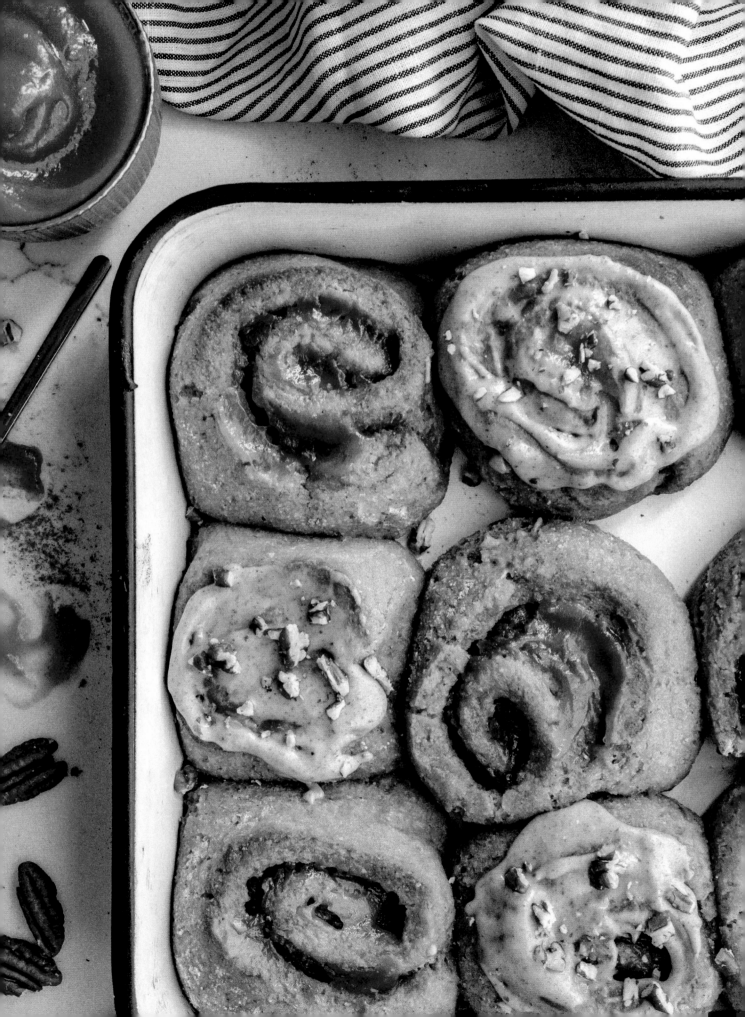

Apple Butter Pecan Rolls

prep: *30 min*   **bake:** *25-30 min*   **cool:** *15-20 min*   **serves:** *6-8 rolls*

Dry ingredients:

- 168g *(1 1/2 cups)* almond flour
- 46g *(1/3 cup)* coconut flour
- 33g *(3 tablespoons)* psyllium husk powder
- 56g *(1/2 cup)* organic collagen *grass-fed*
- 152g *(3/4 cup)* sweetener
    monk fruit, erythritol, xylitol
- 1 teaspoon baking soda
- 1 teaspoon baking powder
- 2 teaspoons instant yeast
- 1 teaspoon sea salt

Wet ingredients:

- 3 free-run eggs *room temp*
- 118mL *(1/2 cup)* coconut milk *full fat*
- 15mL *(1 tablespoon)* honey *activates yeast*
- 30mL *(2 tablespoons)* apple cider vinegar
- 1 teaspoon pure vanilla extract

Filling:

210g *(3/4 cup)* apple butter
    the recipe found on page 195
- *16g (2 tablespoons)* cinnamon
- 56g *(1/4 cup)* grass-fed butter *softened*
    sub for palm shortening to make DF

Topping:

- 65g *(1/2 cup)* pecan *toasted & chopped*
- 120g *(1 cup)* powdered sweetener
- 120g *(1/2 cup)* pecan butter
- 75mL *(3 tablespoons)* nut milk

Instructions

1. Preheat oven to 350°F/180°C. Prep an 8x8 inch pan with parchment paper, and toast whole pecans for 7 minutes. Set aside.
2. In a medium bowl, measure all dry ingredients. Whisk together well and set aside.
3. Measure all wet ingredients in a separate medium bowl. Whisk together until fully incorporated. Pour the wet ingredients on the dry ingredients; Using a rubber spatula, mix well until completely integrated.
4. Place a piece of saran wrap to cover the bowl, and place the dough in the fridge for about 15 minutes to firm up.
5. Place the apple butter and cinnamon in a small bowl, and mix well. Set aside *(for the filling).*
6. Place a large piece of saran wrap on your countertop.
7. Place the chilled dough on the saran-wrapped surface. Take another piece of saran wrap, place it on top of the dough and press down.
8. Using a rolling pin, roll the dough out into a 16x8-inch rectangle.
9. **Filling:** Spread the softened grass-fed butter all over the surface of the dough and spread the apple butter-cinnamon mixture on top of the butter.
10. Roll the dough and fold the saran wrap under it until it rolls into a big log roll.
11. Cut the roll in half using a sharp knife, then cut each half into 3-4 pieces, leaving you with 6-8 even rolls. Place rolls in buttered baking pans.
12. Bake the rolls for 25-35 minutes or until lightly golden brown on top.
13. **Topping:** Add all the topping ingredients into a small bowl. Whisk/stir until silky smooth. Add more or less milk if needed.
14. Let rolls cool down for about 20 min. Once cinnamon rolls are cooled, it's time to drizzle the topping all over your rolls. Enjoy!
15. Store in the fridge in an airtight container for four to five days or freeze for up to three months.

Note

- **It is best to prep the apple butter one day in advance. If you are pressed for time, buy some at your local grocery store. Make sure it's organic & unsweetened.**

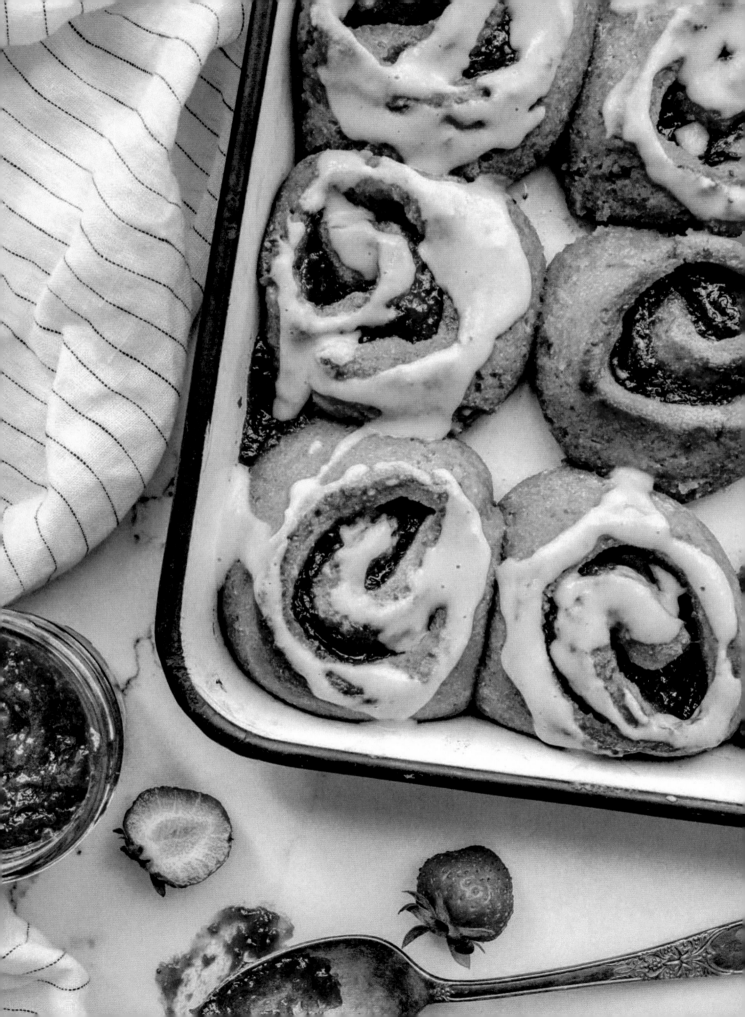

Strawberry Cream Cheese Rolls

prep: *25 min*   **bake:** *25-30 min*   **cool:** *15-20 min*   **serves:** *6-8 rolls*

Dry ingredients:
- 168g *(1 1/2 cups)* almond flour
- 46g *(1/3 cup)* coconut flour
- 33g *(3 tablespoons)* psyllium husk powder
- 56g *(1/2 cup)* organic collagen *grass-fed*
- 152g *(3/4 cup)* sweetener
    monk fruit, erythritol, xylitol
- 1 teaspoon baking soda
- 1 teaspoon baking powder
- 2 teaspoons instant yeast
- 1 teaspoon sea salt

Wet ingredients:
- 3 free-run eggs *room temp*
- 118mL *(1/2 cup)* coconut milk *full fat*
- 15mL *(1 tablespoon)* honey *activates yeast*
- 30mL *(2 tablespoons)* apple cider vinegar
- 1 teaspoon pure vanilla extract

Filling:
- *265g (1 cup)* strawberry jam
    the recipe is found on page 193
- 56g *(1/4 cup)* grass-fed butter *softened*
    *sub for palm shortening to make **DF***

Cream cheese glaze:
- 120g *(1 cup)* powdered sweetener
- 120g *(1/2 cup)* cashew cream cheese
    the recipe is found on page 226
- 75mL *(3 tablespoons)* nut milk

Instructions

1. **Preheat oven to 350°F/180°C.** Prep an 8x8-inch pan with parchment paper.
2. In a medium bowl, measure all dry ingredients. Whisk together well and set aside.
3. Measure all wet ingredients in a separate medium bowl. Whisk together until fully incorporated. Pour the wet ingredients on the dry ingredients; Using a rubber spatula, mix well until completely integrated.
4. Place a piece of saran wrap to cover the bowl, and place the dough in the fridge for about 15 minutes to firm up.
5. In a small saucepot, measure out the pre-made jam. Turn it on to low heat, and let the jam simmer to reduce the moisture for 20-30 minutes; string it every few minutes *(for the filling)*.
6. Place a large piece of saran wrap on your countertop.
7. Place the chilled dough on the saran-wrapped surface. Take another piece of saran wrap, place it on top of the dough and press down.
8. Using a rolling pin, roll the dough out into a 16x8-inch rectangle.
9. **Filling**: Spread the softened grass-fed butter all over the surface of the dough, then spread the jam on top of the butter.
10. Roll the dough and fold the saran wrap under it until it rolls into a big log roll.
11. Cut the roll in half using a sharp knife, then cut each half into 3-4 pieces, leaving you with 6-8 even rolls. Place rolls in buttered baking pans.
12. Bake the rolls for 25-35 minutes or until lightly golden brown on top.
13. **Cream cheese glaze**: Add all the glaze ingredients into a small bowl. Whisk/stir until silky smooth. Add more or less milk if needed.
14. Let rolls cool down for about 20 min. Once cinnamon rolls are cooled, it's time to drizzle the glaze all over your rolls. Enjoy!
15. Store in the fridge in an airtight container for four to five days or freeze for up to three months.

Note

- You can be creative with this recipe. Try any jam flavour you desire! I have even made a peanut butter glaze at one point. I added a few tablespoons of peanut butter into the glaze, and it worked beautifully!
- To give these rolls a festive flavour, I loved making them with cranberry jam and adding orange zest into the cream cheese glaze.

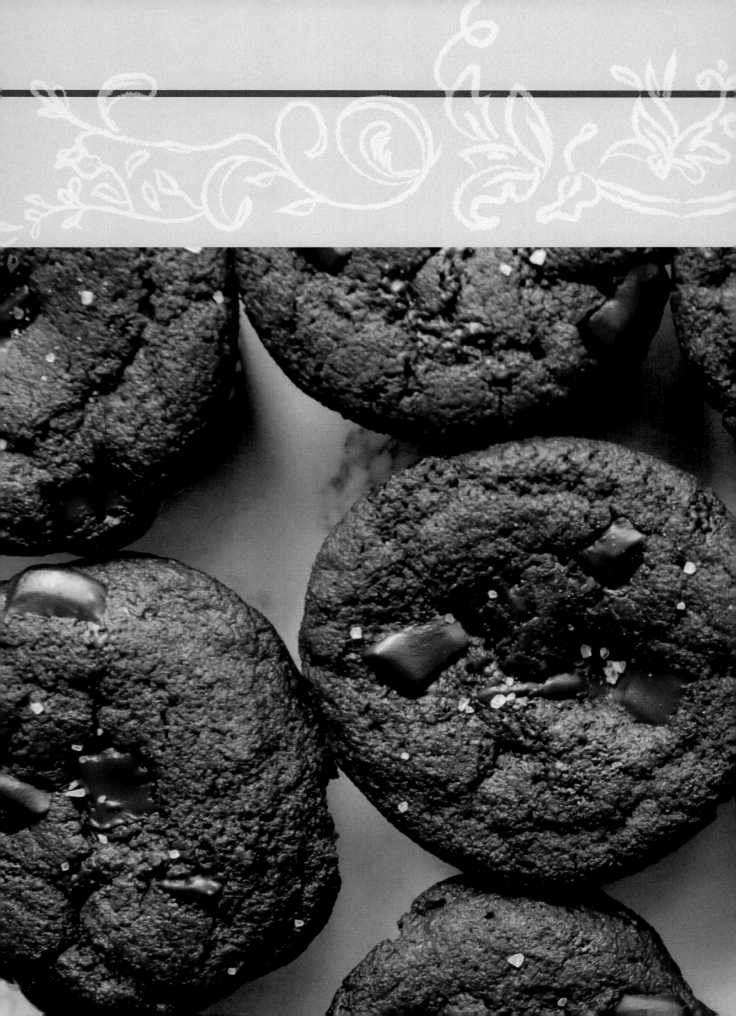

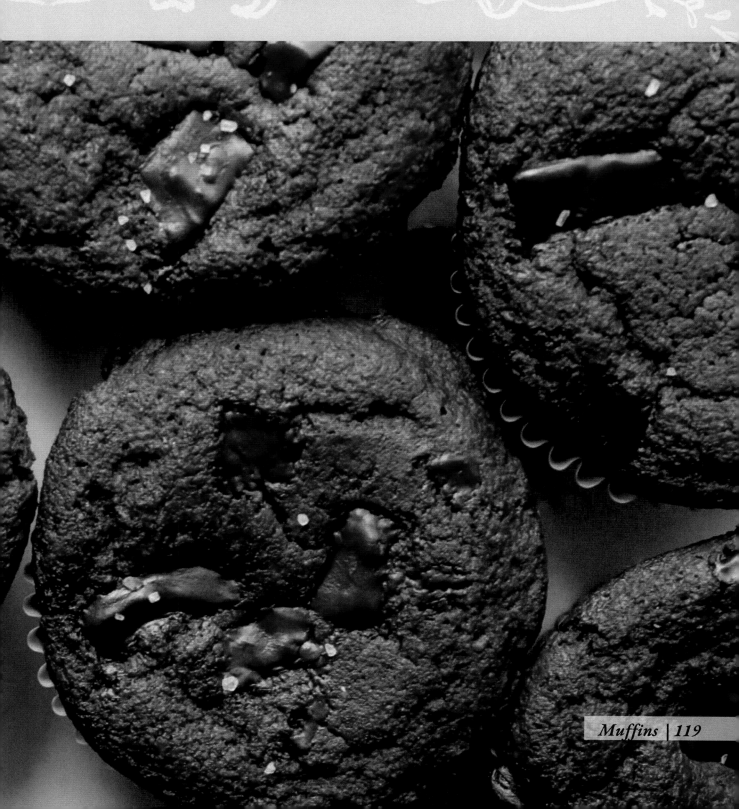

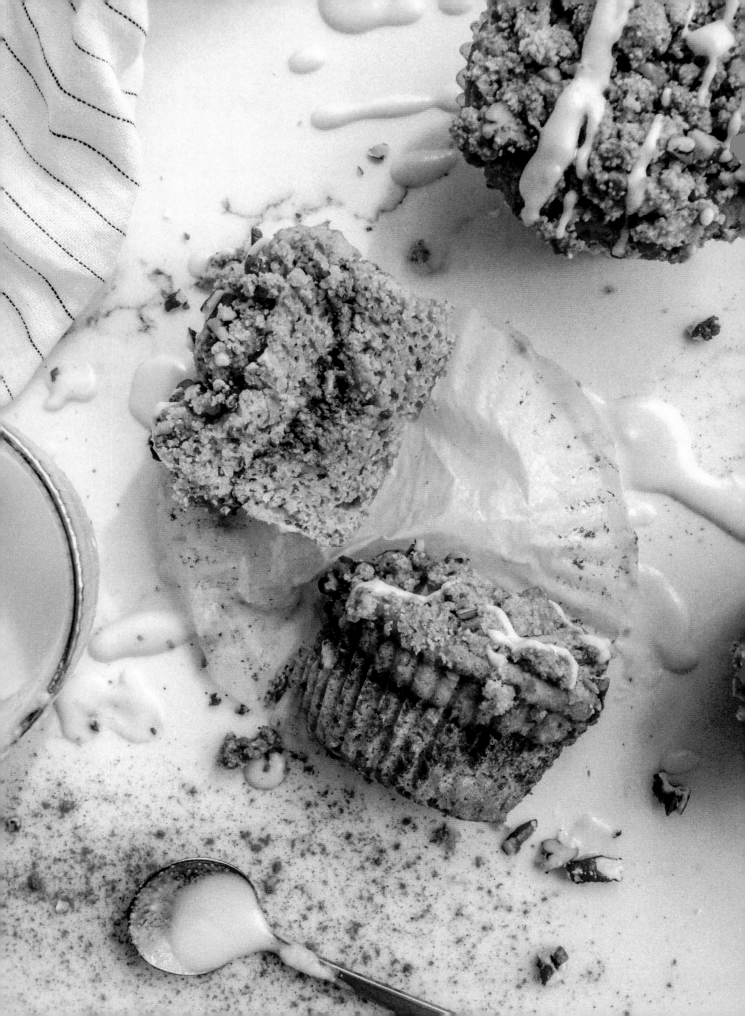

Pumpkin Coffee Cake Muffins

prep: *20 min*   **bake:** *25-30 min*   **cool:** *10-15 min*   **serves:** *12 medium*

*I never understood why coffee cake was called **"coffee cake"** until I had it with a cup of coffee, and I was hooked! My favourite way to start the day is just like that, with a coffee and a "coffee cake" muffin. I love the added pumpkin in these muffins since it adds so much moisture to pair with the streusel topping.*

Dry ingredients:
- 112g *(1 cup)* almond flour
- 68g *(1/2 cup)* coconut flour
- 33g *(3 tablespoons)* psyllium husk powder
- 56g *(1/2 cup)* organic collagen *grass-fed*
- 152g *(3/4 cup)* sweetener
  monk fruit, erythritol, xylitol
- 1 teaspoon baking soda
- 1 teaspoon baking powder
- 1 teaspoon sea salt

Wet ingredients:
- 4 eggs *room temp*
- 120mL *(1/2 cup)* pumpkin purée *unsweet.*
- 118mL *(1/2 cup)* avocado oil
- 59mL *(1/4 cup)* coconut milk *in can*
- 15mL *(1 tablespoon)* apple cider vinegar
- 1 teaspoon pure vanilla extract

Cinnamon layer
- 152g (3/4 cup) sweetener
  monk fruit, erythritol, xylitol
- 1 tablespoon cinnamon

Streusel ingredients:
- 45g *(3 tablespoons)* grass-fed butter
- 112g *(1 cup)* almond flour
- 55g *(1/2 cup)* pecans *chopped fine*
- 40g *(3 tablespoons)* sweetener
- 1 teaspoon cinnamon
- 1 teaspoon pure vanilla extract

Glaze ingredients:
- 30mL *(2 tablespoons)* lemon juice
- 120g *(1 cup)* powdered sweetener
  monk fruit, erythritol, xylitol

Instructions
1. **Preheat oven to 350°F/180°C.**
2. In a medium bowl, measure all dry ingredients, mix and set aside.
3. In a separate medium bowl, add all wet ingredients, whisk together, and pour onto dry ingredients. Using a rubber spatula, mix until well incorporated.
4. **Streusel:** In a small bowl, add all the streusel ingredients. Using your hand, mix everything until it creates a crumbly texture.
5. Line a muffin tray with non-stick parchment liners.
6. Using a medium cookie scoop, scoop out one level scoop into each cup. This should fill about 1/2 of the muffin liner.
7. **Cinnamon layer:** In a small bowl, mix the sweetener and cinnamon. Sprinkle 2 teaspoons of cinnamon sugar on top of each muffin batter.
8. Scoop a few teaspoons of the remainder of the batter on top of the cinnamon-sugar layer in each muffin until there is no batter left.
9. Using your hand, sprinkle the streusel topping on each muffin.
10. Bake the muffins for 25-30 minutes or until lightly golden brown on top.
11. **Glaze:** Mix the lemon juice and powdered sweetener in a small bowl to make the glaze.
12. Cool muffins for 10-15 minutes on a cooling rack. Then drizzle with glaze.
13. Store in the fridge in an airtight container for four to five days or freeze for up to three months.

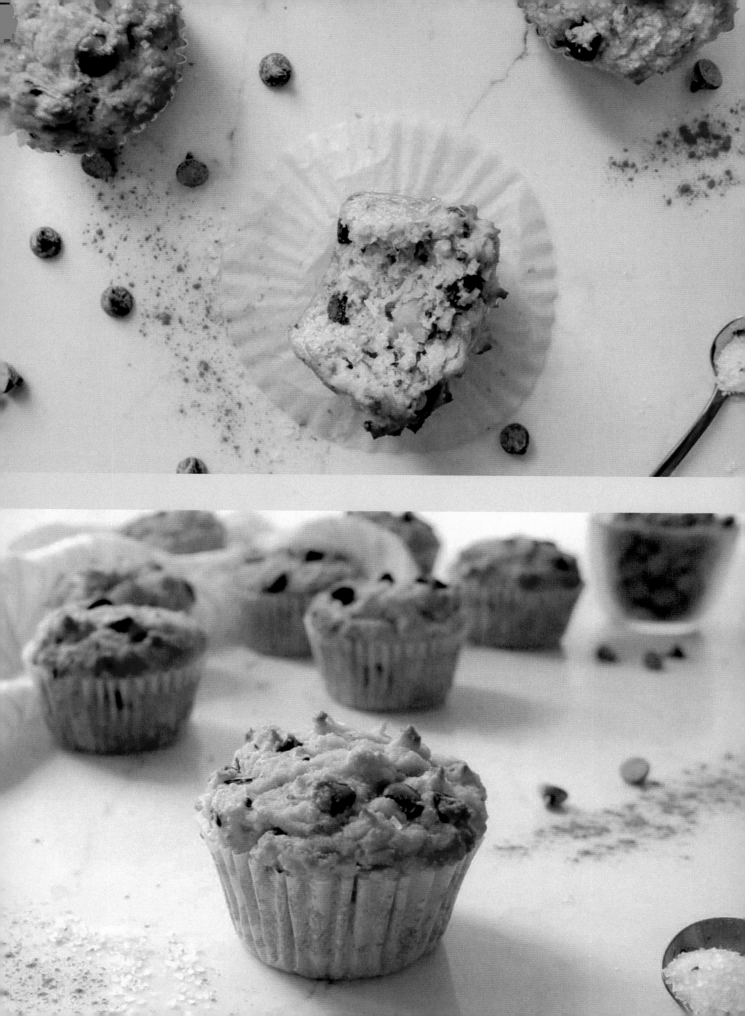

Zucchini Banana Muffins

prep: *20 min*   **bake:** *25-30 min*   **cool:** *10-15 min*   **serves:** *12 medium*

Yes, bananas are not considered keto-friendly. However, adding one ripe banana to this recipe creates a lovely banana flavour without adding too many carbs. Each muffin contains about 5 grams of net carbs.

Dry ingredients

- 112g *(1 cup)* almond flour
- 68g *(1/2 cup)* coconut flour
- 55g (1/2 cup) walnuts *chopped*
- 11g *(1 tablespoon)* psyllium husk powder
- 110g *(1/2 cup)* chocolate chips
  the recipe is found on page 223
- 200g *(1 1/2 cups) zucchini grated*
- 56g *(1/2 cup)* organic collagen *grass-fed*
- 152g *(3/4 cup)* sweetener
  monk fruit, erythritol, xylitol
- 1 teaspoon baking soda
- 1 teaspoon baking powder
- 2 teaspoons cinnamon
- 1 teaspoon sea salt

Wet ingredients:

- 1 large ripe banana *mashed*
- 4 free-run eggs *room temp*
- 118mL *(1/2 cup)* avocado oil
- 118mL *(1/2 cup)* coconut milk *full fat*
- 15mL *(1 tablespoon)* apple cider vinegar
- 1 teaspoon pure vanilla extract

Instructions

1. Preheat oven to 350°F/180°C.
2. Line a cookie sheet with parchment paper.
3. Chop walnuts and toast them for 7 minutes. Set aside.
4. Grate zucchini with a grater or a food processor, and set aside.
5. In a medium bowl, measure all dry ingredients, including toasted walnuts and grated zucchini. Mix and set aside. Make sure the zucchini is not stuck together.
6. In another medium bowl, mash the banana, then add all other wet ingredients. Whisk together and pour onto the dry ingredients. Using a rubber spatula, mix the batter until well incorporated.
7. Line a muffin tray with non-stick parchment liners.
8. Using a large cookie scoop, scoop out one level scoop into each cup. If you have extra remaining, add a few teaspoons to the top of each muffin until there is no batter left.
9. Bake the muffins for 25-30 minutes or until lightly golden brown on top.
10. Cool muffins on a cooling rack for 10-15 minutes, and enjoy them with your morning coffee!
11. Store in the fridge in an airtight container for four to five days or freeze for up to three months.

Note

- **If you don't want to use a banana, add an extra cup of zucchini to add the extra needed moisture.**

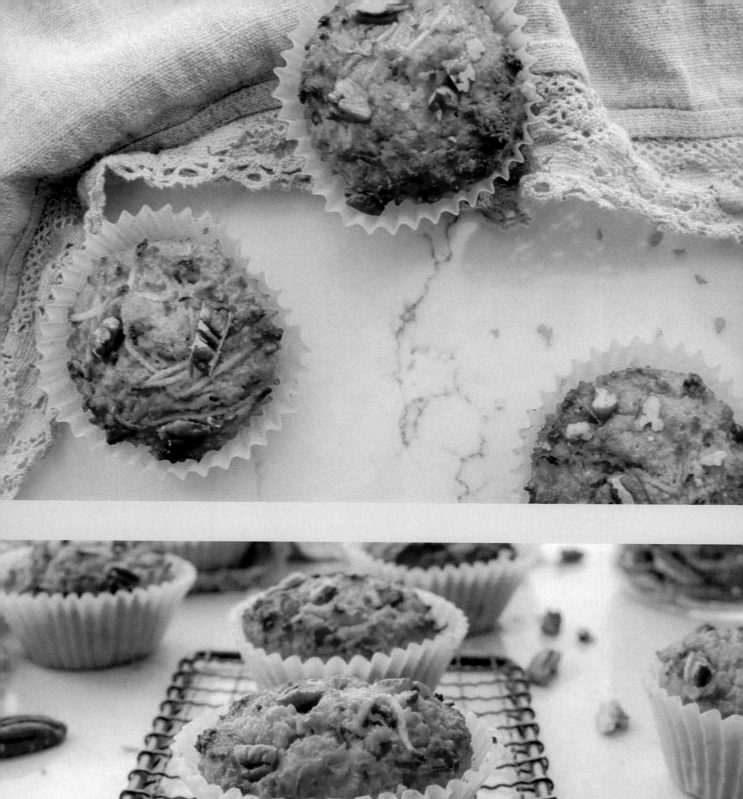
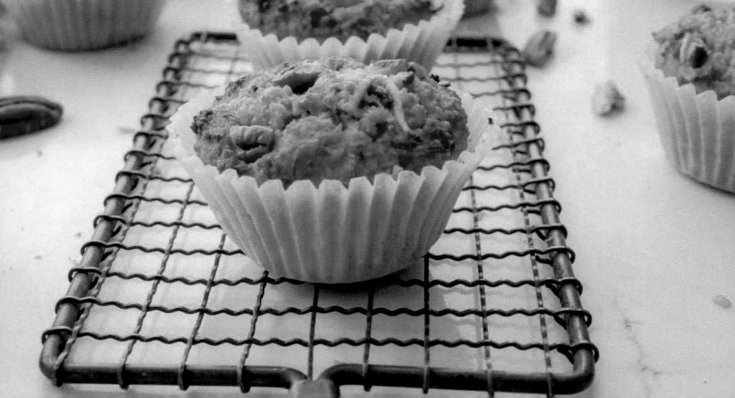

Morning Glory Muffins

prep: *20 min*   **bake:** *25-30 min*   **cool:** *10-15 min*   **serves:** *12 medium*

Good morning muffin! The flavours are delightful in these muffins: the apple, carrots, nuts, and cinnamon make for a glorious morning! You'll be amazed at what these nutrient-packed muffins will do for your morning.

Dry ingredients

- 112g *(1 cup)* almond flour
- 68g *(1/2 cup)* coconut flour
- 42g *(1/2 cup)* coconut flakes *unsweetened*
- 55g *(1/2 cup)* pecans *chopped*
- 11g *(1 tablespoon)* psyllium husk powder
- 110g *(1 cup)* carrots *shredded*
- 120g *(1 large)* tart apple *shredded*
- 56g *(1/2 cup)* organic collagen *grass-fed*
- 152g *(3/4 cup)* sweetener
    monk fruit, erythritol, xylitol
- 1 teaspoon baking soda
- 1 teaspoon baking powder
- 2 teaspoons cinnamon
- 1 teaspoon ginger
- 1 teaspoon sea salt

Wet ingredients:

- 4 free-run eggs *room temp*
- 122g *(1/2 cup)* apple butter
    the recipe is found on page 195
- 118mL *(1/2 cup)* avocado oil
- 59mL *(1/4 cup)* coconut milk *full fat*
- 15mL *(1 tablespoon)* lemon juice
- 1 teaspoon pure vanilla extract

Instructions

1. **Preheat oven to 350°F/180°C.**
2. Prep two small baking sheets with parchment paper.
3. Toast the coconut flakes for 4-5 minutes. Set aside.
4. Toast the chopped pecans for 7 minutes. Set aside.
5. Grate the apples and carrots with a grater or food processor. Set them aside.
6. In a medium bowl, measure all dry ingredients *(including toasted pecans, coconut flakes, and grated apples & carrots). Mix and set aside.* Make sure apples and carrots are not stuck together.
7. In a separate medium bowl, add all wet ingredients. Whisk together and pour onto dry ingredients. Using a rubber spatula, mix until well incorporated.
8. Line a muffin tray with non-stick parchment liners
9. Using a large cookie scoop, scoop out one level scoop into each cup. If you have extra remaining, add a few teaspoons to the top of each muffin until there is no batter left.
10. Bake the muffins for 25-30 minutes or until lightly golden brown on top.
11. Cool muffins on a cooling rack for 10-15 minutes and enjoy them with your morning coffee!
12. Store in the fridge in an airtight container for four to five days or freeze for up to three months.

Note

- It is best to prep the apple butter one day in advance. If you are pressed for time, buy some at your local grocery store. Make sure it's organic & unsweetened.

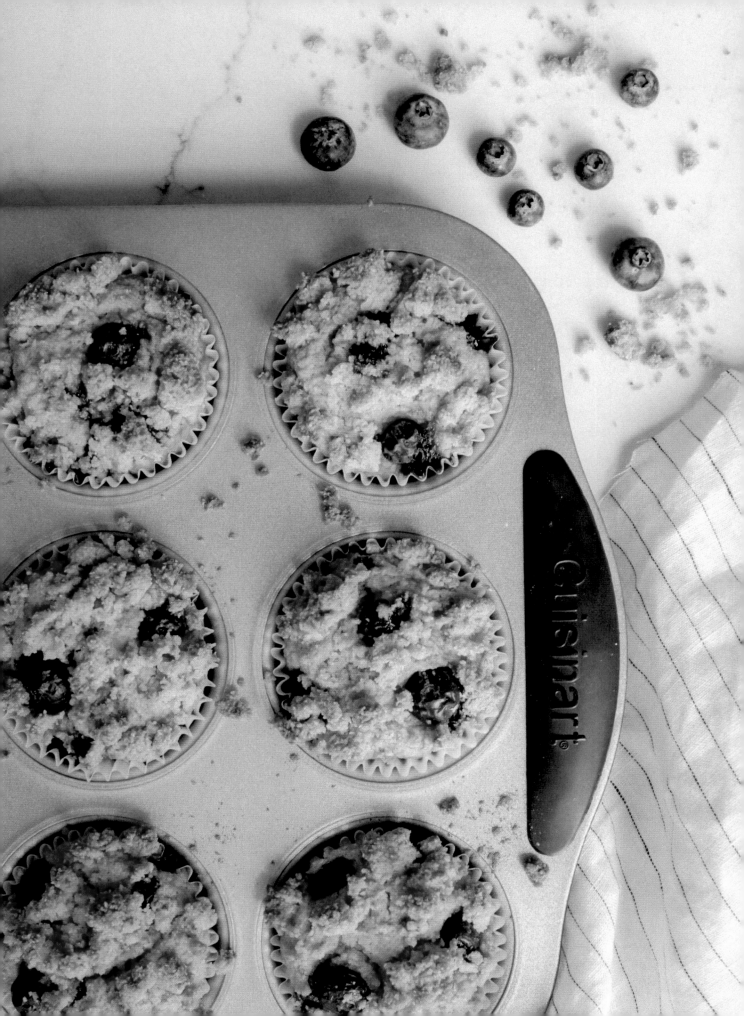

Blueberry Crumble Muffins

prep: *20 min*   **bake:** *25-30 min*   **cool:** *10-15 min*   **serves:** *12 medium*

Nothing is better than a freshly-baked blueberry crumble muffin.
In this recipe, any fresh berry or fruit will make a heavenly pair with the crumble topping.
Chopped granny smith apples are another one of my favorite combinations for this recipe!

Dry ingredients
- 112g *(1 cup)* almond flour
- 68g *(1/2 cup)* coconut flour
- 33g *(2 tablespoons)* psyllium husk powder
- 125g *(2 cups)* fresh blueberries
- 56g *(1/2 cup)* organic collagen *grass-fed*
- 152g *(3/4 cup)* sweetener
  monk fruit, erythritol, xylitol
- 1 teaspoon baking soda
- 1 teaspoon baking powder
- 1 teaspoon sea salt

Wet ingredients:
- 4 free-run eggs *room temp*
- 118mL *(1/2 cup)* avocado oil
- 118mL *(1/2 cup)* coconut milk *full fat*
- 15mL *(1 tablespoon)* apple cider vinegar
- 1 teaspoon pure vanilla extract

Crumble ingredients:
- 45g *(3 tablespoons)* grass-fed butter *room temp*
- 112g *(1/2 cup)* almond flour
- 16g *(2 tablespoons)* coconut flour
- 40g *(3 tablespoons)* sweetener
- 1 teaspoon cinnamon
- 1 teaspoon pure vanilla extract

Instructions
1. Preheat oven to 350°F/180°C.
2. In a medium bowl, measure all dry ingredients, including fresh blueberries. Mix and set aside.
3. In a separate medium bowl, add all wet ingredients. Whisk together, and pour onto dry ingredients. Using a rubber spatula, mix until well incorporated.
4. **Crumble:** In a small bowl, add all the crumble ingredients. Using your hands, mix everything until it creates a crumbly texture.
5. Line a muffin tray with non-stick parchment liners
6. Using a large cookie scoop, scoop out one level scoop into each cup. If you have extra remaining, add a few teaspoons to the top of each muffin until there is no batter left.
7. Using your hand, sprinkle the crumble topping on each muffin.
8. Bake the muffins for 25-30 minutes or until lightly golden brown on top.
9. Cool muffins on a cooling rack for 10-15 minutes, and enjoy them with your morning coffee!
10. Store in the fridge in an airtight container for four to five days or freeze for up to three months.

Note
- **Frozen blueberries can work as well. However, they may change the colour of the batter when mixing. Fresh berries are always the best.**

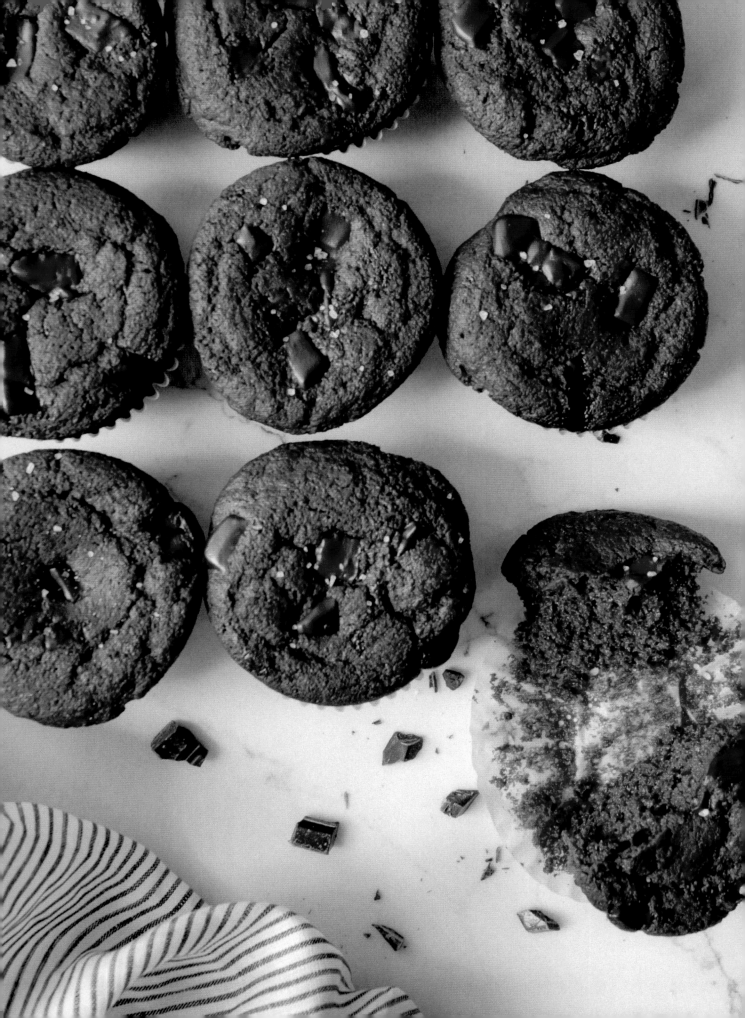

Timeless Triple Chocolate Muffins

prep: *20 min*   **bake:** *25-30 min*   **cool:** *10-15 min*   **serves:** *12 medium*

Who could ever go wrong with such a rich, moist, chocolate muffin that is not only delicious but is also good for your tummy!

Dry ingredients:

- 140g *(1 ¼ cups)* almond flour
- 34g *(1/4 cup)* coconut flour
- 28g *(1/4 cup)* cacao powder
- 11g *(1 tablespoon)* psyllium husk powder
- 56g *(1/2 cup)* organic collagen *grass-fed*
- 152g *(3/4 cup)* sweetener
  monk fruit, erythritol, xylitol
- 1 teaspoon baking soda
- 1 teaspoon baking powder
- 1 teaspoon sea salt

Wet ingredients:

- 110g *(1/2 cup)* chocolate chips *melted*
  the recipe is found on page 223
- 4 free-run eggs *room temp*
- 59mL *(1/4 cup)* avocado oil
- 118mL *(1/2 cup)* coconut milk *full fat*
- 15mL *(1 tablespoon)* apple cider vinegar
- 1 teaspoon pure vanilla extract

Garnish:

- 85g *(1 full)* chocolate bar
  the recipe is found on page 223
- flaky sea salt

Instructions

1. **Preheat oven to 350°F/180°C.**
2. In a medium bowl, measure all dry ingredients. Mix and set aside.
3. Place chocolate chips in a heat-proof bowl and melt using the microwave in 10-sec intervals (mixing every time) or in a water bath on a double boiler.
4. Add all wet ingredients, including the melted chocolate chips, to another medium bowl. Whisk together and pour onto dry ingredients.
5. Using a rubber spatula, mix the batter until well incorporated.
6. Line a muffin tray with non-stick parchment liners
7. Using a large cookie scoop, scoop out one level scoop into each cup. If you have extra remaining, add a few teaspoons to the top of each muffin until there is no batter left.
8. **Garnish:** Chop up the chocolate bar, and garnish each muffin with a few pieces
9. Bake the muffins for 25-30 minutes.
10. Cool muffins for 10-15 minutes on a cooling rack. Garnish with flaky sea salt and enjoy with your morning coffee!
11. Store in the fridge in an airtight container for four to five days or freeze for up to three months.

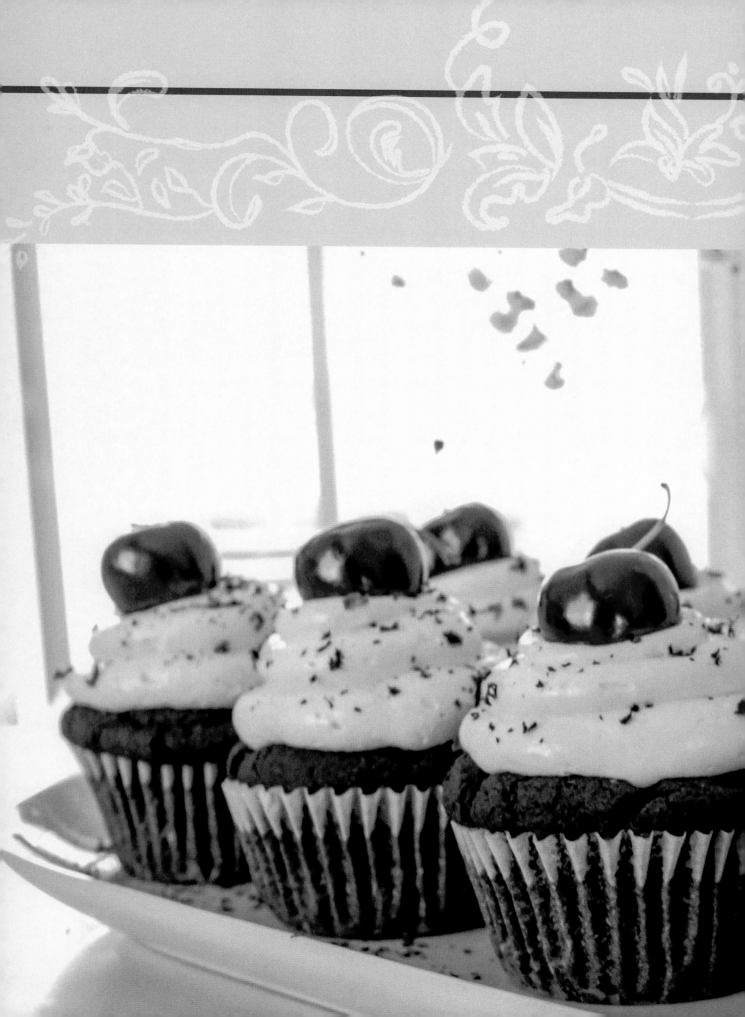

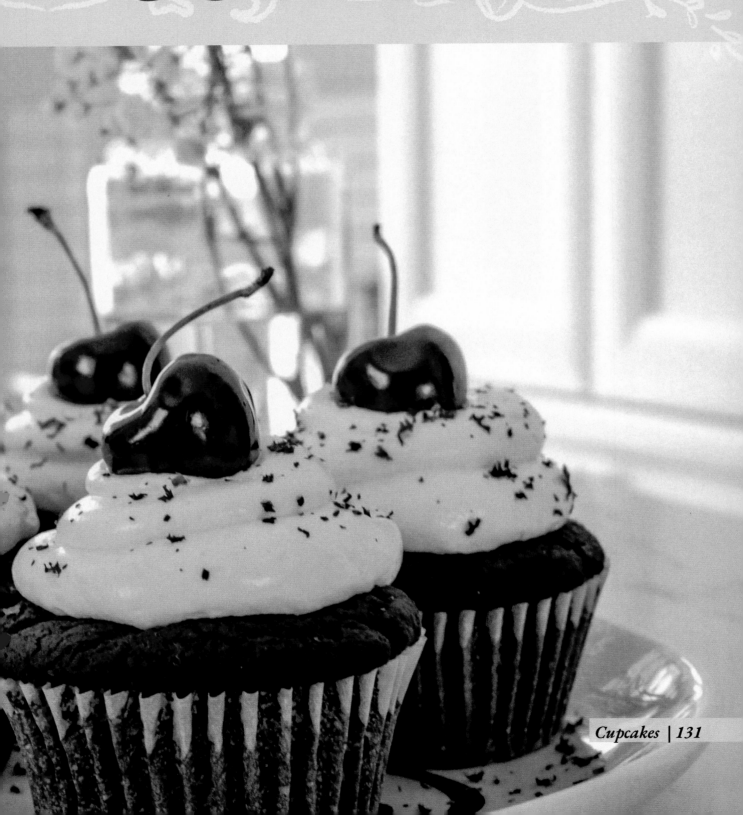

Chapter Six

CUPCAKES

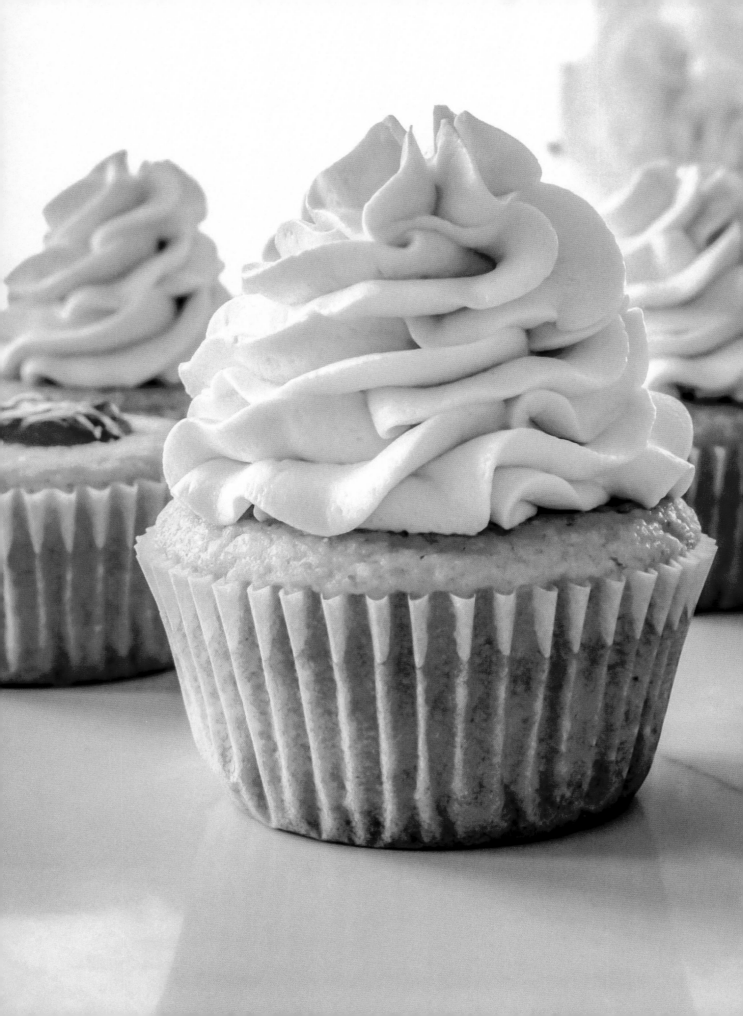

Strawberry & Cream Cupcakes

prep: *20 min*   **bake:** *25-30 min*   **cool:** *10-15 min*   **serves:** *12 medium*

My cupcakes were the number one most requested item on my menu, especially for special occasions like birthdays, Valentine's Day, or any other type of celebration. Oh, and don't forget the surprise inside of each cupcake!

Dry ingredients
- 140g *(1¼ cups)* almond flour
- 46g *(1/3 cup)* coconut flour
- 11g *(1 tablespoon)* psyllium husk powder
- 105g *(1/2 cup)* sweetener
  monk fruit, erythritol, xylitol
- 1 teaspoon baking soda
- 1 teaspoon baking powder
- 1 teaspoon sea salt

Wet ingredients:
- 4 free-run eggs *room temp*
- 118mL *(1/2 cup)* avocado oil
- 118mL *(1/2 cup)* coconut milk *full fat*
- 15mL *(1 tablespoon)* lemon juice
- 1 teaspoon pure vanilla extract

Jam Filling ingredients:
- 175g *(1 cup)* strawberry jam
  the recipe is found on page 193

Vanilla Buttercream:
- 1 batch Vanilla Buttercream + **DF option**
  the recipe is found on page 185

Instructions

1. **Preheat oven to 325°F/163°C.**
2. In a medium bowl, sift coconut flour and measure all remaining dry ingredients. Mix well and set aside.
3. In a separate medium bowl, place all wet ingredients. Whisk together and pour onto dry ingredients. Using a rubber spatula, mix the batter until well incorporated.
4. Line a muffin/cupcake tray with 12 non-stick parchment liners
5. Using a large cookie scoop, scoop out one level scoop into each cup. If you have extra remaining, add a few teaspoons to the top of each cupcake until there is no batter left.
6. Bake the cupcake for 25-30 minutes or until lightly golden brown on top.
7. **Jam Filling:** While baking cupcakes, prepare the jam in a small bowl and have it ready *(best to make the jam the day before)*.
8. Using a stand mixer bowl *(whisk attachment)* or an electric hand mixer, make the **Vanilla Buttercream frosting** on page 185.
9. Cool cupcakes for 10-15 minutes on a cooling rack.
10. Use a cupcake coring tool to core out the center of each cupcake. Add approx two tablespoons of jam filling into each hole!
11. Add buttercream frosting into a piping bag with a piping tip. Starting at the edge of the cupcakes, swirl the buttercream into a mountain two and a half times to the top.
12. When serving the cupcakes, ensure the frosting is at room temperature since it will harden when cool. Take cupcakes out of the fridge 20-min before eating.
13. Store in the fridge in an airtight container for four to five days or freeze for up to two months.

Note

- **Cupcakes have always been tricky in creating that perfect round top. My number one recommendation is to make sure all liquids are warm or at room temp.**
- **You may make these cupcakes 100% dairy-free with my DF frosting option on page 185.**

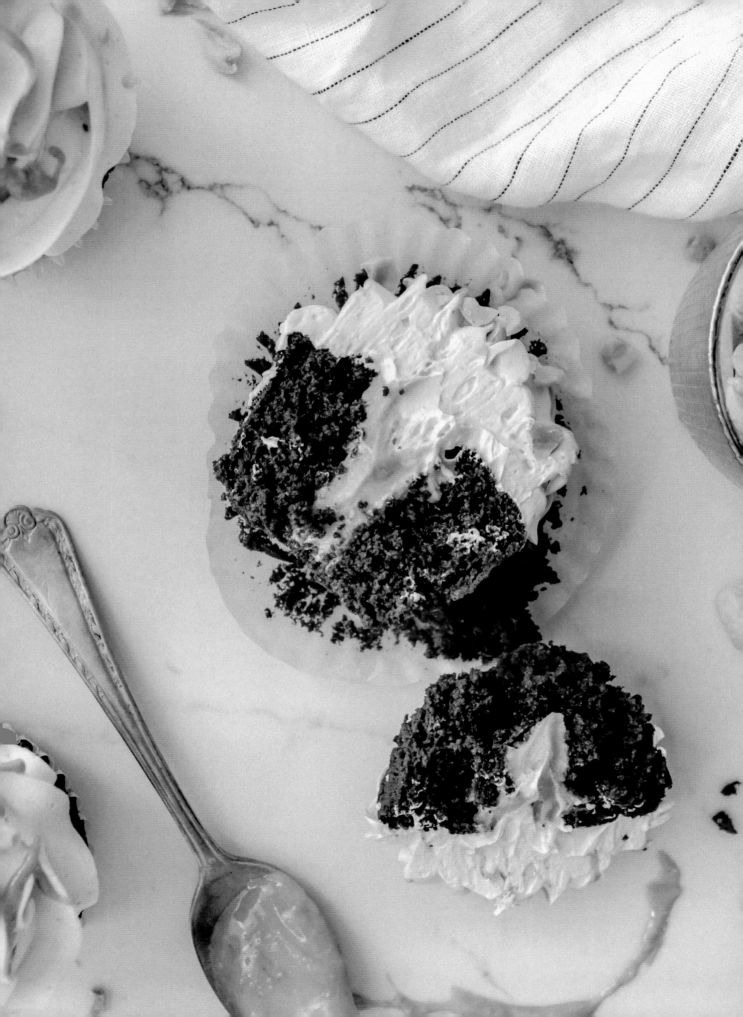

Reese's Pieces Stuffed Cupcakes

prep: *20 min*   **bake:** *25-30 min*   **cool:** *10-15 min*   **serves:** *12 medium*

Reese's Pieces seems to always be a favourite flavour, try these cupcake out for your next gathering!

Dry ingredients:
- 112g *(1 cup)* almond flour
- 34g *(1/4 cup)* coconut flour
- 56g *(1/2 cup)* cacao powder
- 11g *(1 tablespoon)* psyllium husk powder
- 152g *(3/4 cup)* sweetener
  monk fruit, erythritol, xylitol
- 1 teaspoon baking soda
- 1 teaspoon baking powder
- 1 teaspoon sea salt

Wet ingredients:
- 4 free-run eggs *room temp*
- 118mL *(1/2 cup)* avocado oil
- 118mL *(1/2 cup)* coconut milk *full fat*
- 15mL *(1 tablespoon)* apple cider vinegar
- 1 teaspoon pure vanilla extract

Reese's filling ingredients:
- 175g *(3/4 cup)* peanut butter *natural*
- 120g *(1 cup)* powdered sweetener
  monk fruit, erythritol, xylitol
- 60mL *(1/4 cup)* coconut milk *full fat*

Vanilla Buttercream:
- 1 batch Vanilla Buttercream + **DF option**
  the recipe is found on page 185
- 120g *(1/2 cup)* peanut butter *natural*
- 150g *(1 cup)* dry-roasted peanuts *to garnish*

Instructions

1. **Preheat oven to 325°F/163°C.**
2. In a medium bowl, sift coconut flour and cacao powder. Measure all remaining dry ingredients. Mix and set aside.
3. In a separate medium bowl, place all wet ingredients, whisk together and pour onto dry ingredients.
4. Using a rubber spatula, mix the batter until well incorporated.
5. Line a cupcake tray with non-stick parchment liners
6. Using a large cookie scoop, scoop out one level scoop into each cup. If you have extra remaining, add a few teaspoons to the top of each cupcake until there is no batter left.
7. Bake the cupcakes for 25-30 minutes or until lightly golden brown on top.
8. **Reese's filling:** Mix Reese's filling ingredients and set them aside in a small bowl.
9. Using a stand mixer bowl *(whisk attachment)* or an electric hand mixer, make the **Vanilla Buttercream frosting** on page 185.
10. Add 1/2 cup natural peanut butter and whisk for an additional 5 minutes.
11. Cool cupcakes for 10-15 minutes on a cooling rack.
12. Use a cupcake coring tool to core out the center of each cupcake.
13. Add approx two tablespoons of Reese's filling into each hole!
14. Add buttercream frosting into a piping bag with a piping tip. Starting at the edge of the cupcakes, swirl the buttercream into a mountain two and a half times to the top.
15. When serving the cupcakes, ensure the frosting is at room temperature since it will harden when cool. Take cupcakes out of the fridge 20-min before eating.
16. Store in the fridge in an airtight container for four to five days or freeze for up to two months.

Note

- **Cupcakes have always been tricky to create that perfect round top. My number one recommendation is to make sure all liquids are warm or at room temp.**
- **You may make these cupcakes 100% dairy-free with my DF frosting option on page 185.**

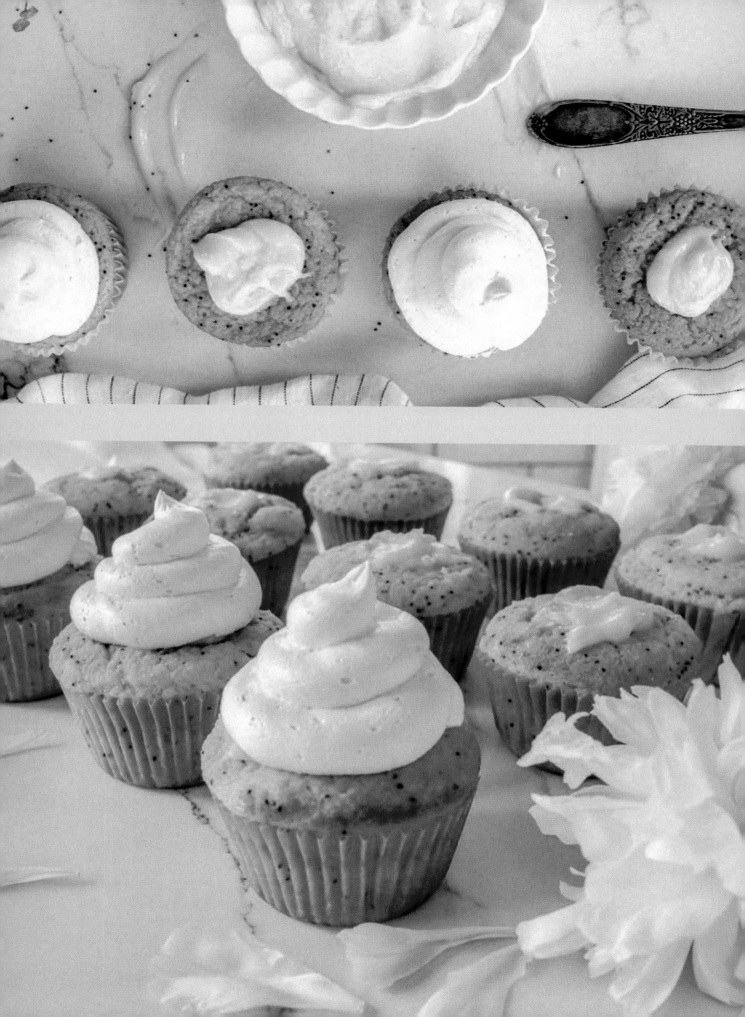

Lemon Poppy Seed Custard Cupcakes

prep: *20 min* **bake:** *25-30 min* **cool:** *10-15 min* **serves:** *12 medium*

Truthfully, I was never a lemon fan when it came to desserts. However, when I made these cupcakes, I found a new love for lemon, especially when it is combined with a creamy custard to smooth out the tartness.

Dry ingredients:
- 140g *(1¼ cups)* almond flour
- 46g *(1/3 cup)* coconut flour
- 11g *(1 tablespoon)* psyllium husk powder
- 105g *(1/2 cup)* sweetener
  monk fruit, erythritol, xylitol
- 1 tablespoon poppy seeds
- 1 teaspoon baking soda
- 1 teaspoon baking powder
- 1 teaspoon sea salt

Wet ingredients:
- 4 free-run eggs *room temp*
- 118mL *(1/2 cup)* avocado oil
- 118mL *(1/2 cup)* coconut milk *full fat*
- 15mL *(1 tablespoon)* lemon juice
- 1/2 teaspoon pure lemon oil extract
- 1 teaspoon pure vanilla extract

Lemon Custard:
- 1 batch Lemon Custard
  the recipe is found on page 197

Vanilla Buttercream:
- 1 batch Vanilla Buttercream + **DF option**
  the recipe is found on page 185

Instructions

1. Make sure the custard is pre-made to cool the custard when it's time to fill the cupcakes.
2. **Preheat oven to 325°F/163°C.**
3. In a medium bowl, sift coconut flour and measure all remaining dry ingredients. Mix and set aside.
4. In a separate medium bowl and add wet ingredients, whisk together and pour onto dry ingredients.
5. Using a rubber spatula, mix the batter until well incorporated.
6. Line a cupcake tray with non-stick parchment liners
7. Using a large cookie scoop, scoop out one level scoop into each cup. If you have extra remaining, add a few teaspoons to the top of each cupcake until there is no batter left.
8. Bake the muffins for 25-30 minutes or until lightly golden brown on top.
9. Using a stand mixer bowl *(whisk attachment)* or an electric hand mixer, make the **Vanilla Buttercream frosting** on page 185.
10. Cool cupcakes for 10-15 minutes on a cooling rack.
11. Use a cupcake coring tool to core out the center of each cupcake.
12. **Lemon Custard:** Add approx two tablespoons of custard into each hole!
13. Add buttercream frosting into a piping bag with a piping tip. Starting at the edge of the cupcakes, swirl the buttercream into a mountain two and a half times to the top.
14. When serving the cupcakes, ensure the frosting is at room temperature since it will harden when cool. Take cupcakes out of the fridge 20-min before eating.
15. Store in the fridge in an airtight container for four to five days or freeze for up to two months.

Note

- Cupcakes have always been tricky to create that perfect round top. My number one recommendation is to make sure all liquids are warm or at room temp.
- You may make these cupcakes 100% dairy-free with my DF frosting option on page 185.

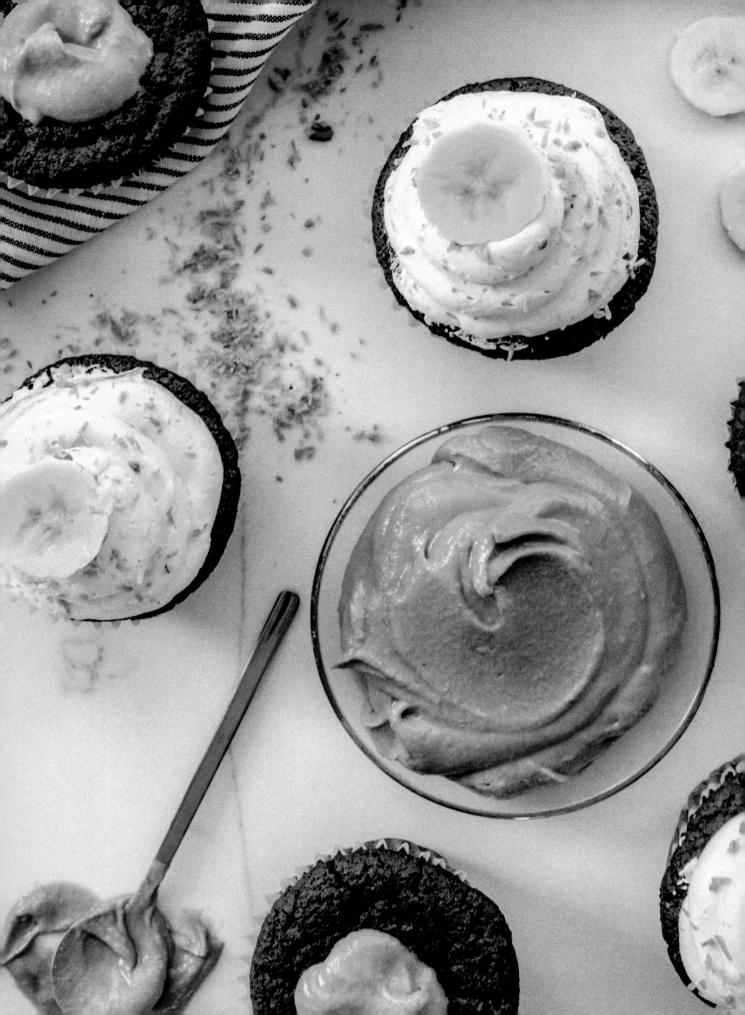

Coconut Banana Custard Cupcakes

prep: *20 min*   **bake:** *25-30 min*   **cool:** *10-15 min*   **serves:** *12 medium*

These cupcakes taste like a heavenly banana coconut cream pie wrapped in a fluffy, moist cake. YUM!

Dry ingredients:

- 112g *(1 cup)* almond flour
- 34g *(1/4 cup)* coconut flour
- 56g *(1/2 cup)* cacao powder
- 11g *(1 tablespoon)* psyllium husk powder
- 152g *(3/4 cup)* sweetener
  monk fruit, erythritol, xylitol
- 1 teaspoon baking soda
- 1 teaspoon baking powder
- 1 teaspoon sea salt

Wet ingredients:

- 4 free-run eggs *room temp*
- 118mL *(1/2 cup)* coconut oil *melted*
- 118mL *(1/2 cup)* coconut milk *full fat*
- 15mL *(1 tablespoon)* apple cider vinegar
- 1 teaspoon pure vanilla extract

Banana Coco Custard:

- 1 batch Chocolate Custard
  the recipe is found on page 197
- 1 medium ripe banana *mashed*
- 1 teaspoon pure coconut extract

Vanilla Buttercream:

- 1 batch Vanilla Buttercream + **DF option**
  the recipe is found on page 185
- 1 teaspoon coconut extract
- 21g *(1/4 cup)* toasted coconut flakes *to garnish*

Note

- Cupcakes have always been tricky to create that perfect round top. My number one recommendation is to make sure all liquids are warm or at room temp.
- You may make these cupcakes 100% dairy-free with my DF frosting option on page 185.

Instructions

1. **Custard:** Make sure the custard is pre-made so that when it's time to fill the cupcakes, the custard is cool. Mash a ripe banana and add coconut extract for a more coconut-y punch.
2. **Preheat oven to 325°F/163°C.**
3. In a medium bowl, sift coconut flour and cacao powder. Measure all remaining dry ingredients. Mix and set aside.
4. Melt coconut oil *(ensure it is warm, not hot, as hot oil will curdle the eggs).*
5. In a separate medium bowl, add all wet ingredients. Whisk together and pour onto dry ingredients. Using a rubber spatula, mix the batter well.
6. Line a cupcake tray with parchment liners.
7. Using a large cookie scoop, scoop out one level scoop into each cup. If you have extra remaining, add a few teaspoons to the top of each cupcake until there is no batter left.
8. Bake the cupcakes for 25-30 minutes or until lightly golden brown on top.
9. Toast coconut flakes on a small baking sheet lined with parchment paper for 4 minutes.
10. Using a stand mixer bowl *(whisk attachment)* or an electric hand mixer, make the **Vanilla Buttercream frosting** on page 185.
11. Add coconut extract, and whisk for an additional 5 minutes.
12. Cool cupcakes for 10-15 minutes on a cooling rack.
13. Use a cupcake coring tool to core out the center of each cupcake. Add approx two tablespoons of custard into each hole!
14. Add buttercream frosting into a piping bag with a piping tip. Starting at the edge of the cupcakes, swirl the buttercream into a mountain two and a half times to the top.
15. Sprinkle with toasted coconut and a slice of banana.
16. Store in the fridge in an airtight container for four to five days or freeze for up to two months.

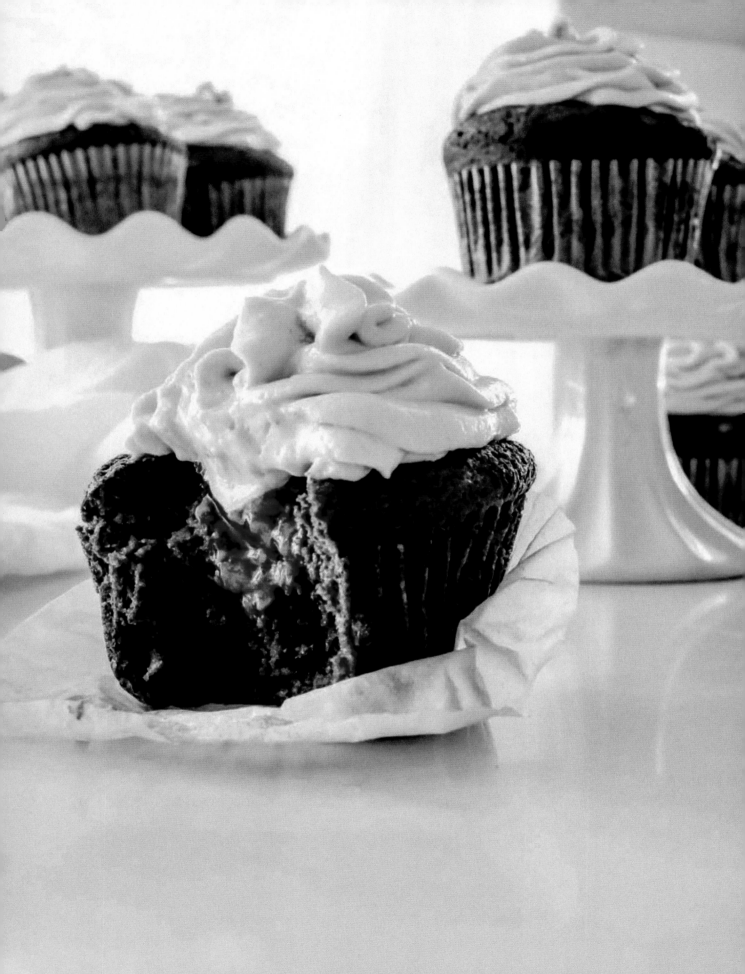

Tart Chocolate Raspberry Cupcakes

prep: *20 min* **bake:** *25-30 min* **cool:** *10-15 min* **serves:** *12 medium*

I made these chocolate raspberry cupcakes my first time for a Valentine's Day Special, and they became a an instant favourite on my menu.

Dry ingredients:

- 112g *(1 cup)* almond flour
- 34g *(1/4 cup)* coconut flour
- 56g *(1/2 cup)* cacao powder
- 11g *(1 tablespoon)* psyllium husk powder
- 152g *(3/4 cup)* sweetener
  monk fruit, erythritol, xylitol
- 1 teaspoon baking soda
- 1 teaspoon baking powder
- 1 teaspoon sea salt

Wet ingredients:

- 4 free-run eggs *room temp*
- 118mL *(1/2 cup)* avocado oil
- 118mL *(1/2 cup)* coconut milk *full fat*
- 15mL *(1 tablespoon)* apple cider vinegar
- 1 teaspoon pure vanilla extract

Jam filling ingredients:

- 175g *(1 cup)* raspberry jam
  the recipe is found on page 193

Raspberry Buttercream:

- 1 batch vanilla buttercream + **DF option**
  the recipe is found on page 185
- 175g *(1 cup)* raspberry jam
  the recipe is found on page 193

Instructions

1. **Preheat oven to 325°F/163°C.**
2. In a medium bowl, sift coconut flour and cacao powder. Measure and add all remaining dry ingredients. Mix and set aside.
3. In a separate medium bowl, add all wet ingredients, whisk together and pour onto dry ingredients.
4. Using a rubber spatula, mix the batter until well incorporated.
5. Line a cupcake tray with non-stick parchment liners.
6. Using a large cookie scoop, scoop out one level scoop into each cup. If you have extra remaining, add a few teaspoons to the top of each cupcake until there is no batter left.
7. Bake the cupcakes for 25-30 minutes or until lightly golden brown on top.
8. **Jam Filling:** While baking cupcakes, prepare the jam in a small bowl and have it ready *(best to make the jam the day before)*.
9. Using a stand mixer bowl *(whisk attachment)* or an electric hand mixer, make the **Vanilla Buttercream frosting** on page 185. Add the jam and whip for another 3min.
10. Cool cupcakes for 10-15 minutes on a cooling rack.
11. Use a cupcake coring tool to core out the center of each cupcake. Add approx two tablespoons of jam filling into each hole!
12. Add buttercream frosting into a piping bag with a piping tip. Starting at the edge of the cupcakes, swirl the buttercream into a mountain two and a half times to the top.
13. When serving the cupcakes, ensure the frosting is at room temperature since it will harden when cool. Take cupcakes out of the fridge 20-min before eating.
14. Store in the fridge in an airtight container for four to five days or freeze for up to two months.

Note

- Cupcakes have always been tricky in creating that perfect round top. My number one recommendation is to make sure all liquids are warm or at room temp.
- You may make these cupcakes 100% dairy-free with my DF frosting option on page 185.

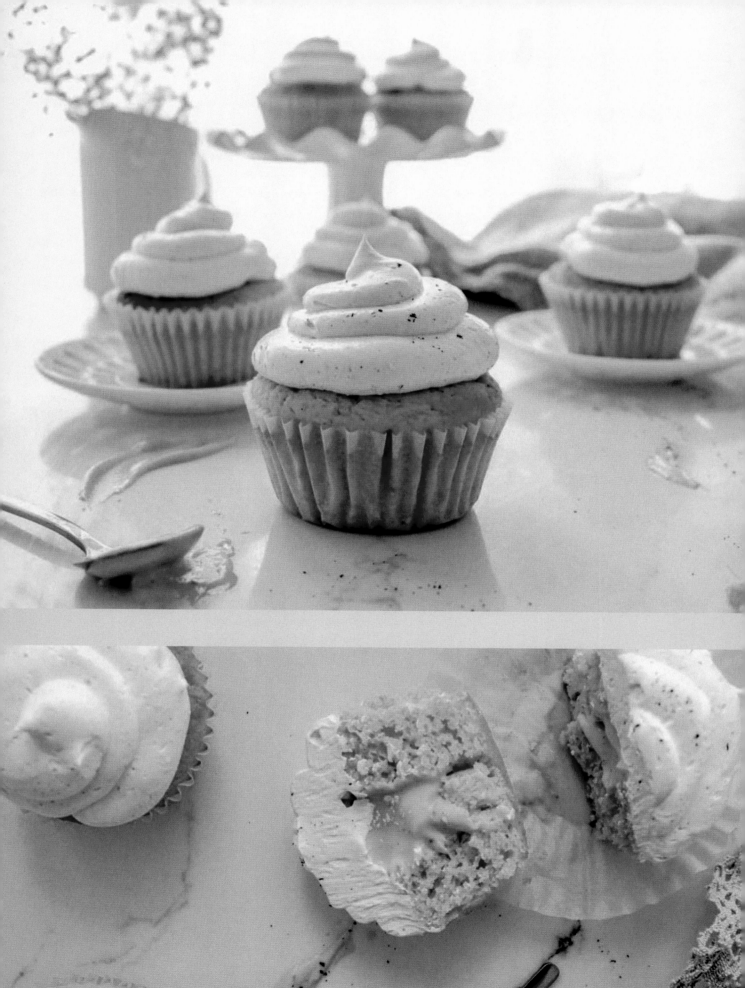

Vanilla Bean Custard Cupcakes

prep: *20 min*   **bake:** *25-30 min*   **cool:** *10-15 min*   **serves:** *12 medium*

These classic Vanilla Bean Custard Cupcakes are so light, refreshing and delightful. The added custard inside brings these vanilla cupcakes to a classy delicacy.

Dry ingredients:

- 140g *(1¼ cups)* almond flour
- 46g *(1/3 cup)* coconut flour
- 11g *(1 tablespoon)* psyllium husk powder
- 105g *(1/2 cup)* sweetener
  monk fruit, erythritol, xylitol
- 1 teaspoon baking soda
- 1 teaspoon baking powder
- 1 teaspoon sea salt

Wet ingredients:

- 4 free-run eggs *room temp*
- 118mL *(1/2 cup)* avocado oil
- 118mL *(1/4 cup)* coconut milk *full fat*
- 15mL *(1 tablespoon)* lemon juice
- 1 teaspoon pure vanilla extract

Vanilla Bean Custard:

- 1 batch Vanilla Bean Custard
  the recipe is found on page 197

Vanilla Buttercream:

- 1 batch vanilla buttercream + **DF option**
  the recipe is found on page 185
- 1/2 teaspoon vanilla bean powder

Instructions

1. Make sure the custard is pre-made to cool when it's time to fill the cupcakes.
2. **Preheat oven to 325°F/163°C.**
3. In a medium bowl, sift coconut flour. Add all remaining dry ingredients. Mix and set aside.
4. In a separate medium bowl, add all wet ingredients, whisk together and pour onto dry ingredients.
5. Using a rubber spatula, mix the batter until well incorporated.
6. Line a cupcake tray with non-stick parchment liners
7. Using a large cookie scoop, scoop out one level scoop into each cup. If you have extra remaining, add a few teaspoons to the top of each cupcake until there is no batter left.
8. Bake the cupcakes for 25-30 minutes or until lightly golden brown on top.
9. Using a stand mixer bowl *(whisk attachment)* or an electric hand mixer, make the **Vanilla Buttercream frosting** on page 185.
10. Cool cupcakes for 10-15 minutes on a cooling rack.
11. Use a cupcake coring tool to core out the center of each cupcake. Add approx two tablespoons of custard into each hole!
12. Add buttercream frosting into a piping bag with a piping tip. Starting at the edge of the cupcakes, swirl the buttercream into a mountain two and a half times to the top.
13. When serving the cupcakes, ensure the frosting is at room temperature since it will harden when cool. Take cupcakes out of the fridge 20-min before eating.
14. Store in the fridge in an airtight container for four to five days or freeze for up to two months.

Note

- **Cupcakes have always been tricky in creating that perfect round top. My number one recommendation is to make sure all liquids are warm or at room temp.**
- **You may make these cupcakes 100% dairy-free with my DF frosting option on page 185.**

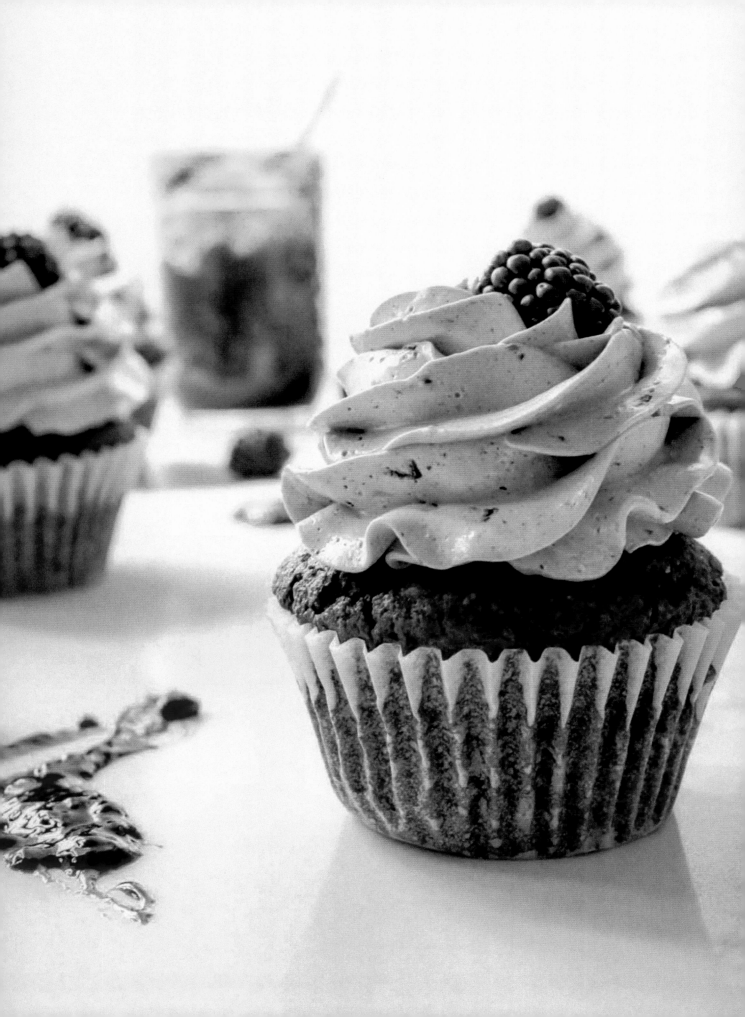

Decadent Blackberry Cupcakes

prep: *20 min*   **bake:** *25-30 min*   **cool:** *10-15 min*   **serves:** *12 medium*

Decadent, delicious, and so divine are these blackberry jam - filled cupcakes!

Dry ingredients:
- 112g *(1 cup)* almond flour
- 34g *(1/4 cup)* coconut flour
- 56g *(1/2 cup)* cacao powder
- 11g *(1 tablespoon)* psyllium husk powder
- 152g *(3/4 cup)* sweetener
  monk fruit, erythritol, xylitol
- 1 teaspoon baking soda
- 1 teaspoon baking powder
- 1 teaspoon sea salt

Wet ingredients:
- 4 free-run eggs *room temp*
- 118mL *(1/2 cup)* avocado oil
- 118mL *(1/2 cup)* coconut milk *full fat*
- 15mL *(1 tablespoon)* apple cider vinegar
- 1 teaspoon pure vanilla extract

Jam filling ingredients:
- 175g *(1 cup)* blackberry jam
  the recipe is found on page 193

Raspberry Buttercream:
- 1 batch Vanilla Buttercream + **DF option**
  the recipe is found on page 185
- 14g *(2 tablespoons)* cacao powder
- 175g *(1 cup)* blackberry jam
  the recipe is found on page 193

Instructions
1. **Preheat oven to 325°F/163°C.**
2. In a medium bowl, sift coconut flour and cacao powder. Add all remaining dry ingredients. Mix and set aside.
3. In a separate medium bowl, add all wet ingredients, whisk together and pour onto dry ingredients.
4. Using a rubber spatula, mix the batter until well incorporated.
5. Line a cupcake tray with non-stick parchment liners
6. Using a large cookie scoop, scoop out one level scoop into each cup. If you have extra remaining, add a few teaspoons to the top of each cupcake until there is no batter left.
7. Bake the cupcakes for 25-30 minutes or until lightly golden brown on top.
8. **Jam Filling**: While baking cupcakes, prepare the jam in a small bowl and have it ready *(best to make the jam the day before)*.
9. Using a stand mixer bowl *(whisk attachment)* or an electric hand mixer, make the **Vanilla Buttercream frosting** on page 185.
10. Once the buttercream has doubled in size, add sifted cacao powder and the jam, and whip for another 3min.
11. Cool cupcakes for 10-15 minutes on a cooling rack.
12. Use a cupcake coring tool to core out the center of each cupcake. Add approx two tablespoons of jam filling into each hole!
13. Add buttercream frosting into a piping bag with a piping tip. Starting at the edge of the cupcakes, swirl the buttercream into a mountain two and a half times to the top.
14. When serving the cupcakes, ensure the frosting is at room temperature since it will harden when cool. Take cupcakes out of the fridge 20-min before eating.
15. Store in the fridge in an airtight container for four to five days or freeze for up to two months.

Note
- **Cupcakes have always been tricky in creating that perfect round top. My number one recommendation is to make sure all liquids are warm or at room temp.**
- **You may make these cupcakes 100% dairy-free with my DF frosting option on page 185.**

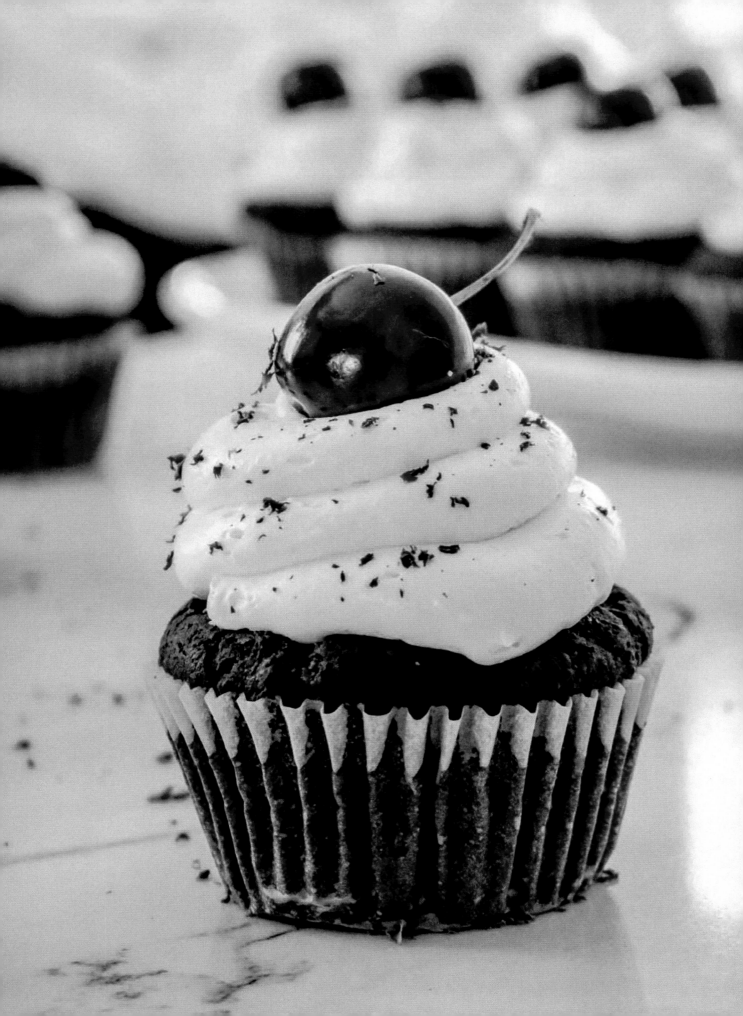

Black Forest Cupcakes

prep: *20 min*   **bake:** *25-30 min*   **cool:** *10-15 min*   **serves:** *12 medium*

These Black Forest Cupcakes taste as divine as they look.

Dry ingredients:
- 112g *(1 cup)* almond flour
- 34g *(1/4 cup)* coconut flour
- 56g *(1/2 cup)* cacao powder
- 11g *(1 tablespoon)* psyllium husk powder
- 152g *(3/4 cup)* sweetener
  monk fruit, erythritol, xylitol
- 1 teaspoon baking soda
- 1 teaspoon baking powder
- 1 teaspoon sea salt

Wet ingredients:
- 4 free-run eggs *room temp*
- 118mL *(1/2 cup)* avocado oil
- 118mL *(1/2 cup)* coconut milk *full fat*
- 15mL *(1 tablespoon)* apple cider vinegar
- 1 teaspoon pure vanilla extract

Jam filling ingredients:
- 175g *(1 cup)* cherry jam
  the recipe is found on page 193

Vanilla Buttercream:
- 1 batch Vanilla Buttercream + **DF option**
  the recipe is found on page 185

Garnish
- 12 large fresh cherry *garnish for the top*
- 85g *(1/4)* chocolate bar *shaved for the top*
  the recipe is found on page 223

Note

- **Cupcakes have always been tricky in creating that perfect round top. My number one recommendation is to make sure all liquids are warm or at room temp.**
- **You may make these cupcakes 100% dairy-free with my DF frosting option on page 185.**

Instructions

1. **Preheat oven to 325°F/163°C.**
2. In a medium bowl, sift coconut flour and cacao powder. Add all remaining dry ingredients. Mix and set aside.
3. In a separate medium bowl, add all wet ingredients, whisk together and pour onto dry ingredients.
4. Using a rubber spatula, mix the batter until well incorporated.
5. Line a cupcake tray with non-stick parchment liners
6. Using a large cookie scoop, scoop out one level scoop into each cup. If you have extra remaining, add a few teaspoons to the top of each cupcake until there is no batter left.
7. Bake the cupcakes for 25-30 minutes or until lightly golden brown on top.
8. **Jam Filling:** While baking cupcakes, prepare the jam in a small bowl and have it ready *(best to make the jam the day before)*.
9. Using a stand mixer bowl *(whisk attachment)* or an electric hand mixer, make the **Vanilla Buttercream frosting** on page 185.
10. Once the buttercream has doubled in size, add the jam and whip for another 3 min.
11. Cool cupcakes for 10-15 minutes on a cooling rack.
12. Use a cupcake coring tool to core out the center of each cupcake. Add approx two tablespoons of jam filling into each hole!
13. Add buttercream frosting into a piping bag with a piping tip. Starting at the edge of the cupcakes, swirl the buttercream into a mountain two and a half times to the top.
14. **Garnish:** Shave chocolate on top, and add a gorgeous cherry.
15. When serving the cupcakes, ensure the frosting is at room temperature since it will harden when cool. Take cupcakes out of the fridge 20-min before eating.
16. Store in the fridge in an airtight container for four to five days or freeze for up to two months.

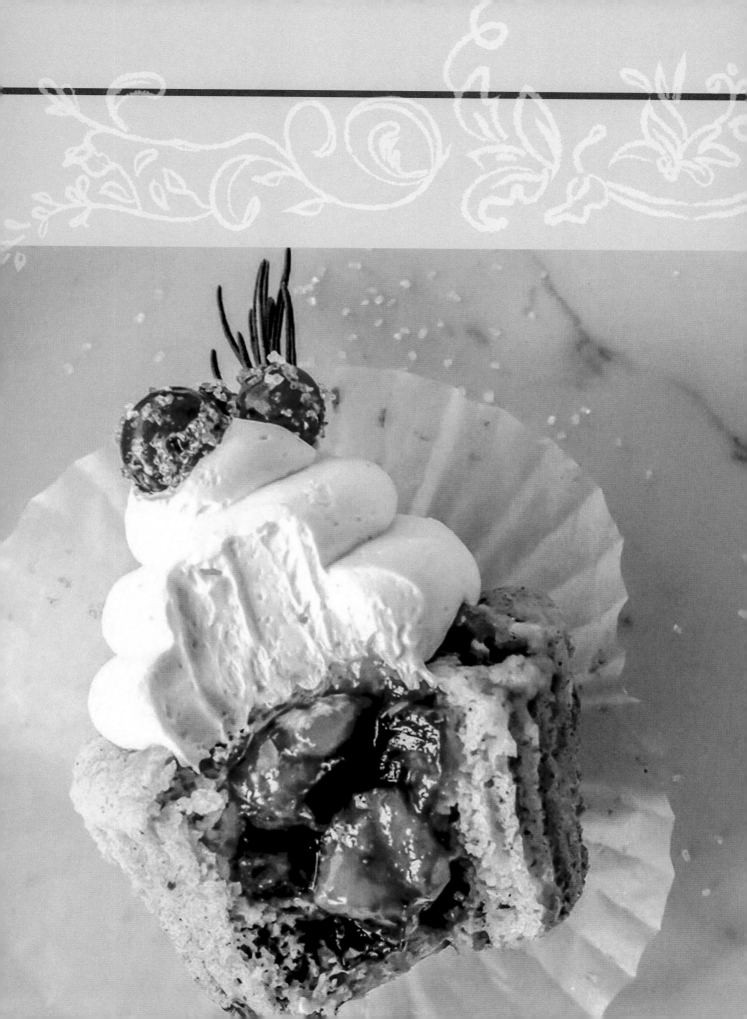

CUPCAKES
Christmas

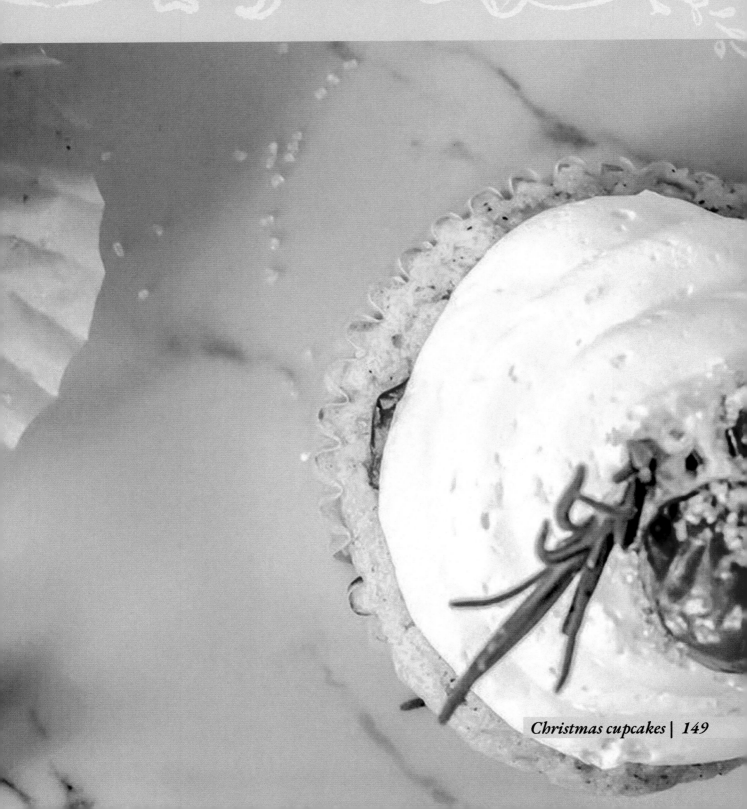

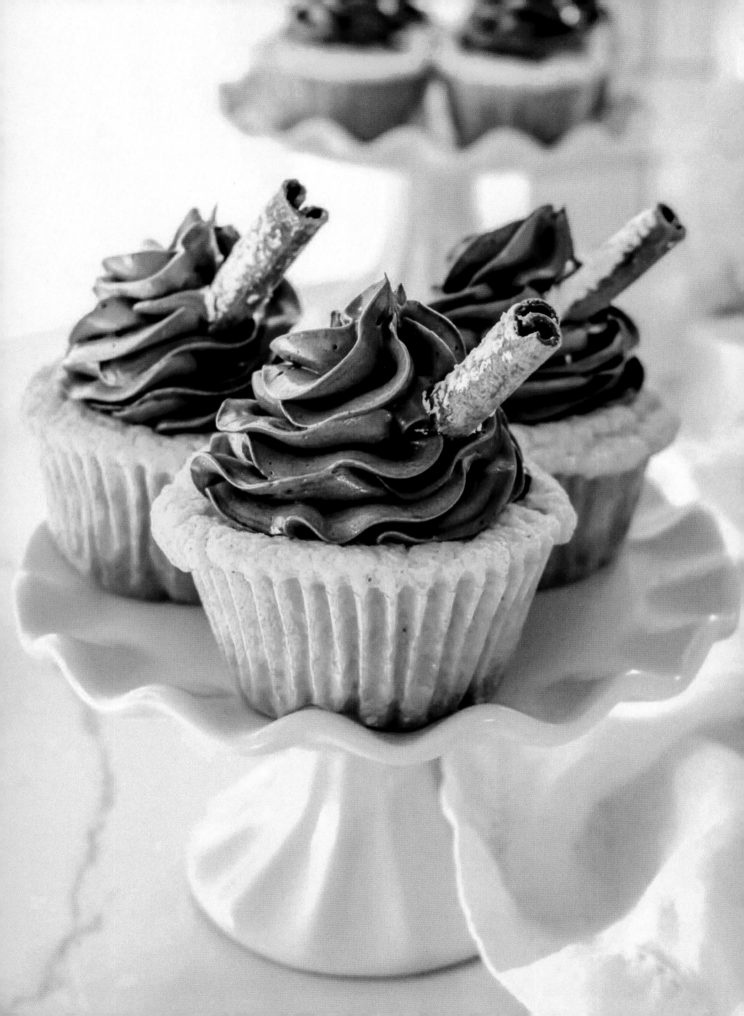

Spiced Eggnog Custard Cupcakes

prep: *20 min*   **bake:** *25-30 min*   **cool:** *10-15 min*   **serves:** *12 medium*

Eggnog custard-filled cupcakes are such a treat around Christmas time. The spiced vanilla cupcake base, combined with the rich chocolate buttercream, is to die for.

Dry ingredients:
140g *(1¼ cups)* almond flour
- 46g *(1/4 cup)* coconut flour
- 11g *(1 tablespoon)* psyllium husk powder
- 105g *(1/2 cup)* sweetener
  monk fruit, erythritol, xylitol
- 1 teaspoon cinnamon
- 1/2 teaspoon nutmeg
- 1 teaspoon baking soda
- 1 teaspoon baking powder
- 1 teaspoon sea salt

Wet ingredients:
- 4 free-run egg *room temp*
- 118mL *(1/2 cup)* avocado oil
- 118mL *(1/2 cup)* coconut milk *full fat*
- 15mL *(1 tablespoon)* apple cider vinegar
- 1 teaspoon rum extract
- 1 teaspoon pure vanilla extract

Vanilla Bean Custard:
- 1 batch Vanilla Bean Custard
  the recipe is found on page 197
- 1 teaspoon rum extract

Chocolate Buttercream:
- 1 batch Chocolate Buttercream + **DF option**
  the recipe is found on page 187

Garnish:
- 12 small cinnamon sticks *to garnish*
- powdered sweetener *to garnish*

Note

- Cupcakes have always been tricky in creating that perfect round top. My number one recommendation is to make sure all liquids are warm or at room temp.
- You may make these cupcakes 100% dairy-free with my DF frosting option on page 185.

Instructions

1. **Custard:** Make sure the custard is pre-made so that the custard is cool when it's time to fill the cupcakes.
2. **Preheat oven to 325°F/163°C.**
3. In a medium bowl, sift coconut flour and add all remaining dry ingredients. Mix and set aside.
4. In a separate medium bowl, add all wet ingredients.
5. Whisk together and pour onto dry ingredients.
6. Using a rubber spatula, mix the batter until well incorporated.
7. Line a cupcake tray with non-stick parchment liners.
8. Using a large cookie scoop, scoop out one level scoop into each cup. If you have extra remaining, add a few teaspoons to the top of each cupcake until there is no batter left.
9. Bake the cupcake for 25-30 minutes or until lightly golden brown on top.
10. Using a stand mixer bowl *(whisk attachment)* or an electric hand mixer, make the **Buttercream frosting** on page 187.
11. Cool cupcakes on a cooling rack for 10-15 minutes, and use a cupcake coring tool, core out each center of the cupcakes, and add approximately two tablespoons of custard into each hole!
12. Add buttercream frosting into a piping bag with a piping tip. Starting at the edge of the cupcakes, swirl the buttercream into a mountain two and a half times to the top.
13. **Garnish:** Add a small cinnamon stick to the icing, dusting it with powdered sweetener.
14. When serving the cupcakes, ensure the frosting is at room temperature since it will harden when cool. Take cupcakes out of the fridge 20-min before eating.
15. Store in the fridge in an airtight container for four to five days or freeze for up to two months.

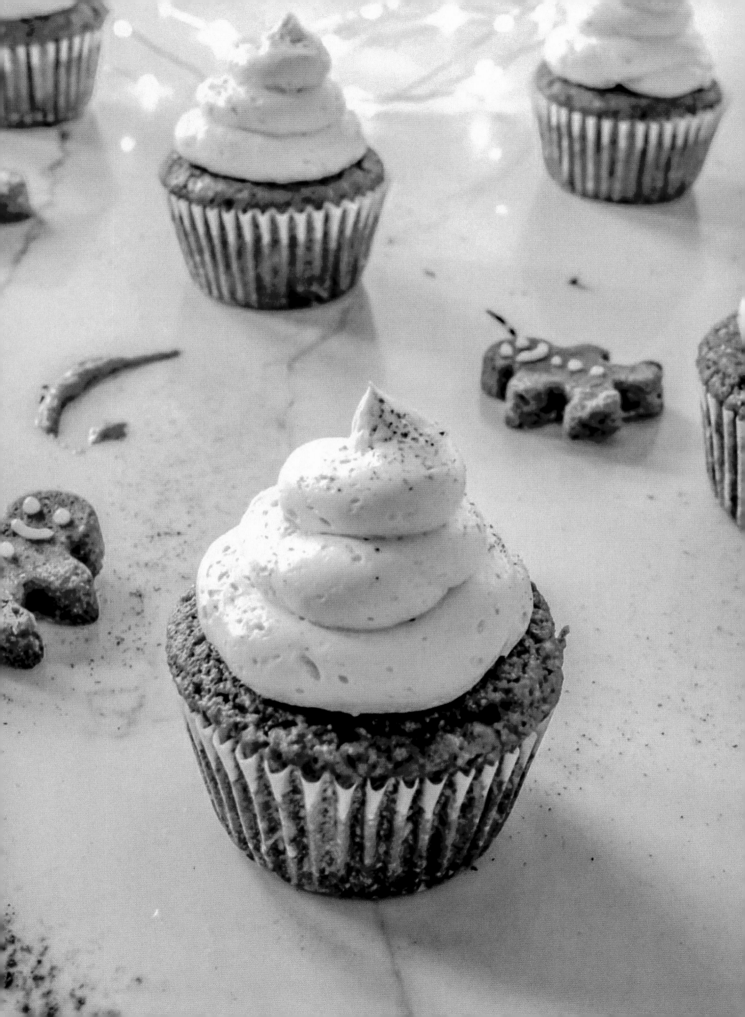

Gingerbread Caramel Cupcakes

prep: *20 min*   **bake:** *25-30 min*   **cool:** *10-15 min*   **serves:** *12 medium*

Gingerbread is always a must when the holidays roll around. The surprise caramel filling makes these a decadent dessert for hosting a memorable Christmas gathering.

Dry ingredients
- 140g *(1¼ cups)* almond flour
- 46g *(1/4 cup)* coconut flour
- 11g *(1 tablespoon)* psyllium husk powder
- 105g *(1/2 cup)* sweetener
   monk fruit, erythritol, xylitol
- 1 teaspoon cinnamon
- 1 tablespoon fresh ginger *grated*
- 1/2 teaspoon nutmeg
- 1/2 teaspoon allspice
- 1 teaspoon baking soda
- 1 teaspoon baking powder
- 1 teaspoon sea salt

Wet ingredients:
- 4 eggs *room temp*
- 118mL *(1/2 cup)* avocado oil
- 118mL *(1/2 cup)* coconut milk *full fat*
- 15mL *(1 tablespoon)* apple cider vinegar
- 40g *(1 tablespoon)* blackstrap molasses
- 1 teaspoon pure vanilla extract

Caramel Sauce:
- 245g *(1 cup)* Caramel Sauce
   the recipe is found on page 219

Vanilla Buttercream:
- 1 batch Vanilla Buttercream + **DF option**
   the recipe is found on page 185
- 1 dash of cinnamon *to garnish*

Instructions
1. **Caramel:** Make sure caramel sauce is pre-made, so it is cooled when it's time to fill the cupcakes.
2. **Preheat oven to 325°F/163°C.**
3. In a medium bowl, sift coconut flour and measure all remaining dry ingredients. Mix and set aside
4. Whisk together and pour onto dry ingredients in a separate medium bowl and all wet ingredients.
5. Using a rubber spatula, mix the batter until well incorporated.
6. Line a cupcake tray with non-stick parchment liners.
7. Using a large cookie scoop, scoop out one level scoop into each cupcake. If you have extra remaining, add a few teaspoons to the top of each cupcake.
8. Bake the cupcakes for 25-30 minutes or until lightly golden brown on top.
9. In a stand mixer bowl with a whisk attachment, make **Vanilla buttercream frosting** on page 185.
10. Cool cupcakes on a cooling rack for 10-15 minutes, and use a cupcake coring tool, core out each center of the cupcakes, and add approximately two tablespoons of caramel into each hole!
11. Add buttercream frosting into a piping bag with a piping tip. Starting at the edge of the cupcakes, swirl the buttercream into a mountain two and a half times to the top.
12. When serving the cupcakes, ensure the frosting is at room temperature since it will harden when cool. Take cupcakes out of the fridge 20-min before eating.
13. Store in the fridge in an airtight container for four to five days or freeze for up to two months.

Note

- Cupcakes have always been tricky in creating that perfect round top. My number one recommendation is to make sure all liquids are warm or at room temp.
- You may make these cupcakes 100% dairy-free with my DF frosting option on page 185.

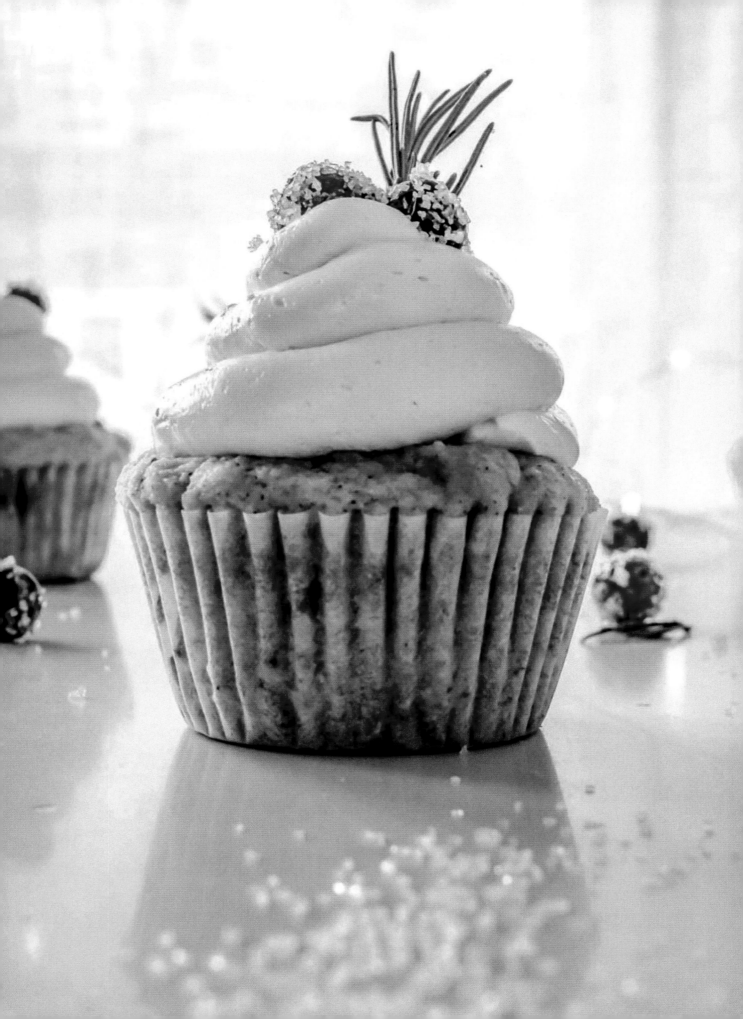

Sparkling Cranberry Cupcakes

prep: *20 min*   **bake:** *25-30 min*   **cool:** *10-15 min*   **serves:** *12 medium*

These are my personal favourite Christmas cupcakes! Not only are they absolutely stunning and so Christmasy; The spiced orange cupcake base paired with the tarty cranberry jam and smoothed out with the vanilla buttercream frosting tastes like a magical Christmas celebration.

Dry ingredients
- 140g *(1¼ cups)* almond flour
- 46g *(1/4 cup)* coconut flour
- 11g *(1 tablespoon)* psyllium husk powder
- 105g *(1/2 cup)* sweetener
  monk fruit, erythritol, xylitol
- 1 tablespoon *(medium)* orange zest *fresh*
- 1 teaspoon cinnamon
- 1 teaspoon baking soda
- 1 teaspoon baking powder
- 1 teaspoon sea salt

Wet ingredients:
- 4 free-run eggs *room temp*
- 118mL *(1/2 cup)* avocado oil
- 118mL *(1/2 cup)* coconut milk *full fat*
- 15mL *(1 tablespoon)* lemon juice
- 1 teaspoon pure vanilla extract

Jam filling ingredients:
- 175g *(1 cup)* cranberry jam
  the recipe is found on page 193

Vanilla Buttercream:
- 1 batch Vanilla Buttercream + **DF option**
  the recipe is found on page 185
- 36 fresh cranberries *-3 for each cupcake*
- 2-3 fresh rosemary stems *to garnish*
- 50g *(1/4 cup)* sweetener *to roll cranberries in*

Note

- **Cupcakes have always been tricky in creating that perfect round top. My number one recommendation is to make sure all liquids are warm or at room temp.**
- **You may make these cupcakes 100% dairy-free with my DF frosting option on page 185.**

Instructions

1. Preheat oven to 325°F/163°C.
2. In a medium bowl, sift coconut flour and measure all remaining dry ingredients. Mix and set aside.
3. Whisk together and pour onto dry ingredients in a separate medium bowl and all wet ingredients. Using a rubber spatula, mix the batter until well incorporated.
4. Line a cupcake tray with non-stick parchment liners.
5. Using a large cookie scoop, scoop out one level scoop into each cup. If you have extra remaining, add a few teaspoons to the top of each cupcake.
6. Bake the cupcakes for 25-30 minutes or until lightly golden brown on top.
7. **Jam filling:** While cupcakes are baking in a small bowl, ensure your jam is ready to go *(best to make the jam the day before).*
8. Using a stand mixer bowl *(whisk attachment)* or an electric hand mixer, make the **Vanilla Buttercream frosting** on page 185.
9. Cool cupcakes on a cooling rack for 10-15 minutes, and use a cupcake coring tool, core out each center of the cupcakes, and add approximately two tablespoons of jam filling into each hole!
10. Add buttercream frosting into a piping bag with a piping tip. Starting at the edge of the cupcakes, swirl the buttercream into a mountain two and a half times to the top.
11. When serving cupcakes, ensure the buttercream is at room temperature since it will harden when cool.
12. Slightly dampen cranberries to help the sweetener stick, and roll in granulated sweetener *(I like to use Classic monk fruit by Lakanto).* Place three sparkling cranberries on top of the buttercream frosting.
13. Cut the rosemary stem into 12 pieces. Stick rosemary stems in each of the buttercream toppings besides the cranberries.
14. When serving the cupcakes, ensure the frosting is at room temperature since it will harden when cool. Take cupcakes out of the fridge 20-min before eating.
15. Store in the fridge in an airtight container for four to five days or freeze for up to two months. *Cupcakes* | **155**

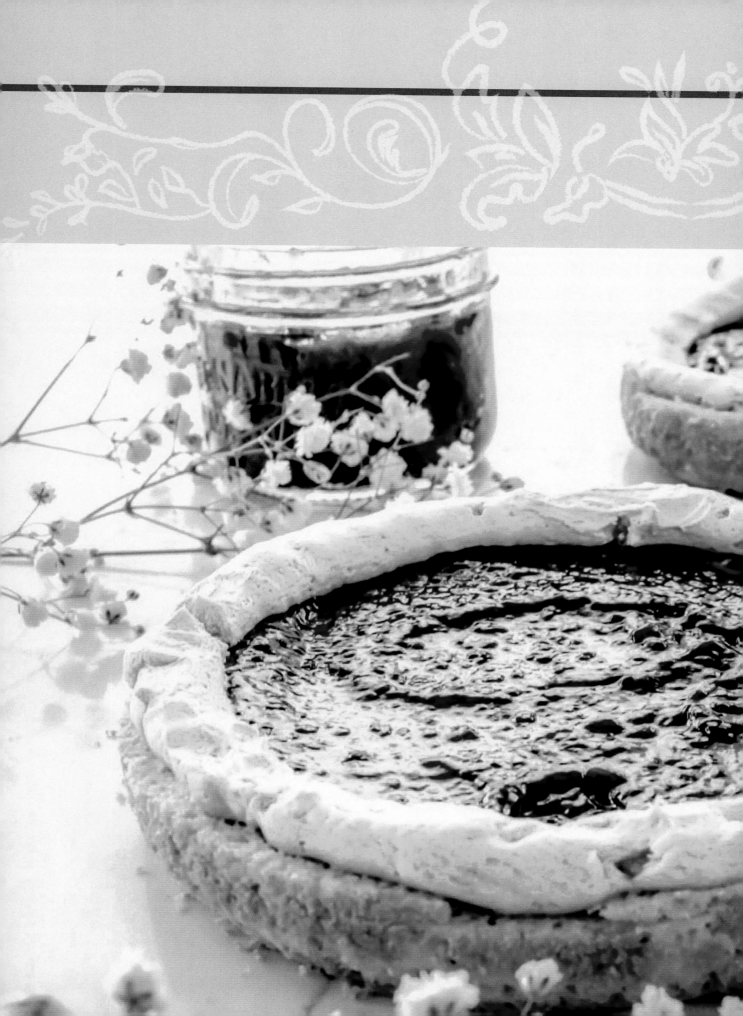

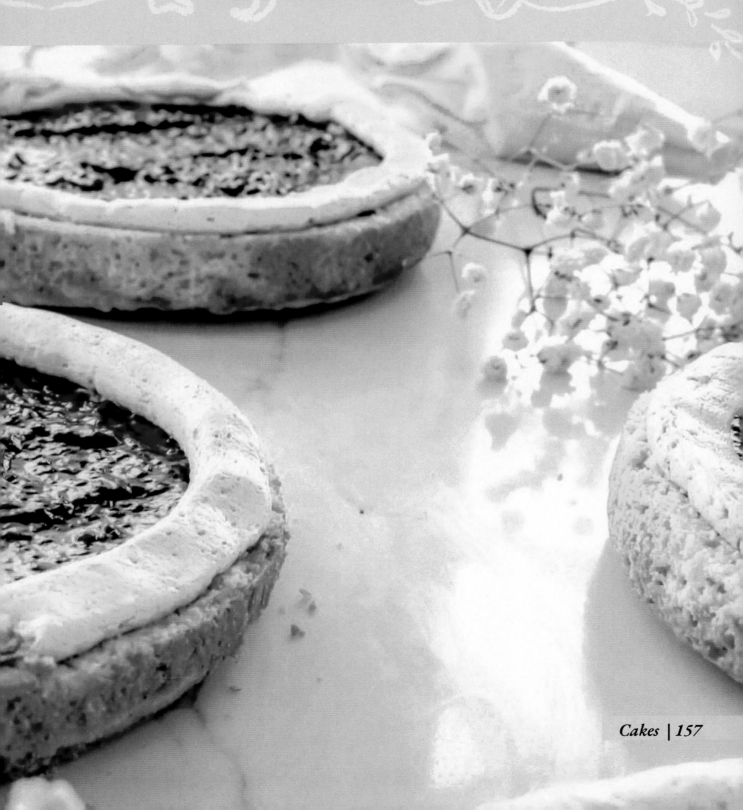

Chapter Seven
CAKES

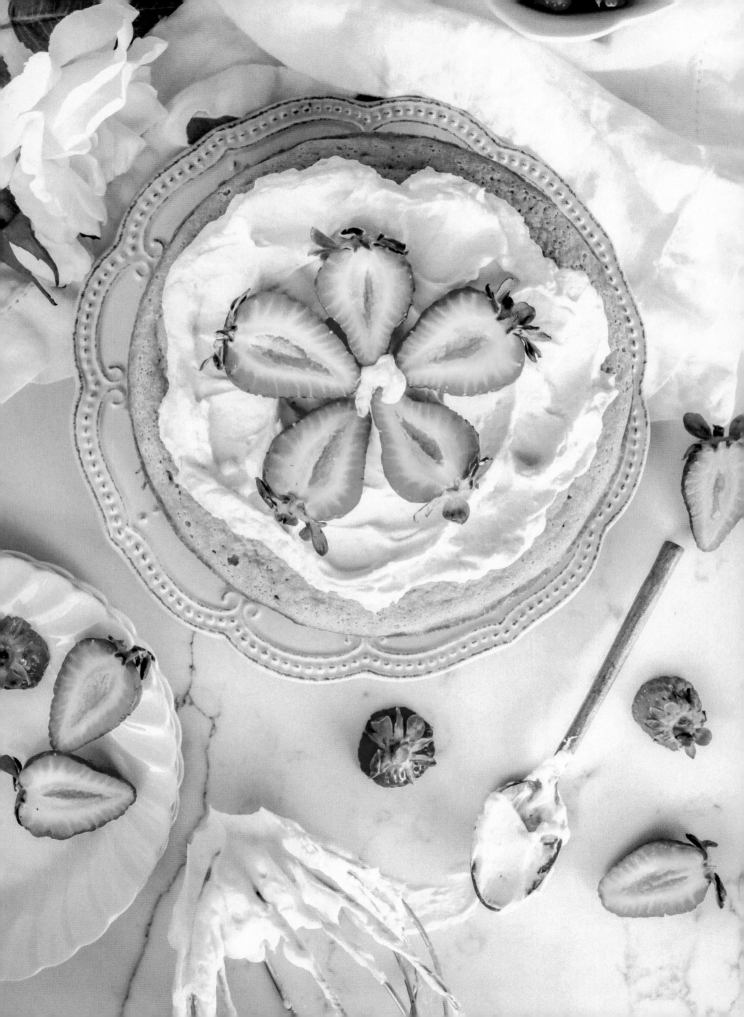

Strawberry Shortcake

prep: *25 min*   **bake:** *40-50 min*   **cool:** *30-45 min*   **serves:** *1 six inch cake*

If you love a refreshing, light and airy cake, then this strawberry shortcake will be your new go-to recipe. I love this recipe because it is 100% dairy-free since the whipped cream is a homemade coconut whipped cream.

Dry ingredients
- 168g *(1½ cups)* almond flour
- 68g *(1/2 cup)* coconut flour
- 11g *(1 tablespoon)* psyllium husk powder
- 155g *(3/4 cup)* sweetener
  - *monk fruit, erythritol, xylitol*
- 1 teaspoon baking soda
- 1 teaspoon baking powder
- 1 teaspoon sea salt

Wet ingredients:
- 5 free-run eggs *room temp*
- 118mL *(1/2 cup)* avocado oil
- 118mL *(1/2 cup)* coconut milk *full fat*
- 56mL *(1/4 cup)* lemon juice
- 1 teaspoon pure vanilla extract

Coconut Whipped Cream:
- 1 batch Coconut Whipped Cream
  - *the recipe is found on page 189*
- 300g *(2 cups)* fresh strawberries *chopped*
leave 3 whole strawberries to garnish the top

Instructions

1. **Preheat oven to 325°F/163°C.**
2. In a medium bowl, sift coconut flour and measure all remaining dry ingredients. Mix and set aside.
3. Whisk together and pour onto dry ingredients in a separate medium bowl and all wet ingredients. Using a rubber spatula, mix the batter until well incorporated.
4. In two 6-inch springform cake pans, grease/spray with avocado oil, and trace cake pan bottoms on parchment paper, cut out and place parchment rounds in the bottom of the cake pan.
5. Using a food scale, place the cake pan on top of the food scale, tare to 0, and add roughly 480 grams of cake batter to each prepped cake pan. Or, you may use measuring cups to evenly measure the same amount of batter in each cake pan.
6. Bake the cakes for 40-50 minutes, depending on the oven, or until lightly golden brown on top.
7. Make coconut whipped cream in a stand mixer bowl with a whisk attachment on page 189. *(coconut milk must be chilled in the can for up to 6 hours for the best result)*
8. In a small bowl, chop fresh strawberries into little pieces, leaving 3 whole strawberries for the top to garnish the cake.
9. Add half the coconut cream to the small bowl with chopped strawberries, and leave the remainder for the top of the cake. *(add more whipped cream for the chopped strawberries if you want to make a four-layer cake instead of a two-layer cake)*
10. Before using, cool the cake for 45 minutes to 1 full hour on a cooling rack.
11. You may cut the cake round in half with a serrated knife *(bread knife)* to make four layers, or you may serve it just how it is as a two-layer cake.
12. Add whipped cream strawberry filling to each layer *(1-3 layers)*, using an offset cake spatula, spread to the edges of the cake, and repeat.
13. For the top of the cake, add the remainder of the plain coconut whipped cream and spread it to the edges. Slice strawberries in half and decorate the top of the cake.
14. Best to keep the cake in the fridge right before serving.
15. Store in the fridge in an airtight container for four to five days or freeze for up to two months.

Note

- **This cake requires a dairy-free coconut whipped cream, which means that the coconut milk must be chilled in the fridge for up to 6 hours before using it. to allow all the fat to harden at the top of the can.**

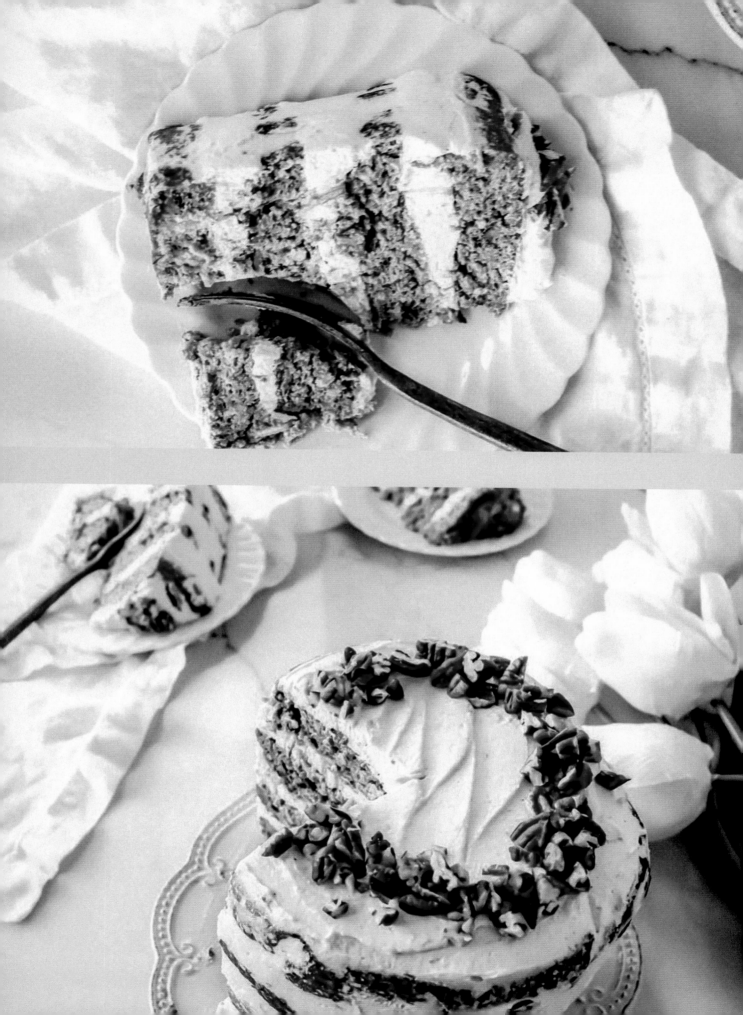

Harvest Carrot Cake

prep: *25 min*   **bake:** *40-50 min*   **cool:** *30-45 min*   **serves:** *1 six inch cake*

Ever since I was a little girl, I could never turn down carrot cake, especially homemade carrot cake!
Enjoy this cake any time of the season, and your energy and belly will enjoy it too!

Dry ingredients

- 140g *(1¼ cups)* almond flour
- 68g *(1/2 cup)* coconut flour
- 22g *(2 tablespoons)* psyllium husk powder
- 42g *(1/2 cup)* coconut flakes *unsweetened*
- 55g *(1/2 cup)* pecans *chopped*
- 220g *(2 cups)* carrots *shredded*
- 80g *(1/2 cup)* raisins *optional if on paleo*
- 152g *(3/4 cup)* sweetener
   monk fruit, erythritol, xylitol
- 1 teaspoon baking soda
- 1 teaspoon baking powder
- 2 teaspoons cinnamon
- 1 teaspoon ginger
- 1/2 teaspoon clove
- 1 teaspoon sea salt

Wet ingredients:

- 5 free-run eggs *room temp*
- 118mL *(1/2 cup)* avocado oil
- 118mL *(1/2 cup)* apple sauce
- 59mL *(1/4 cup)* coconut milk *full fat*
- 56mL *(1/4 cup)* lemon juice
- 1 teaspoon pure vanilla extract

Cashew cream cheese frosting:

- 1 batch Cashew Cream Cheese Frosting
   the recipe is found on page 188
- 55g *(1/2 cup)* pecans *garnish*

Instructions

1. **Preheat oven to 325°F/163°C.** Prep a cookie sheet with two small pieces of parchment paper side by side,
2. Toast coconut flakes for 4-5 minutes, and toast chopped pecans (*1 cup inside the cake & garnish)* for 7 minutes, set aside.
3. With a grater or food processor, grate carrots and set them aside.
4. Sift coconut flour and measure all remaining dry ingredients, including toasted nuts and carrots. Make sure carrots are not stuck together. Mix and set aside
5. In a separate medium bowl, add all the wet ingredients, whisk together and pour onto the dry ingredients. Using a rubber spatula, mix the batter until well incorporated.
6. In two 6-inch springform cake pans, grease/spray with avocado oil, and trace cake pan bottoms on parchment paper, cut out and place parchment rounds in the bottom of the cake pan.
7. Using a food scale, place the cake pan on top of the food scale, tare to 0, and add roughly 650 grams of cake batter to each prepped cake pan. Or, you may use measuring cups to evenly measure the same amount of batter in each cake pan.
8. Bake the cakes for 55-65 minutes, depending on the oven, or until lightly golden brown on top.
9. In a stand mixer bowl with a whisk attachment, make **cashew cream cheese frosting** on page 188.
10. Cool cake for 45 minutes to 1 full hour on a cooling rack.
11. You may cut the cake round in half with a serrated knife *(bread knife)* to make 4 layers, or you may serve it just how it is as a 2 layer cake.
12. Add cashew cream cheese frosting to each layer (*1-4 layers),* using an offset cake spatula, spread to the edges of the cake, and repeat. Placing each cake layer on top of the other when iced.
13. Add the remainder of the icing and spread it to the edges and sides.
14. Take the cake out of the fridge 20-min before eating. Decorate the cake with chopped toasted pecans. Place in the refrigerator until it's time to eat.
15. Store in the fridge in an airtight container for four to five days or freeze for up to two months.

Note

- **Cashew cream cheese frosting is best to make a day prior to icing the cake, to allow it to cool and harden in the fridge.**

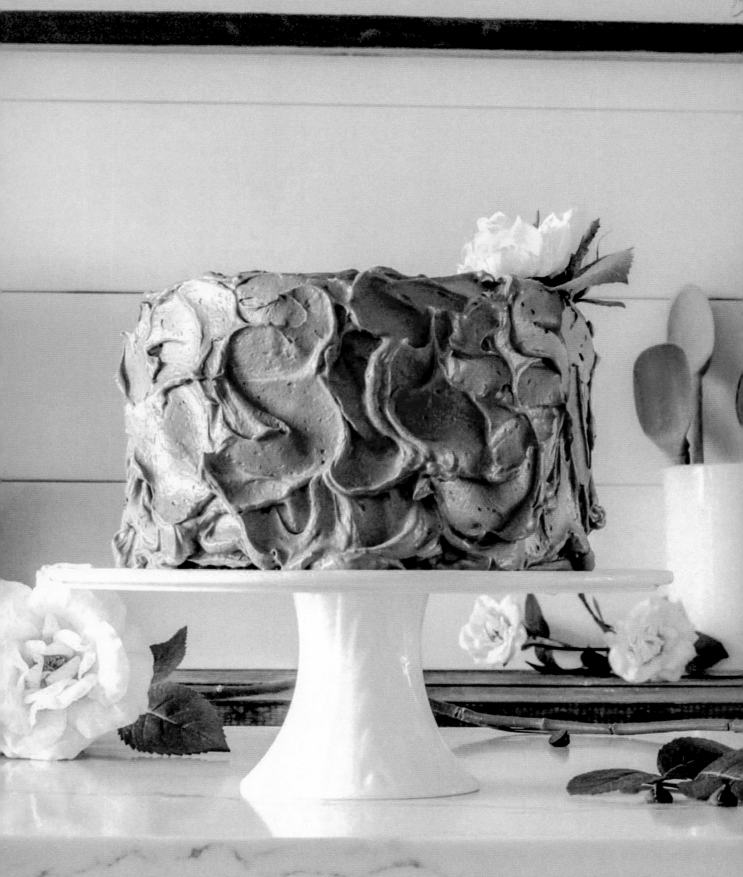

Classic Chocolate Cake

prep: *25 min*   **bake:** *40-50 min*   **cool:** *30-45 min*   **serves:** *1 six inch cake*

This cake recipe is my number one viewed video on my YouTube channel! However, I even made it better by tweaking some of the ratios. I can't wait for you to dig into this decadent chocolate cake!

Dry ingredients
- 168g *(1 ½ cups)* almond flour
- 34g *(1/4 cup)* coconut flour
- 56g *(1/2 cup)* cacao powder
- 22g *(2 tablespoons)* psyllium husk powder
- 210g *(1 cup)* sweetener
  monk fruit, erythritol, xylitol
- 1 teaspoon baking soda
- 1 teaspoon baking powder
- 1 teaspoon sea salt

Wet ingredients:
- 5 free-run eggs *room temp*
- 118mL *(1/2 cup)* avocado oil
- 110g *(1 cup)* chocolate bar *melted*
  the recipe is found on page
- 118mL *(1/2 cup)* coconut milk *in can*
- 15g *(2oz)* double shot of espresso *organic*
- 56mL *(1/4 cup)* apple cider vinegar
- 1 teaspoon pure vanilla extract

Chocolate Buttercream:
- 1 batch Chocolate Buttercream + **DF option**
  the recipe is found on page 187

Note
- **If you don't have an espresso machine, I recommend purchasing a high-quality instant espresso powder. Add 1tbsp of espresso powder, and dissolve into 2oz of warm water.**
- **You can make this cake 100% dairy-free with my DF frosting option on page 187.**

Instructions
1. Preheat oven to 325°F/163°C.
2. In a medium bowl, sift cacao powder and coconut flour and measure all remaining dry ingredients. Mix and set aside.
3. In a small heat-proof bowl, melt chocolate chips in the microwave at 10-sec intervals and stir in between intervals or on a double boiler with simmering water.
4. Whisk all wet ingredients *(including melted chocolate)* together in a separate medium bowl and pour onto dry ingredients. Using a rubber spatula, mix the batter until well incorporated.
5. In two 6-inch springform cake pans, grease/spray with avocado oil, and trace cake pan bottoms on parchment paper, cut out and place parchment rounds in the bottom of the cake pan.
6. Using a food scale, place the cake pan on top of the food scale, tare to 0, and add roughly 850 grams of cake batter to each prepped cake pan. Or, you may use measuring cups to evenly measure the same amount of batter in each cake pan.
7. Bake the cakes for 55-65 minutes, depending on the oven, or until lightly golden brown on top.
8. In a stand mixer bowl with a whisk attachment, make the **chocolate buttercream frosting** on page 187.
9. Cool cakes for 45 minutes to 1 full hour on a cooling rack.
10. You may cut the cake round in half with a serrated knife *(bread knife)* to make 4 layers, or you may serve it just how it is as a 2 layer cake.
11. Add buttercream frosting to each layer *(1-4 layers)*, using an offset cake spatula, spread to the edges of the cake, and repeat. Placing each layer on top of each other when iced.
12. For the top of the cake, add the remainder of the icing and spread to the edges and down the sides. Decorate the cake in any style you desire. In the picture, I just used a small offset cake spatula.
13. Place in the fridge until it's time to eat. Best to take the cake out of the fridge 30 min - 1 hour before slicing and serving.
14. Store in the fridge in an airtight container for four to five days or freeze for up to two months.

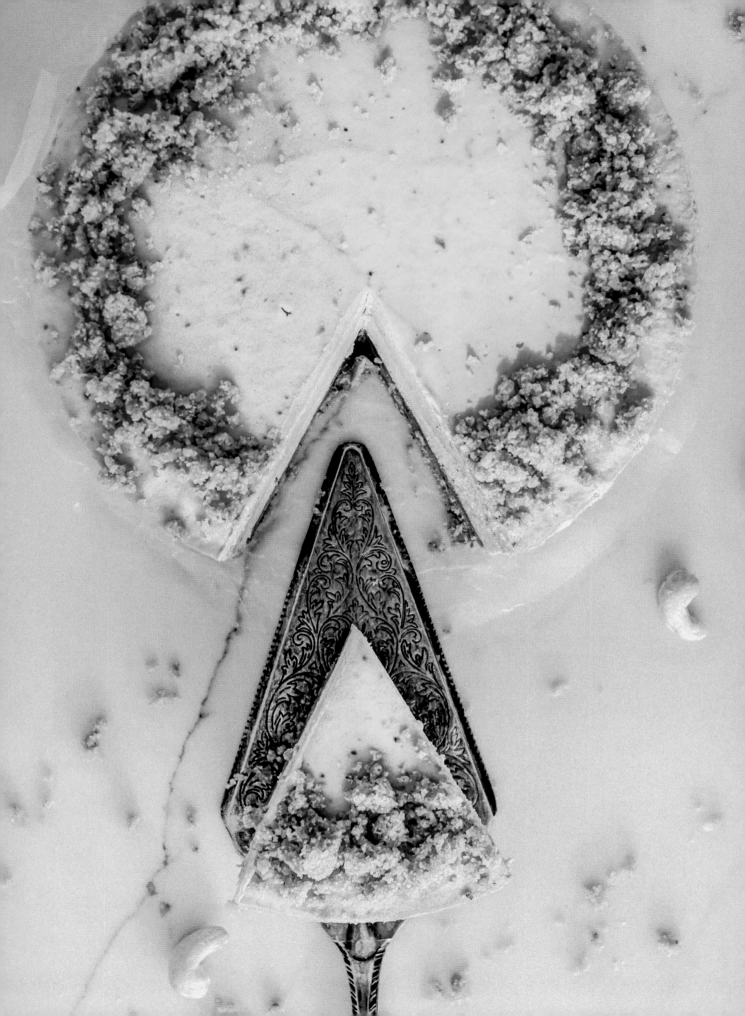

Raw Strawberry Crumble Cheesecake

prep: *40 min*   **cool:** *4 hours*   **serves:** *1 six inch cake*

Going dairy-free was a breeze for me since cashews make such an incredible alternative. This recipe is my hubby's favourite cake; I make sure I have the time to make it every anniversary!

Graham crust ingredients

- 224g *(2 cups)* almond flour
- 46g *(1/3 cup)* coconut flour
- 14g *(2 tablespoons)* flaxseed meal *ground*
- 118mL *(1/2 cup)* coconut oil *melted*
- 105g *(1/2 cup)* sweetener
  monk fruit, erythritol, xylitol
- 2 teaspoons cinnamon
- 30mL *(1-2 tablespoons)* cold water
- 1 teaspoon sea salt

Cheesecake Ingredients:

- 225g *(1½ cups)* strawberries *fresh or frozen*
  see step 9
- 420g *(3 cups)* raw cashews *soaked overnight*
- 118mL *(1/2 cup)* coconut oil *melted*
- 235mL *(1 cup)* coconut milk *full fat*
- 210g *(1 cup)* sweetener
  monk fruit, erythritol, xylitol
- 56mL *(1/4 cup)* lemon juice
- 1 teaspoon pure vanilla extract
- 2 teaspoon sea salt

Crumble ingredients:

- 40g *(2-3 tablespoons)* coconut oil *room temp*
- 84g *(3/4 cup)* almond flour
- 40g *(3 tablespoons)* sweetener
- 1 teaspoon cinnamon
- 1 teaspoon pure vanilla extract
- 1/8 teaspoon sea salt

Instructions

1. Grease a 6" springform pan with coconut oil and line a 6" cake pan with parchment paper *(cut in a circle)*.
2. **Graham crust:** Add all the crust ingredients into a medium bowl *(or stand mixer bowl with paddle attachment)*. Using your hands, mix/beat until it forms a solid softball of dough.
3. Press the rest of the graham crust dough evenly along the bottom of the prepared pan.
4. Place the crust in the freezer while preparing the cheesecake filling.
5. **Cheesecake:** To make the first vanilla layer of cheesecake, In a high-powered blender, combine all of the cheesecake *(not the strawberries)* filling ingredients & make sure coconut oil is melted. Blend for about 2 minutes until the mixture is smooth and creamy.
6. Scrape down the sides as necessary. You may need to add a bit more coconut milk or lemon juice to get it to blend smoothly if your blender isn't super high-powered.
7. Once it's smooth, taste the mixture and adjust the sweetness/tartness levels, if desired.
8. Pour ½ of the cheesecake filling into the prepared pan over the crust. Smooth the top and tap the pan hard against the counter a few times to release air bubbles. Place in the freezer.
9. **Strawberry layer:** Add the strawberries to the remainder of the cashew cream, and blend on high until you see no chunks of strawberries.
10. Take the cake from the freezer, and pour the entire strawberry filling on top. Again, smooth out the top and tap the pan hard against the counter a few times to release air bubbles.
11. Place in the freezer to set for at least 3-4 hours or until completely firm.
12. **Crumble:** Add all crumble ingredients in a small bowl, mix with hands, and press together until it reaches a soft yet crumbly texture.
13. If storing in the freezer, let it thaw in the refrigerator for a few hours before serving or let it thaw at room temperature for 15 minutes before serving.
14. Add extra graham crumble on top!
15. Before slicing & serving, I recommend running your knife under hot water to warm it up before cutting the cheesecake with the still-hot *(dried)* knife.
16. Store leftovers in an airtight container in the freezer for three months.

Note

- **Cashew blend the best for this recipe when you soak it overnight, or at least 6 hours in warm water.**

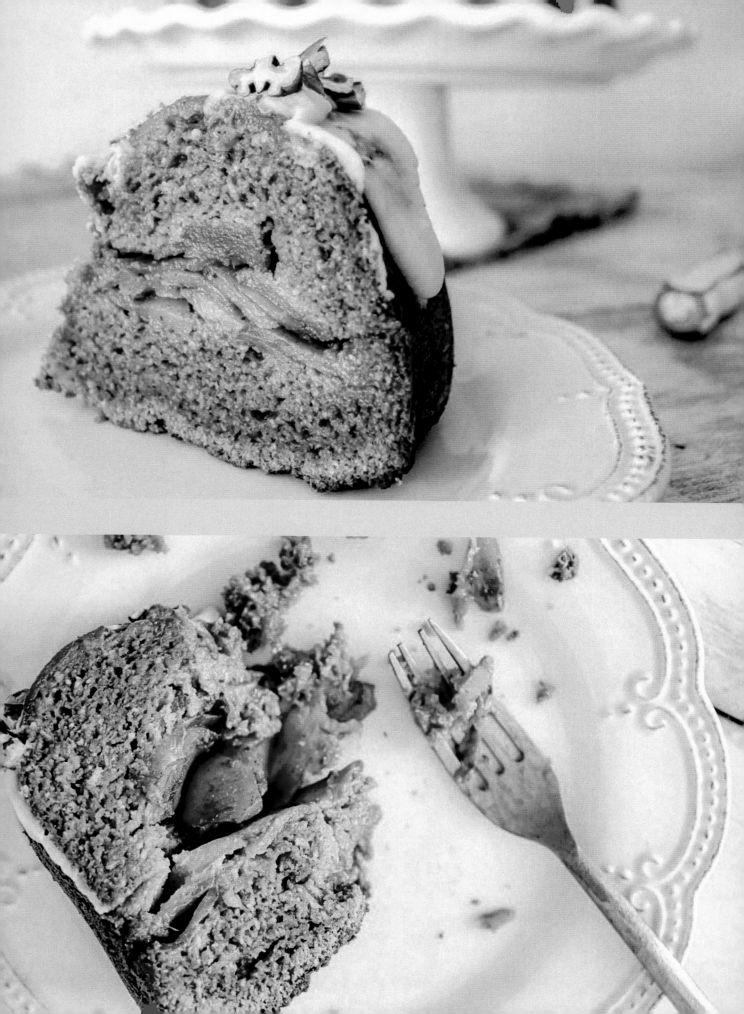

Heavenly Apple Bundt Cake

prep: *25 min*   **bake:** *60-95 min*   **cool:** *30-45 min*   **serves:** *1 ten inch cake*

Apple in any dessert always has a massive place in my heart. This cake is to die for since every bit is filled with apple goodness. This cake is perfect in the cooler weather since it brings a simple warmness to the soul.

Dry ingredients

- 168g *(1½ cups)* almond flour
- 102g *(1/4 cup)* coconut flour
- 22g *(2 tablespoons)* psyllium husk powder
- 220g *(1 cup)* sweetener
  monk fruit, erythritol, xylitol
- 1 teaspoon baking soda
- 1 teaspoon baking powder
- 2 teaspoons cinnamon
- 1 teaspoon sea salt

Apple Layer

- apples *(4 medium)* Granny Smith
- 1 tablespoon cinnamon
- 105g *(1/2 cup)* sweetener
  monk fruit, erythritol, xylitol

Wet ingredients:

- 6 free-run eggs *room temp*
- 118mL *(1/2 cup)* avocado oil
- 118mL *(1/2 cup)* apple butter
  the recipe is found on page 195
- 118mL *(1/2 cup)* coconut milk *full fat*
- 56mL *(1/4 cup)* lemon juice
- 1 teaspoon pure vanilla extract

Glaze:

- 56mL *(1/4 cup)* lemon juice
- 58mL *(1/4 cup)* coconut milk *full fat*
- 180g *(1 1/2 cups)* powdered sweetener
  monk fruit, erythritol, xylitol
- 1 teaspoon pure vanilla extract
- 55g *(1/2 cup)* pecans *garnish*

Instructions

1. Preheat oven to 325°F/163°C. Grease/spray with avocado oil in a 10-inch tube pan *(or large bundt pan)*.
2. Sift coconut flour and measure all remaining dry ingredients. Mix and set aside
3. Whisk together and pour onto dry ingredients in a separate medium bowl and all wet ingredients.
4. Using a rubber spatula, mix/fold the batter until well incorporated.
5. **Apple layer:** Peel, cut & remove the core of the apples. Place apples in a large enough bowl that you can mix sugar & spice! Slice apples into thin slices, about 4-5mm.
6. Add the sugar & spice ingredients on top of the thin-sliced apples and toss to coat.
7. Scoop out ½ of the cake batter in the bottom of the prepared pan. Layer all the remaining apples on top. Scoop out the remaining cake batter on top of the apple layer.
8. Bake the cakes for 1 hour to 1 hour & 15 minutes, depending on the oven, or until lightly golden brown on top.
9. **Glaze:** In a small bowl, mix powdered sweetener, coconut milk, lemon juice, & vanilla until the mixture becomes light & thin *(I used about 1/4 cup of warm coconut milk, you can add more if needed)*. Pour the sugar-free glaze over the top of the cake.
10. Decorate the cake with chopped toasted pecans. Place in the fridge until it's time to eat.
11. Place in the fridge until it's time to eat—best to take the cake out of the refrigerator for 30 min slicing, and serving.
12. Store in the fridge in an airtight container for four to five days or freeze for up to two months.

Note

- **You can use any apple for this cake. However, be aware that granny smith is not only great for their tartness, but they also tend to stay more tender after baking.**

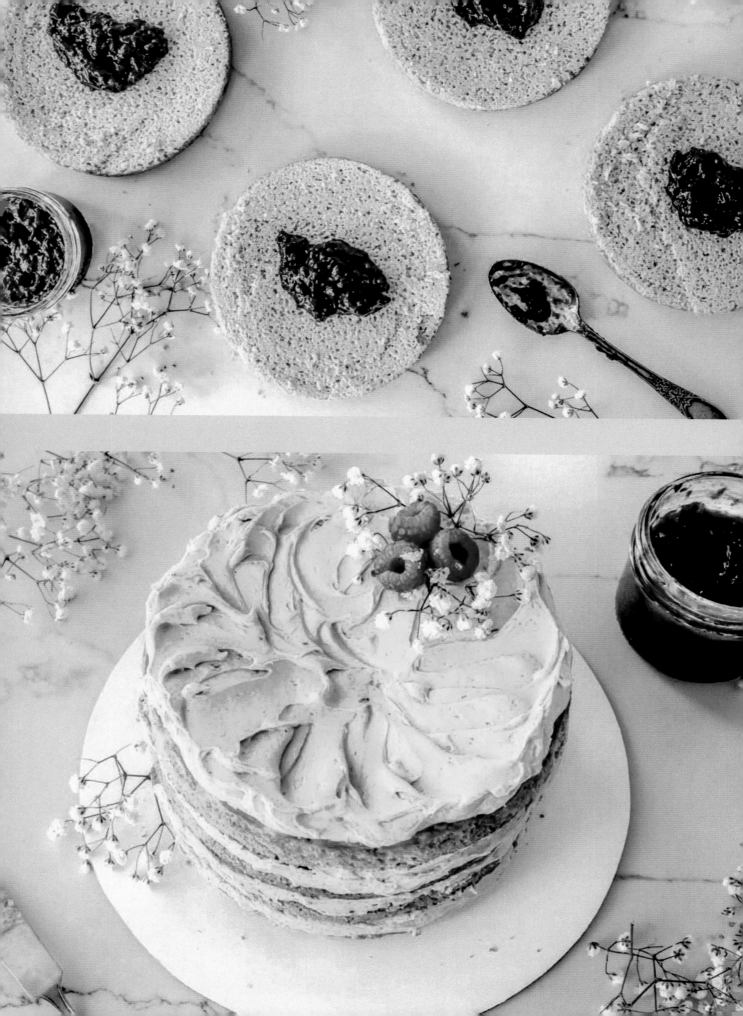

Raspberry Lemon Cake

prep: *25 min*   **bake:** *55-60 min*   **cool:** *30-45 min*   **serves:** *1 six inch cake*

This cake sings springtime with its fresh tartness! Raspberries and lemon pair together so well with a light, airy vanilla sponge cake.

Dry ingredients
- 168g *(1½ cups)* almond flour
- 68g *(1/2 cup)* coconut flour
- 11g *(1 tablespoon)* psyllium husk powder
- 152g *(3/4 cup)* sweetener
  monk fruit, erythritol, xylitol
- 1 zest of a whole large lemon
- 1 teaspoon baking soda
- 1 teaspoon baking powder
- 1 teaspoon sea salt

Wet ingredients:
- 5 free-run eggs *room temp*
- 118mL *(1/2 cup)* avocado oil
- 118mL *(1/2 cup)* coconut milk *full fat*
- 56mL *(1/4 cup)* lemon juice
- 1 teaspoon pure lemon oil
- 1 teaspoon pure vanilla extract

Jam filling ingredients:
- 175g *(1 cup)* raspberry jam
  the recipe is found on page 193

Vanilla Buttercream:
- 1 batch Vanilla Buttercream + **DF option**
  the recipe is found on page 185
- 1 handful of fresh raspberries - *optional*

Note
- **Make sure all wet ingredients are not chilled/cold when making cakes and cupcakes for the best fluffy consistency.**
- **This recipe works beautifully in a Vanilla Raspberry Cake when you omit the lemon oil.**
- **You may make this cake 100% dairy-free with my DF frosting option on page 185.**

Instructions

1. **Jam filling:** Make the raspberry jam ahead of time so that it is called when you are ready to assemble and decorate the cake.
2. **Preheat oven to 325°F/163°C.**
3. In a medium bowl, sift coconut flour and measure all remaining dry ingredients. Mix and set aside.
4. Whisk together and pour onto dry ingredients in a separate medium bowl and all wet ingredients. Using a rubber spatula, mix the batter until well incorporated.
5. In two 6-inch springform cake pans, grease/spray with avocado oil, and trace cake pan bottoms on parchment paper, cut out and place parchment rounds in the bottom of the cake pan.
6. Using a food scale, place the cake pan on top of the food scale, tare to 0, and add roughly 475 grams of cake batter to each prepped cake pan. Or, you may use measuring cups to evenly measure the same amount of batter in each cake pan.
7. Bake the cakes for 55-60 minutes, depending on the oven, or until lightly golden on top.
8. Once your cake is completely cooled to room temperature, it's time to slice them in half with a bread knife.
9. Using a stand mixer bowl *(whisk attachment)* or an electric hand mixer, make the **Vanilla Buttercream frosting** on page 185.
10. Start decorating the cake layers in that raspberry jelly, spread 1/3 cup of jelly on three layers, and pipe the buttercream frosting around the edges of each cake layer.
11. Stack the three jam-filled layers on top of each other, and add the last cake layer for the top of the cake.
12. Lastly, add a dollop of buttercream to the top of the cake; using an offset cake spatula, try to get the buttercream close to the edge of the cake.
13. Once the cake is iced, add some pretty little flowers and fresh raspberries on top.
14. Place in the fridge until it's time to eat. Best to take the cake out of the fridge 30 min - 1 hour before slicing and serving.
15. Store in the fridge in an airtight container for four to five days or freeze for up to two months.

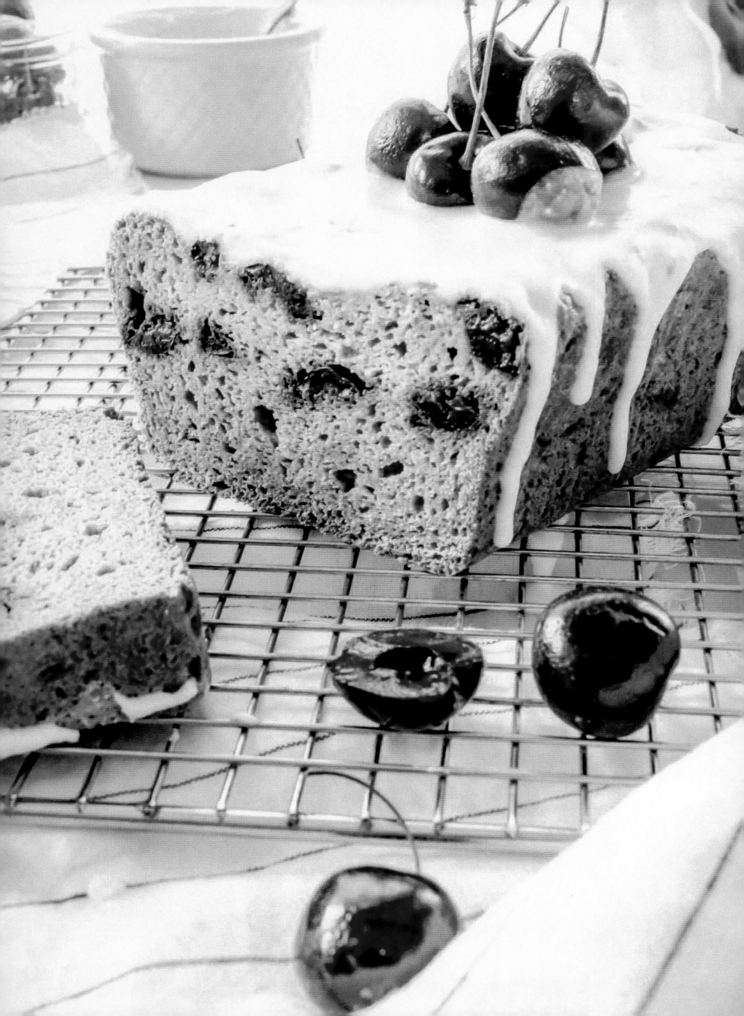

Sour Cherry Pound Cake

prep: *25 min*   **bake:** *75-80 min*   **cool:** *55 min*   **serves:** *1 loaf/pound cake*

Adding the yogurt into this pound cake creates a beautifully moist and denser cake while adding a slight tang.

Dry ingredients

- 112g *(1 cup)* almond flour
- 100g *(3/4 cup)* coconut flour
- 11g *(1 tablespoon)* psyllium husk powder
- 260g *(2 cups)* fresh cherries *deseeded & chopped see step 5*
- 152g *(3/4 cup)* sweetener
  monk fruit, erythritol, xylitol
- 1 teaspoon baking soda
- 1 teaspoon baking powder
- 1 teaspoon sea salt

Wet ingredients:

- 6 free-run eggs *room temp*
- 118mL *(1/2 cup)* avocado oil
- 180mL *(3/4 cup)* coconut yogurt
  the recipe is found on page 232
  you may use greek yogurt if you can tolerate dairy
- 56mL *(1/4 cup)* lemon juice
- 1 teaspoon pure vanilla extract

Glaze:

- 56mL *(1/4 cup)* lemon juice
- 58mL *(1/4 cup)* coconut milk - *in a can*
- 180g *(1½ cups)* powdered sweetener
  monk fruit, erythritol, xylitol
- 1 teaspoon pure vanilla extract
- fresh whole cherries *to garnish*

Instructions

1. **Preheat oven to 325°F/163°C.** Grease and line the loaf pan with parchment paper. **Loaf pan Optimal size: 8"x 4"x 3" (L x W x H)**
2. Slice each cherry using a sharp knife, twist each half to open, and remove the seed.
3. Once all the seeds are removed, chop cherries into quarters.
4. Place chopped cherries into a small bowl, and add 2tsp of coconut flour to ensure your berries don't sink to the bottom. Mix until coated with the dust of coconut flour and set aside
5. **NOTE:** do not add the cherries to the dry ingredients because the cherries will be added in a separate layer.
6. In a medium bowl, sift coconut flour and measure all remaining dry ingredients. Mix and set aside.
7. Whisk together and pour onto dry ingredients in a separate medium bowl and all wet ingredients. Using a rubber spatula, mix the batter until well incorporated.
8. Once the cake batter is done, taking a measuring cup, scoop 2 cups of cake batter into the bottom of the loaf pan.
9. Add half of the cherries evenly to the first layer.
10. Next, add the rest of the batter on top of the first cherry layer and the remainder of the cherries evenly over the top layer.
11. Bake the cakes for 75-80 minutes, depending on the oven, or until lightly golden brown on top.
12. Once the pound cake is thoroughly cooled, you can make the glaze.
13. **Glaze:** In a small bowl, mix powdered sweetener, coconut milk, lemon juice, & vanilla until the mixture becomes light & thin. Pour the sugar-free glaze over the top of the cake.
14. Once the cake is finished, add some fresh cherries on top to garnish.
15. Place in the fridge until it's time to eat. Best to take the cake out of the fridge 30 min - 1 hour before slicing and serving.
16. Store in the fridge in an airtight container for four to five days or freeze for up to two months.

Note

- It's always good to have wet ingredients on the warmer side before mixing them with the dry ingredients, for the best cake batter consistency.
- You may use any fresh berry for this recipe!

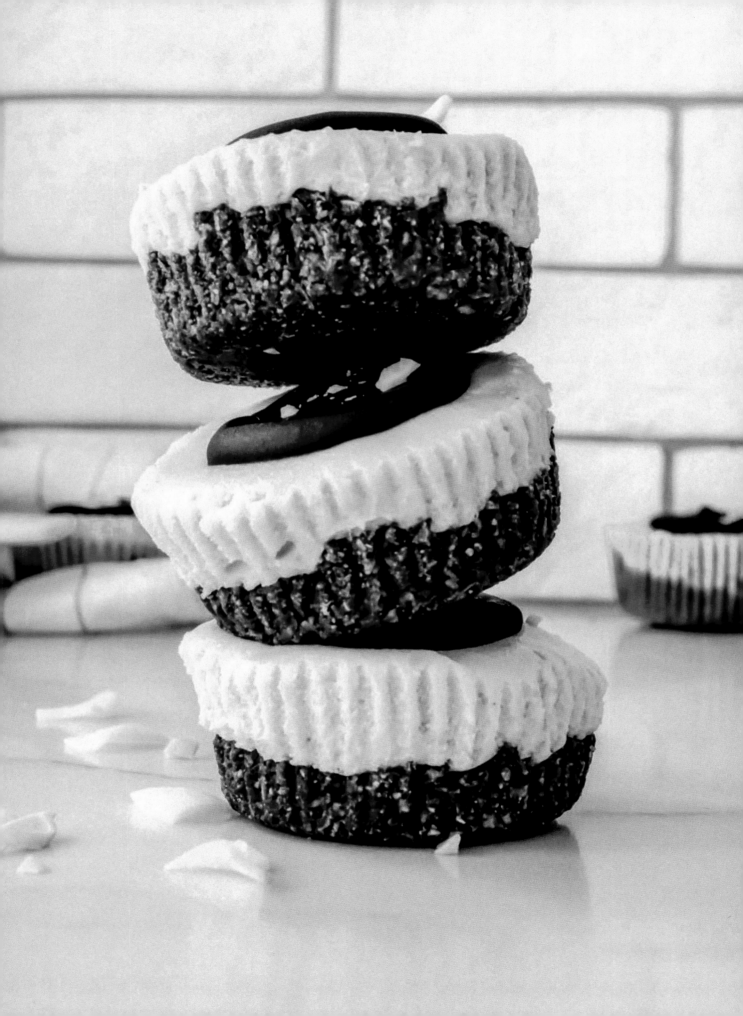

Raw Almond Joy Mini Cheesecake

prep: *35 min*   **cool:** *30-45 min*   **serves:** *9-12 mini cakes*

There is nothing cuter and more delicious than these raw dairy-free cheesecake cups. You can make this recipe a larger cake, like the raw strawberry cheesecake on page 165 or turtle cheesecake on page 181.

Chocolate crust ingredients

- 168g *(1½ cups)* almond flour
- 56g *(1/2 cup)* cacao powder
- 34g *(1/4 cup)* coconut flour
- 42g *(1/2 cup)* coconut flakes *unsweetened*
- 118mL *(1/2 cup)* coconut oil *melted*
- 105g *(1/2 cup)* sweetener
    monk fruit, erythritol, xylitol
- 1 teaspoon sea salt

Cheesecake ingredients:

- 280g *(2 cups)* raw cashews *soaked overnight*
- 118mL *(1/2 cup)* coconut oil - melted
- 59mL *(1/2 cup)* coconut milk *full fat*
- 152g *(3/4 cup)* sweetener
    monk fruit, erythritol, xylitol
- 56mL *(1/4 cup)* lemon juice
- 1 teaspoon pure almond extract
- 1 teaspoon pure vanilla extract
- 2 teaspoons sea salt

Ganache Ingredients:

- 45g *(2 tablespoons)* coconut oil *melted*
- 110g *(1 cup)* chocolate chips *melted*
    the recipe is found on page 223
- coconut flakes or almond *garnish*

Instructions

1. Line a cupcake tray with non-stick parchment liners.
2. **Crust:** Add all the crust ingredients into a medium bowl *(or stand mixer bowl with paddle attachment).* Using your hands, mix/beat until it forms a solid softball of dough.
3. Press about 2-3 tablespoons of the chocolate coconut crust dough evenly in each of the bottoms of the liners.
4. Place the crust in the freezer while preparing the cheesecake filling.
5. **Cheesecake:** In a high-powered blender, combine all the cheesecake filling ingredients & make sure the coconut oil is melted. Blend for about 2-3 minutes or until the mixture is smooth and creamy.
6. Scrape down the sides as necessary. You may need to add a bit more coconut milk to get it to blend smoothly if your blender isn't super high-powered.
7. Once it's smooth, taste the cheesecake mixture and adjust the sweetness levels if desired.
8. Pour/scoop 1/4 cup *(using a large cookie scoop)* of the cheesecake filling each crust. Smooth the top and tap the pan hard against the counter a few times to release any air bubbles. Place in the freezer.
9. Place in the freezer to set for at least 2 hours or until completely firm.
10. **Ganache:** In a small heat-proof bowl, melt chocolate chips in the microwave at 10-sec intervals and stir in between each interval - or on a double boiler with simmering water.
11. Add 2 teaspoons of melted chocolate to the top.
12. Before the chocolate hardens, garnish with coconut flakes or chopped almonds.
13. When storing in the freezer, let it thaw in the refrigerator for one hour before serving or let it thaw at room temperature for 15 minutes before serving.
14. Store leftovers in an air-tight container in the freezer for three months.

Note

- **Cashew blends the best for this recipe when you soak it overnight or at least 6 hours in warm water.**

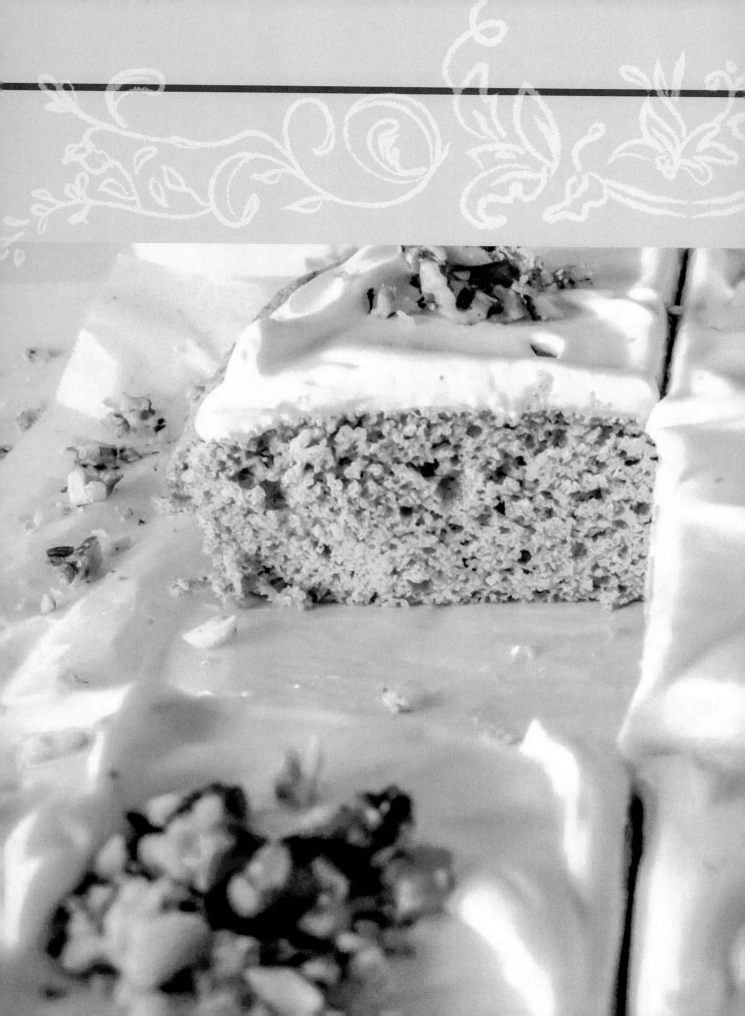

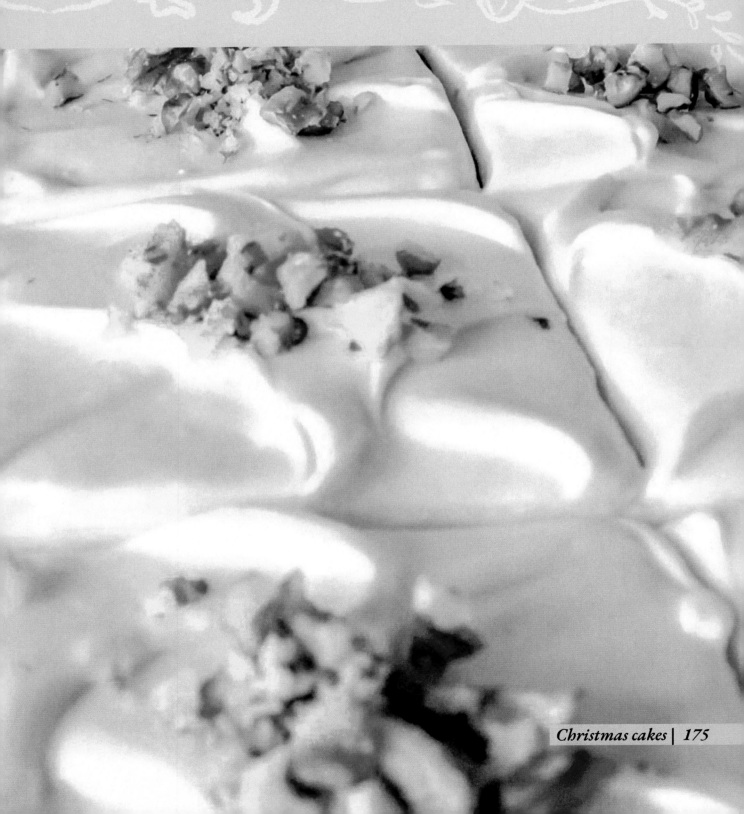

Christmas
CAKES

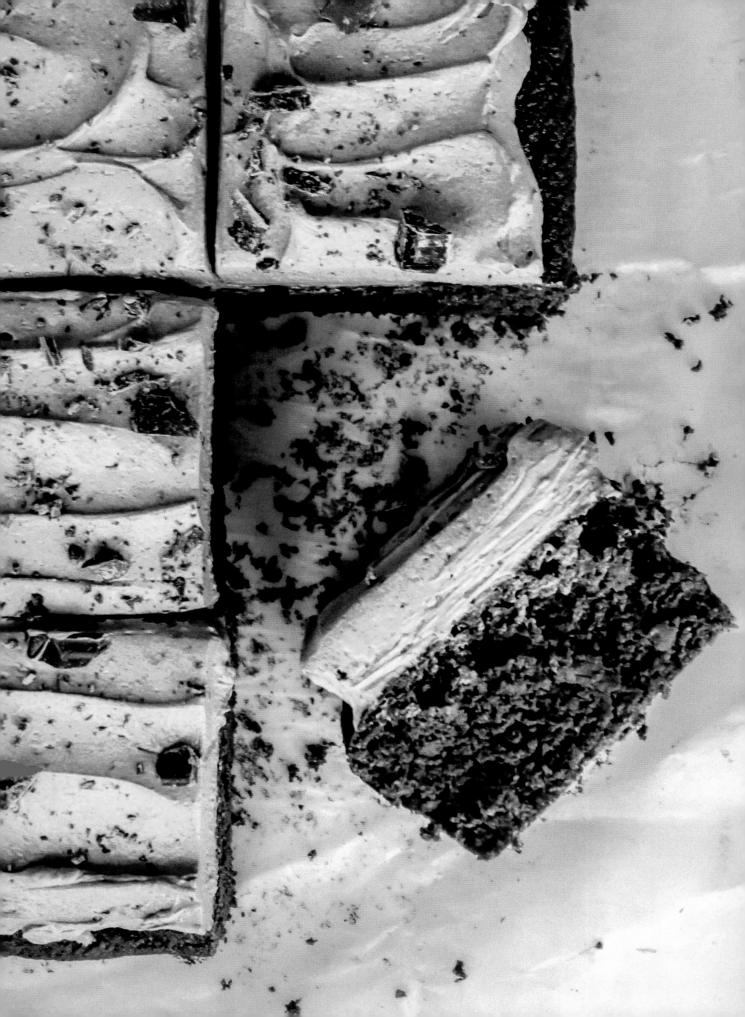

Coco Peppermint Sheet Cake

prep: *25 min*   **bake:** *35-40 min*   **cool:** *30-45 min*   **serves:** *9-12 slices*

There is something so magical around Christmas time when chocolate and peppermint meet together in your mouth. This cake is straightforward to make, yet it makes for a worthy dessert for any Christmas celebration.

Dry ingredients
- 140g *(1½ cups)* almond flour
- 34g *(1/4 cup)* coconut flour
- 56g *(1/2 cup)* cacao powder
- 11g *(1 tablespoon)* psyllium husk powder
- 210g *(1 cup)* sweetener
  monk fruit, erythritol, xylitol
- 1 teaspoon baking soda
- 1 teaspoon baking powder
- 1 teaspoon sea salt

Wet ingredients:
- 5 free-run eggs *room temp*
- 118mL *(1/2 cup)* avocado oil
- 118mL *(1/2 cup)* coconut milk *full fat*
- 56mL *(1/4 cup)* apple cider vinegar
- 1 teaspoon pure peppermint oil
- 1 teaspoon pure vanilla extract

Chocolate Buttercream:
- 1 batch chocolate buttercream + **DF option**
  the recipe is found on page 187
- 1 teaspoon pure peppermint oil
- 85g *(1 full)* chocolate bar *chopped*
  the recipe is found on page 223

Instructions
1. **Preheat oven to 325°F/163°C.**
2. In a medium bowl, sift cacao powder and coconut flour and measure all remaining dry ingredients. Mix and set aside.
3. Whisk together and pour onto dry ingredients in a separate medium bowl and all wet ingredients. Using a rubber spatula, mix the batter until well incorporated.
4. Grease one square 9-inch X 12-inch cake/sheet pan with non-stick cooking spray and line it with parchment paper.
5. Bake on the oven's centre rack for 30-35 minutes or until a toothpick inserted in the centre comes out clean or with some crumb remaining.
6. In a stand mixer bowl, with a whisk attachment, make **chocolate buttercream frosting** on page 187, and add the peppermint oil.
7. Cool the cake on a cooling rack for 45 minutes to 1 full hour.
8. Add buttercream frosting on the top of the cake, and spread it to the edges of the cake using an offset cake spatula.
9. Chop up chocolate par, and sprinkle on top of the cake.
10. Place in the fridge until it's time to eat. Best to take the cake out of the fridge 30 min - 1 hour before slicing and serving.
11. Store in the fridge in an airtight container for four to five days or freeze for up to two months.

Note
- If you don't have an espresso machine, I recommend purchasing a high-quality instant espresso powder. Add 1tbsp of espresso powder, and dissolve into 2oz of warm water.
- You may make this cake 100% dairy-free with my DF frosting option on page 187.

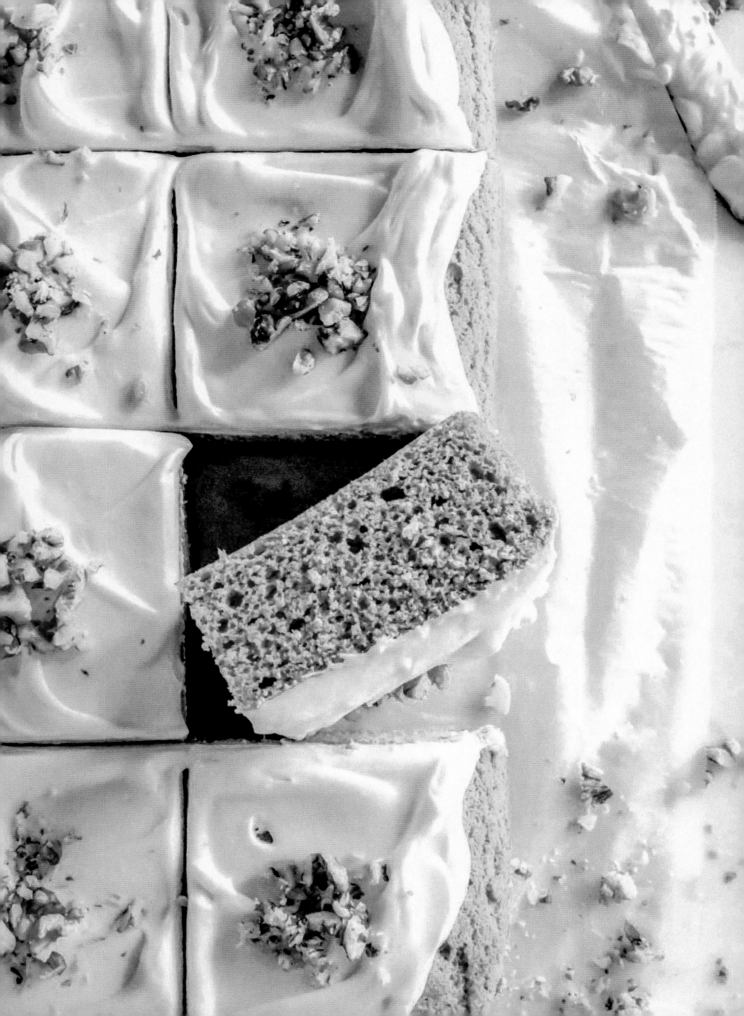

Pumpkin Spice Sheet Cake

prep: *25 min*   **bake:** *55-60 min*   **cool:** *30-45 min*   **serves:** *1 six inch cake*

This cake sings springtime with its fresh tartness! Raspberries and lemon pair together so well with a light, airy vanilla sponge cake.

Dry ingredients

- 140g *(1¼ cups)* almond flour
- 68g *(1/2 cup)* coconut flour
- 22g *(2 tablespoons)* psyllium husk powder
- 155g *(3/4 cup)* sweetener
  monk fruit, erythritol, xylitol
- 1 tablespoon pumpkin spice
- 1 teaspoon baking soda
- 1 teaspoon baking powder
- 1 teaspoon sea salt

Wet ingredients:

- 5 free-run eggs *room temp*
- 118mL *(1/2 cup)* avocado oil
- 120mL *(1/2 cup)* pumpkin purée *unsweetened*
- 118mL *(1/2 cup)* coconut milk *full fat*
- 56mL *(1/4 cup)* apple cider vinegar
- 1 teaspoon pure vanilla extract

Cream cheese frosting:

- 1 batch Cashew Cream Cheese Frosting
  the recipe is found on page 188
- 55g *(1/2 cup)* walnuts *toasted & chopped*

Instructions

1. **Preheat oven to 325°F/163°C.**
2. In a medium bowl, sift coconut flour and measure all remaining dry ingredients. Mix and set aside.
3. Whisk together and pour onto dry ingredients in a separate medium bowl and all wet ingredients. Using a rubber spatula, mix the batter until well incorporated.
4. Grease one square 9-inch X 12-inch cake/sheet pan with non-stick cooking spray and line it with parchment paper.
5. Bake on the oven's centre rack for 30-35 minutes or until a toothpick inserted in the centre comes out clean or with some crumb remaining.
6. Bake walnuts for garnish for 5-6minutes. Chop, and set aside to cool.
7. In a stand mixer bowl with a whisk attachment, make **cashew cream cheese frosting** on page 188.
8. Cool the cake on a cooling rack for 45 minutes to 1 full hour.
9. Add buttercream frosting on the top of the cake, and spread it to the edges of the cake using an offset cake spatula.
10. Scrape cashew frostings on the cooled cake, use an offset cake spatula, and spread frosting to the edges.
11. Sprinkle chopped walnuts on top of the cashew cream cheese frosting.
12. Place in the fridge until it's time to eat. Best to take the cake out of the fridge 30 min - 1 hour before slicing and serving.
13. Store in the fridge in an airtight container for four to five days or freeze for up to two months.

Note

- **If you don't have pumpkin spice use:**
  1 teaspoon cinnamon
  1/2 teaspoon ginger
  1/8 teaspoon cloves
  1/8 teaspoon nutmeg

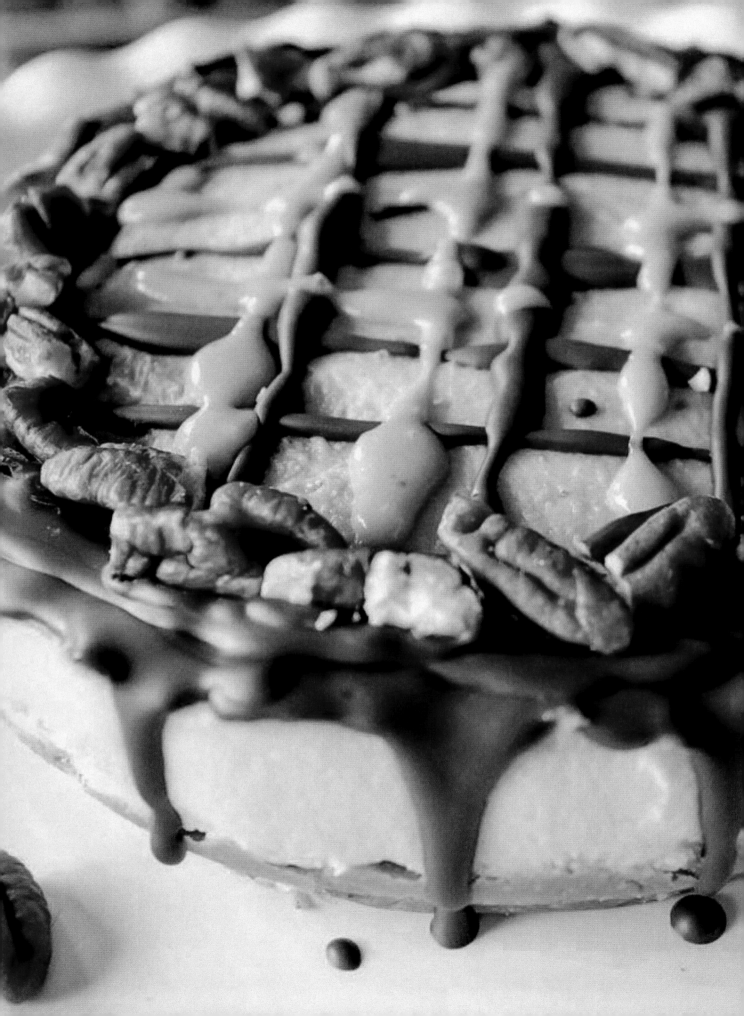

Raw Turtle Cheesecake

prep: *40 min*   **cool:** *4 hours*   **serves:** *1 six inch cake*

Turtles must be celebrated around Christmas time! Impress your guests with making this cake, and they won't believe you that it's 100% dairy-free, sugar-free and gluten-free! This Raw Trurle Cheesecake is beyond amazing.

Crust ingredients
- 140g *(1¼ cups)* almond flour
- 46g *(1/3 cup)* coconut flour
- 14g *(2 tablespoons)* flaxseed meal *ground*
- 120g *(1/2 cup)* caramel sauce
  the recipe is found on page 219
- 1 teaspoons cinnamon
- 1 teaspoon sea salt

Cheesecake Ingredients:
- 280g *(2 cups)* raw cashews *soaked overnight*
- *240g (1 cup)* caramel sauce
for the top cheesecake layer - see step 8
- 118mL *(1/2 cup)* coconut oil *melted*
- 118mL *(1 cup)* coconut milk *full fat*
- 120g *(1 cup)* powdered sweetener
  monk fruit, erythritol, xylitol
- 56mL *(1/4 cup)* lemon juice
- 1 teaspoon pure vanilla extract
- 2 teaspoons sea salt

Turtle topping ingredients:
- 28g *(2 tablespoons)* coconut oil *melted*
- 110g *(1/2 cup)* chocolate chips *melted*
  the recipe is found on page 223
- 60g *(1/4 cup)* caramel sauce *top layer*
- 55g *(1/2 cup)* pecans *toasted garnish*

Instructions

1. Grease a 6" springform pan with coconut oil and line it with parchment paper *(cut in a circle)*.
2. **Crust:** Add all the crust ingredients into a medium bowl *(or stand mixer bowl with paddle attachment)*. Using your hands, mix/beat until it forms a solid softball of dough.
3. Press the rest of the graham crust dough evenly along the bottom of the prepared pan.
4. Place the crust in the freezer while preparing the cheesecake filling.
5. **Cheesecake:** To make the first vanilla layer of cheesecake, In a high-powered blender, combine all of the cheesecake *(not the caramel)* filling ingredients & make sure coconut oil is melted. Blend for about 2 minutes until the mixture is smooth and creamy.
6. Scrape down the sides as necessary. You may need to add a bit more coconut milk to get it to blend smoothly if your blender isn't super high-powered.
7. Pour 3/4 of the cheesecake filling into the prepared pan over the crust. Smooth the top and tap the pan hard against the counter a few times to release air bubbles. Place in the freezer.
8. Add the caramel to the remainder of the cashew cheesecake filling, and blend on high until smooth.
9. Take the cake from the freezer, and pour the entire caramel cheesecake filling layer on top. Again, smooth out the top and tap the pan hard against the counter a few times to release air bubbles.
10. Place in the freezer to set for at least 4 hours or until completely firm.
11. **Turtle toppings:** In a small heat-proof bowl, melt chocolate chips and coconut oil in the microwave at 10-sec intervals and stir in between intervals. Drizzle melted chocolate around the edges.
12. Warm-up caramel sauce, and drizzle the melted chocolate and caramel sauce in a checkered pattern over the top.
13. Garnish the top with toasted pecans before the chocolate hardens.
14. When storing in the freezer, let it thaw in the refrigerator for a few hours before serving or let it thaw at room temperature for 15 minutes before serving.
15. Before slicing & serving, I recommend running your knife under hot water to warm it up before cutting the cheesecake with the still-hot *(dried)* knife—store leftovers in tight airtight containers in the freezer for three months.

Note

- Cashew blends the best for this recipe when you soak it overnight or at least 6 hours in warm water.

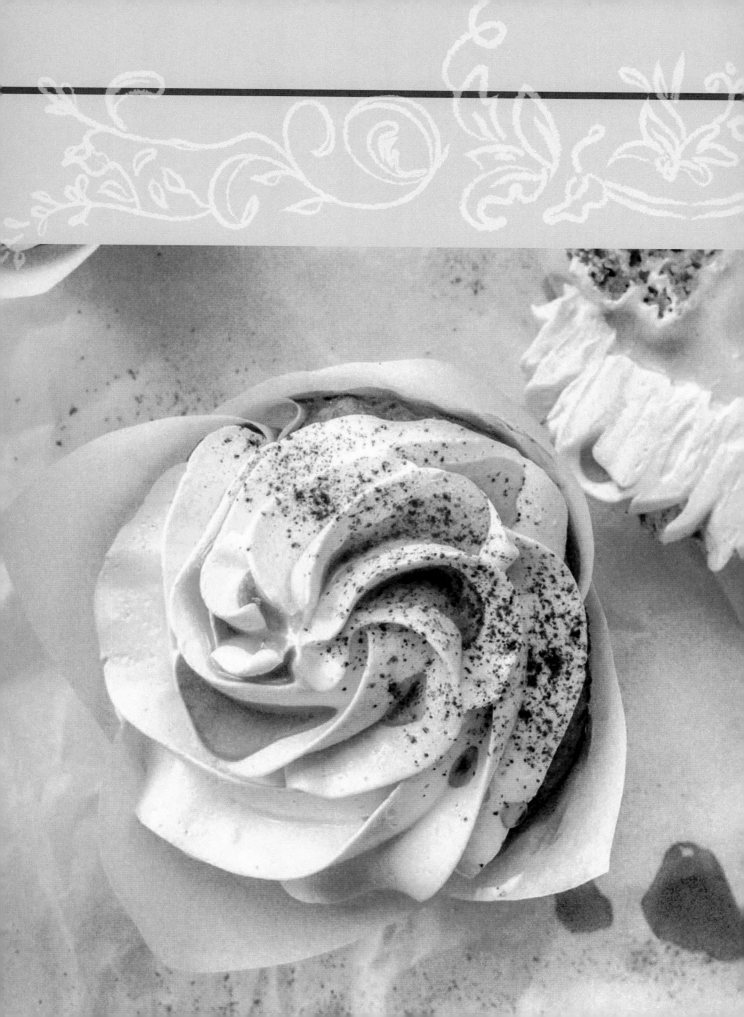

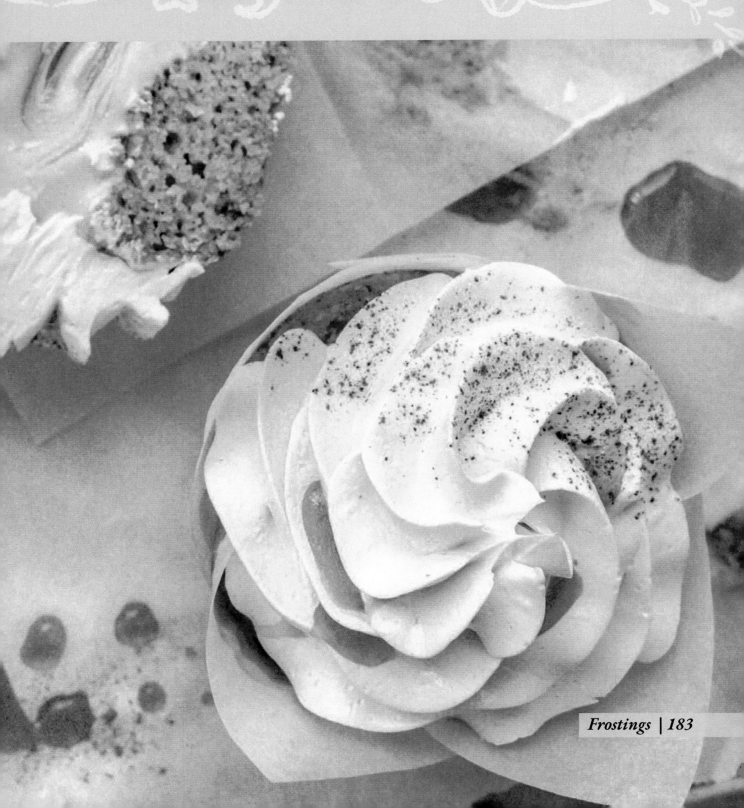

Chapter Eight

FROSTINGS

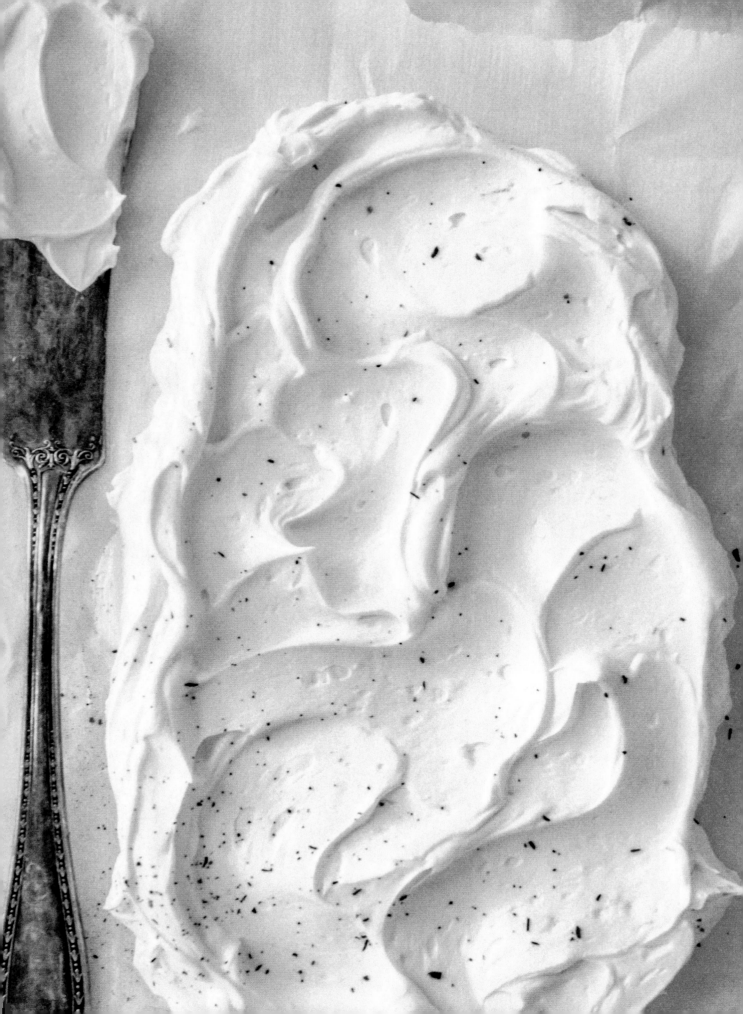

The Perfect Vanilla Buttercream

prep: *15 min*   **serves:** *12 cupcakes - or - 1 six inch cake*

To create a perfect buttercream frosting, there are a few tips and tricks will make the fluffiest, lightest frosting to consider. If you follow the easy steps below, you will be a master frosting whipper!

Ingredients

- 120g *(1 cup)* powdered sweetener
  monk fruit, erythritol, xylitol
- 245g *(1 cup) grass-fed butter* *room temp*
- 10mL *(2 teaspoons)* pure vanilla extract
- 1 teaspoon vanilla bean powder
- 1 teaspoon sea salt *if using unsalted butter*

Dairy-Free Ingredients

- 120g *(1 cup)* powdered sweetener
  monk fruit, erythritol, xylitol
- 245g *(1 cup)* palm shortening *room temp*
- 10mL *(2 teaspoons)* pure vanilla extract
- 1 teaspoon vanilla bean powder
- 1 teaspoon sea salt

Instructions

1. To create the perfect buttercream, it needs to start with the perfect softness of the butter.
2. Leaving the butter out for 12-24 hours at room temperature works excellently. However, ensure it's not too warm and oily, or your buttercream will not hold its structure.
3. In a stand mixer with a whisk attachment or handheld mixer, begin whipping butter at high speed.
4. Whip, and keep whipping for 5-7 minutes until the butter has doubled in size and becomes super pale white in colour.
5. Scrape down the sides and bottom of the bowl with a rubber spatula to ensure no solid stuck butter. And whip again for another 3-4 minutes.
6. Sift in powder sweetener and add the pure vanilla extract and vanilla bean powder; Whip again for another few minutes.
7. Add jam to vanilla buttercream after step 6, whip again twice, and scrape down sides between whisking.
8. Use immediately, or store in an airtight container in the fridge for up to a month and freeze for three months.
9. **NOTE:** If making frosting ahead of time, make sure when you pull it out of the fridge/freezer to thaw it out until it reaches room temperature and whips it again before frosting your cakes/cupcakes.

Note

- **The dairy-free option makes an even lighter/airy frosting. You can also try combining half palm shortening with half butter to create a lighter buttercream frosting, which is actually my favourite combination when making any frosting.**

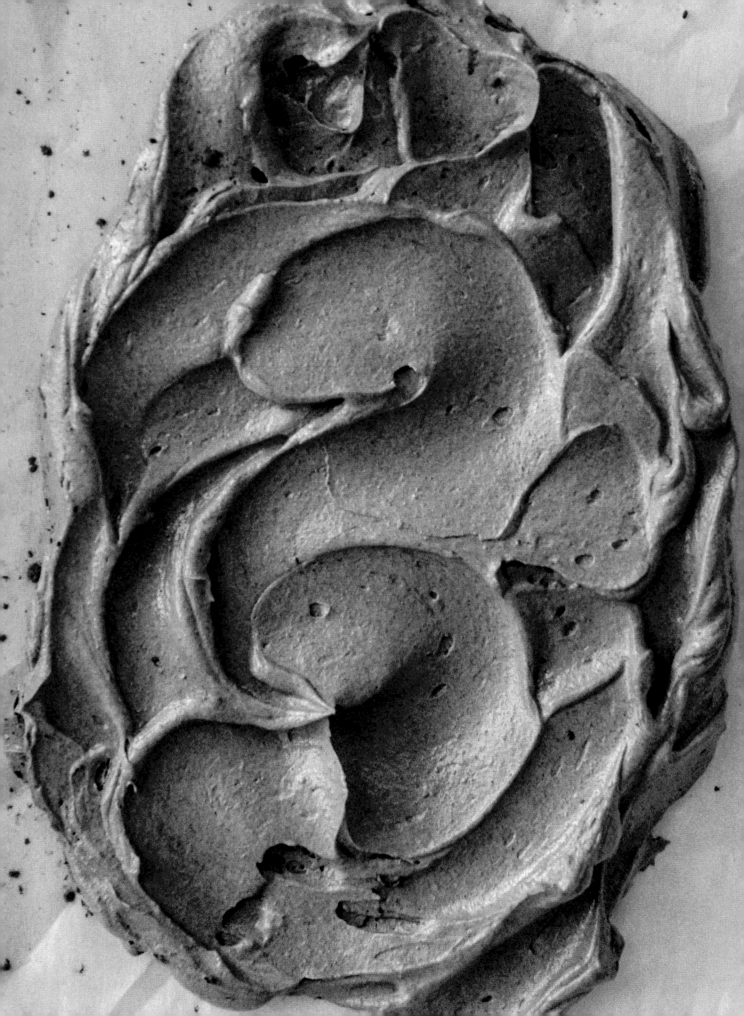

Decadent Chocolate Buttercream

prep: *15 min*   **serves:** *12 cupcakes - or - 1 six inch cake*

To create a perfect chocolate buttercream frosting, there are a few tips and tricks will make the richest, fluffiest, lightest frosting to consider. If you follow the easy steps below, you will be a master frosting whipper!

Ingredients

- 120g *(1 cup)* powdered sweetener
  monk fruit, erythritol, xylitol
- 84g *(3/4 cup)* cacao powder
- 14g *(1 tablespoon)* coconut oil *melted*
- 110g *(1/2 cup)* chocolate chips *melted*
  the recipe is found on page 214
- 245g *(1 cup)* grass-fed butter *room temp*
- 10mL *(1-2 teaspoons)* pure vanilla extract
- 1 teaspoon sea salt *if using unsalted butter*

Dairy-Free Ingredients

- 120g *(1 cup)* powdered sweetener
  monk fruit, erythritol, xylitol
- 84g *(3/4 cup)* cacao powder
- 14g *(1 tablespoon)* coconut oil *melted*
- 110g *(1/2 cup)* chocolate chips *melted*
  the recipe is found on page 214
- 245g *(1 cup)* palm shortening *room temp*
- 10mL *(2 teaspoons)* pure vanilla extract
- 1 teaspoon sea salt

Instructions

1. To create the perfect buttercream, it needs to start with the perfect softness of the butter.
2. Leaving the butter out for 12-24 hours at room temperature works excellently. However, ensure it's not too warm and oily, or your buttercream will not hold its structure.
3. In a stand mixer with a whisk attachment or handheld mixer, begin whipping butter at high speed.
4. Whip, and keep whipping for 5-7 minutes until the butter has doubled in size and becomes super pale white in colour.
5. Scrape down the sides and bottom of the bowl with a rubber spatula to ensure no solid stuck butter. And whip again for another 3-4 minutes.
6. In a small heat-proof bowl, melt chocolate chips and coconut oil in the microwave at 10-sec intervals, and stir in between intervals or on a double boiler with simmering water.
7. Make sure the melted chocolate is not hot but warm to the touch, so it doesn't deflate the buttercream.
8. Slowly drizzle melted chocolate into the buttercream at low speed, frosting as it whips.
9. Sift in cacao powder and powdered sweetener and add the pure vanilla extract; Whip again for another few minutes.
10. Use immediately, or store in an airtight container in the fridge for up to a month and freeze for three months.
11. **NOTE:** If making frosting ahead of time, make sure when you pull it out of the fridge/freezer to thaw it out until it reaches room temperature and whips it again before frosting your cakes/cupcakes.

Note

- The dairy-free option makes an even lighter/airy frosting. You can also try combining half palm shortening with half butter to create a lighter buttercream frosting, which is actually my favourite combination when making any frosting.

Cashew Cream Cheese Frosting

prep: *25 min*   **serves:** *12 cupcakes or a six inch cake*

This is a great alternative to the traditional inflammatory dairy cream cheese frosting. No one will believe you that it is not real cream cheese frosting, and you wont believe it either!

Ingredients

- 120g *(1 cup)* powdered sweetener
  monk fruit, erythritol, xylitol
- 245g *(1 cup)* cashew cream cheese
  the recipe is found on page 235
- 112g *(1/2 cup)* palm shortening *room temp*
- 10mL *(1-2 teaspoons)* pure vanilla extract
- 1 teaspoon sea salt

Note

- Make cashew cream cheese the night before for optimal results. Remember, purchasing pre-made cashew cream cheese costs 4x the price of making it yourself. However, many great brands are available now that make cashew cream cheese. They can usually be found in the dairy section at your local health food grocery store.

Instructions

1. It is best to make the cashew cream cheese a day in advance to allow it to solidify and firm up overnight in the fridge.
2. In a stand mixer with a whisk attachment or handheld mixer, begin whipping cashew cream cheese and palm shortening at high speed.
3. Whip, and keep whipping for a full 5-7 minutes until the frosting has allowed air to fluff it up.
4. Scrape down the sides and bottom of the bowl with a rubber spatula to ensure no solid cream cheese has been stuck to the sides or bottom. And whip again for another 3-4 minutes.
5. Sift in powder sweetener and add the pure vanilla extract. Whip again for another few minutes.
6. Use right away, or store in an airtight container in the fridge for up to a month and freeze for three months.
7. **NOTE:** If making frosting ahead of time, make sure when you pull it out of the fridge/freezer to thaw it out until it reaches room temperature and whip it again before frosting your cakes/cupcakes.

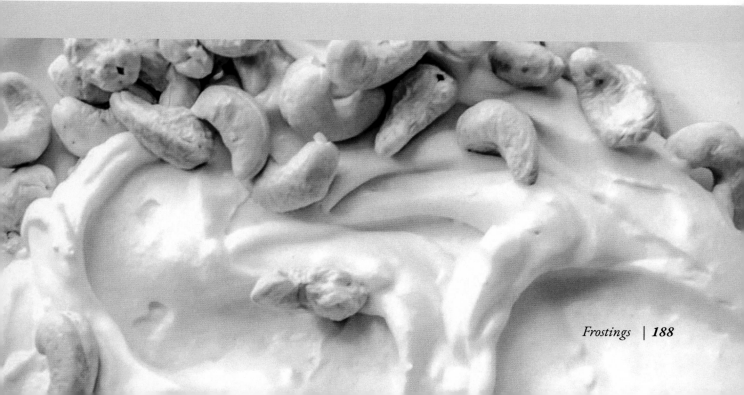

Coconut Whipped Cream

prep: *15 min*   **serves:** *12 cupcakes or a six inch cake*

Who doesn't love whipped cream? This non-dairy coconut whipped cream is even better than the real deal!

Ingredients

- 60g *(1/2 cup)* powdered sweetener
  monk fruit, erythritol, xylitol
- 800mL *(2 cans)* coconut milk
  must be full-fat coconut milk from a can
- 10mL *(1-2 teaspoons)* pure vanilla extract
- 1 teaspoon sea salt

Instructions

1. Remove the chilled bowl and beaters or whisk attachment from the freezer or refrigerator and set them up. Best to chill for at least half an hour.
2. Using a can of coconut milk from the refrigerator, carefully turn it over. Using a can opener, open and pour the coconut water, leaving you with the coconut cream. *(**TIP:** I love saving my coconut water can be saved and added to smoothies or discarded.)*
3. Scoop the solid coconut cream from the can and add it to the bowl. Sift in powdered sweetener and salt. Whisk on high until the coconut cream resembles whipped cream. Add the vanilla and whip again.
4. Use immediately, or store in an airtight container in the fridge for up to a month. This whipped cream is excellent on coffee, pancakes, and waffles!
5. Use immediately, or store in an airtight container in the fridge for up to a month.

Note

- **Leaving a can of coconut milk in the fridge overnight is the best way to ensure that coconut cream will be solidified. Remember, always look for a BPA-free brand. Store-bought coconut whipped cream deflates exceptionally quickly and is loaded with a lot of unwanted sugar.**

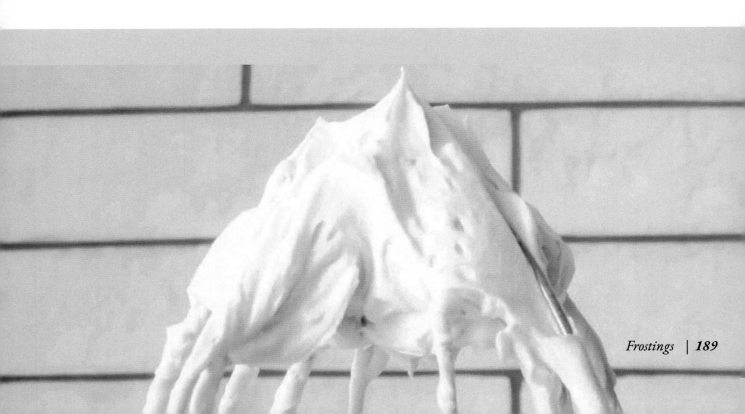

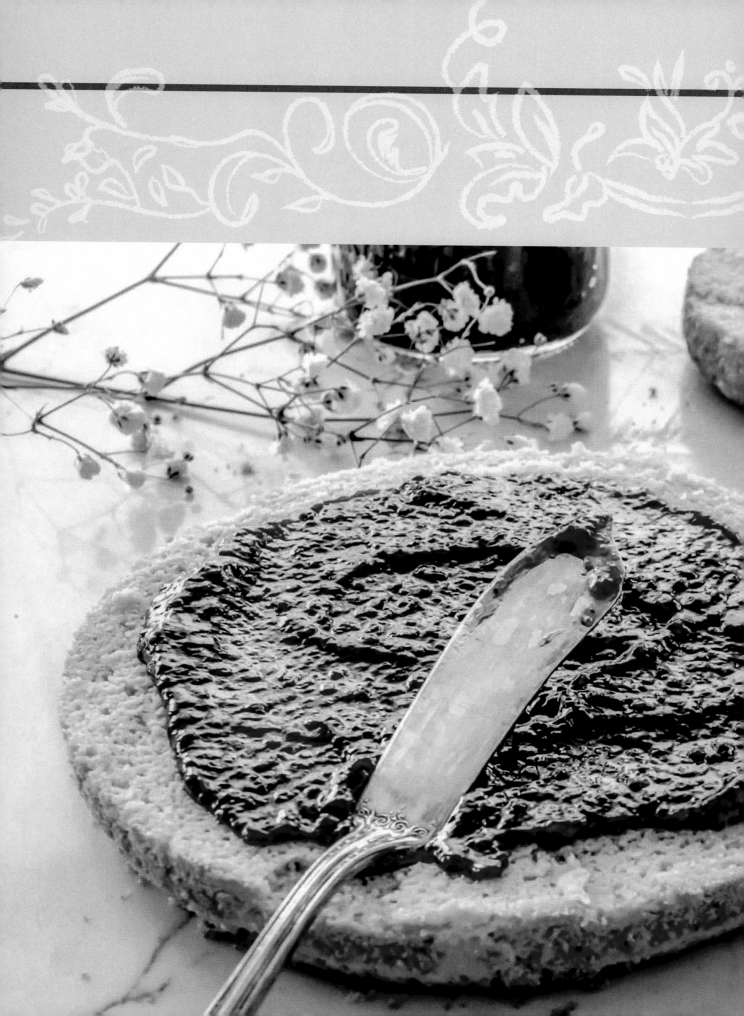

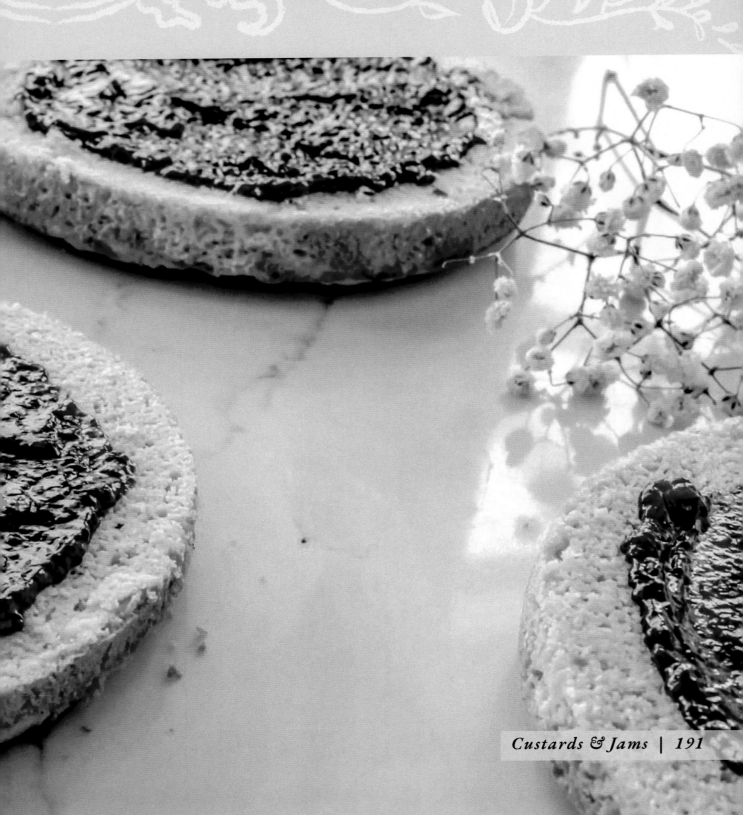

Chapter Nine
CUSTARDS & JAMS

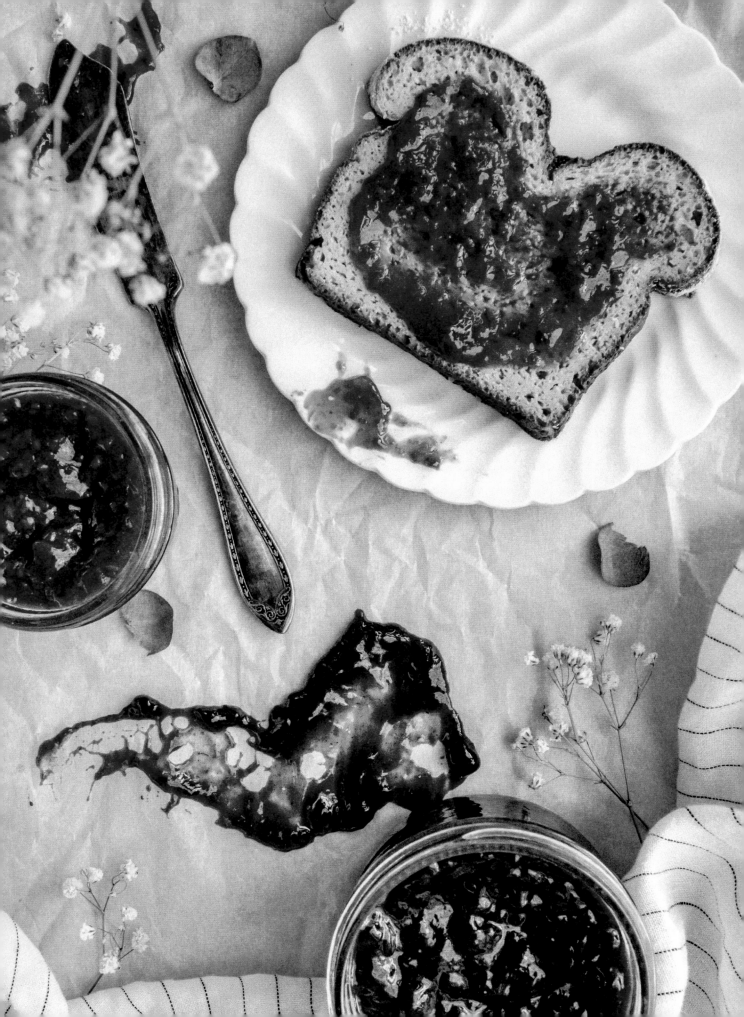

Berry Jams

prep: *5 min* **cook:** *14 min* **cool:** *1 hour* **serves:** *2 cups*

Making homemade sugar-free jam is quite simple. As you have noticed, jam is one of my favourite things to add to many of my baked goods. I have tried many natural ways to thicken my jams without using pectin, and I found that chia seeds and gelatin work wonders. Plus, they both have incredible health benefits!

Berries

best to by organic & local if possible

strawberries

raspberries

blueberries

blackberries

cranberries

Chia jam ingredients

- 280g *(2 cups)* berries *fresh or frozen*
- *24g (2 tablespoons)* chia seeds
- 55g *(1/4 cup)* sweetener
  monk fruit, erythritol, xylitol
- 15mL *(1 tablespoon)* lemon juice

Gelatin jam ingredients

- 280g *(2 cups)* berries *fresh or frozen*
- 28g *(1 tablespoon)* gelatin *grass-fed*
- 55g *(1/4 cup)* sweetener
  monk fruit, erythritol, xylitol
- 30mL *(2 tablespoons)* lemon juice *warm*

bloom gelatin in warmed-up lemon juice

Instructions

1. In a small saucepan/pot, weigh out berries.
2. Cook the desired berries over medium heat until they break down, about 5-7 minutes.
3. If using gelatin to thicken the jam up, warm a cup of lemon juice in a small bowl for about 20 sec in the microwave, and stir in the gelatin.
4. Wait 2 minutes to allow the gelatin to bloom.
5. Stir in the lemon juice *(and gelatin if using)* and sweetener. Using a large fork, mash the berries down or leave them it a chunky texture.
6. Cook for 5 more minutes, and remove from heat.
7. If adding the chia seeds, stir in them now. Let cool until the jam begins to thicken.
8. If the jam becomes too thick, add a small amount of water *(1 tablespoon)* if needed to thin it out until desired consistency is reached.
9. If the jam is too runny, cook down without a lid for another 5 minutes to allow moisture to evaporate.
10. Allow cooling to room temperature and store in mason jars or an airtight container in the fridge for one to two weeks and in the freezer for up to three months.

Note

- **When selecting a berry, make sure the total berries you will be cooking down in the saucepan weigh around 300g for the perfect consistency. Note: volume will be very different from weight** *(ex. 2 cups of whole strawberries will weigh differently than 2 cups full cups of blueberries)*. **So weigh your berries to make sure you end up with the right consistency!**

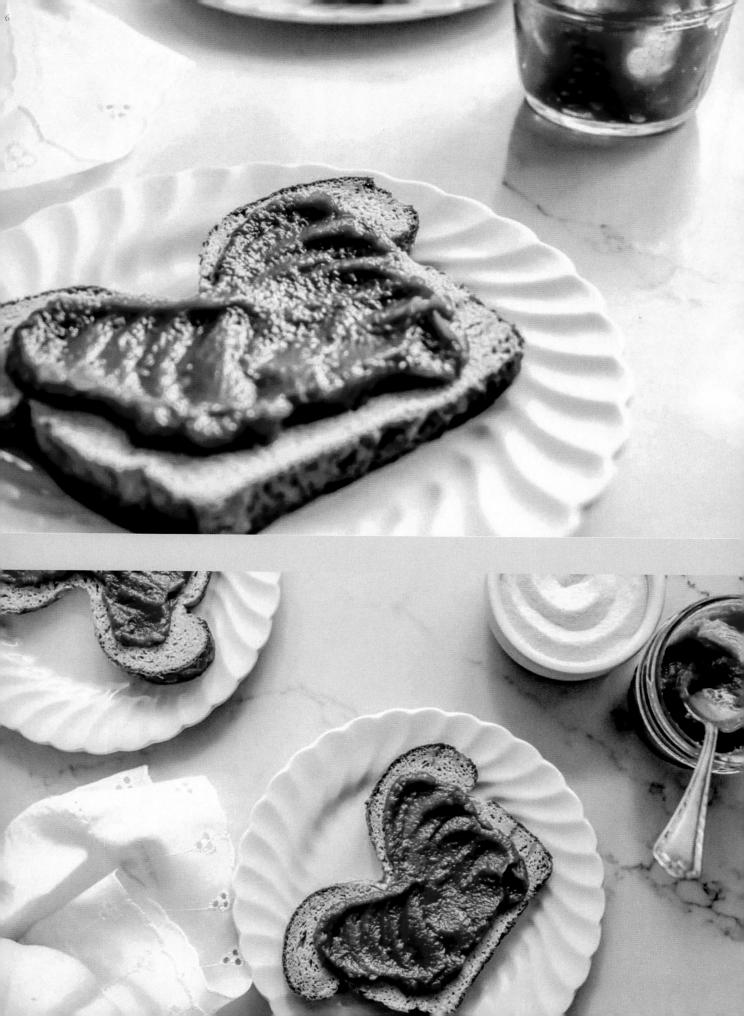

Apple Butter

prep: *5 min*   **cook:** *14 min*   **cool:** *1 hour*   **serves:** *2 cups*

I have always been a huge fan of apple sauce, but I knew there was no way to go back once I tasted apple butter. Apple butter is much creamier, richer in that desired apple taste, and it acts as a beautiful sweet butter into your baked goods, or just even enjoying it spread on a piece of toast, yum!

Ingredients

- 950g *(4 large)* apples *granny smith*
- *15mL (1 tablespoon)* apple cider vinager
- *15mL (1 tablespoon)* lemon juice
- *28g (1 tablespoon)* gelatin *grass-fed*
- 1 teaspoon cinnamon
- 1/2 teaspoon sea salt

Instructions

1. Peel & chop the apples into small pieces; place in a medium saucepot
2. In the same pot with chopped apples & measure out the rest of the ingredients.
3. Place the pot on medium heat with a lid for about 5min; until the apples start to boil & soften.
4. Use a fork and mash down apples.
5. Reduce heat to low & tilt the lid to let the steam and moisture out.
6. Stir occasionally while cooking for 2 hours on low temp!
7. Once apples become beautified deep burgundy in colour, it's time to purée!
8. Use an immersion blender or high-speed blender to purée!
9. Once the apple butter is cooled, transfer it into a small glass jar and store it in the fridge for up to two weeks. *(You can also freeze any extra for a longer shelf life!)*
10. Serve the apple butter on top of some toasted *Bakerlita's Bread*, or it is a great ingredient to add to some healthy baking recipes!
11. Allow cooling to room temperature and store in mason jars or an airtight container in the fridge for one to two weeks and in the freezer for up to three months.

Note

- **The longer you cook down the apples, the thicker, creamier and darker in colour the apple butter will become.**

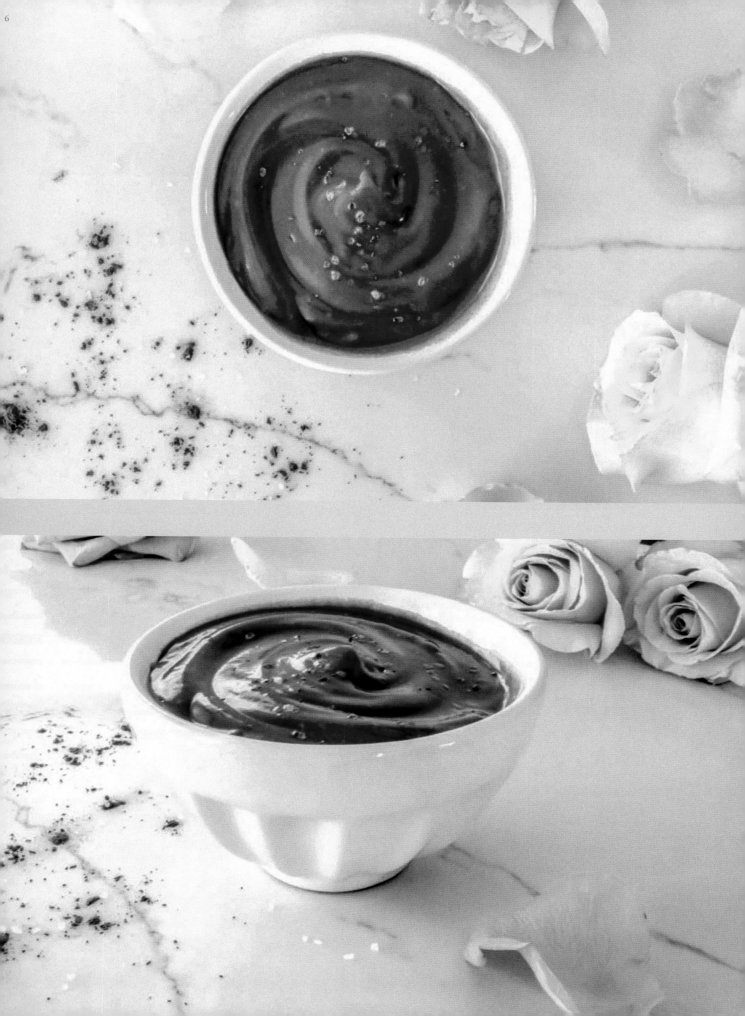

Creamy Custards/Puddings

prep: *10 min* **cook:** *14 min* **cool:** *1 hour* **serves:** *2 cups*

A hidden Surprise in a cupcake or a cake with a creamy custard delight calls for any celebration!

Chocolate Custard

- 75g *(1/3 cup)* grass-fed butter
  sub for palm shortening to make DF
- 70g *(1/3 cup)* coconut oil *extra virgin*
- 56g *(1/4 cup)* cocoa powder
  110g *(1/2 cup)* chocolate chips
  recipe found on page 223
- 80mL *(1/3 cup)* nut milk *unsweetened*
- 152g *(3/4 cup)* sweetener
  monk fruit, erythritol, xylitol
- 4 free-run eggs *room temp*
- 5mL *(1 teaspoon)* pure vanilla extract

Vanilla Custard

- 75g *(1/3 cup)* grass-fed butter
  sub for palm shortening to make DF
- 70g *(1/3 cup)* coconut oil *extra virgin*
- 80mL *(1/3 cup)* nut milk *unsweetened*
- 105g *(1/2 cup)* sweetener
  monk fruit, erythritol, xylitol
- 4 free-run eggs *room temp*
- 10mL *(2 teaspoons)* pure vanilla extract

Lemon Custard

- 75g *(1/3 cup)* grass-fed butter
  sub for palm shortening to make DF
- 70g *(1/3 cup)* coconut oil *extra virgin*
- 80mL *(1/3 cup)* lemon juice
- 105g *(1/2 cup)* sweetener
  monk fruit, erythritol, xylitol
- 4 free-run eggs *room temp*
- 10mL *(2 teaspoons)* pure lemon oil
- 10mL *(2 teaspoons)* pure vanilla extract

Instructions

1. In a small saucepan, combine all the custard ingredients **except the eggs**. Heat on medium-low heat until melted.
2. Turn off the heat.
3. Temper the eggs by adding 1/4 cup of the hot melted creamy custard ingredients from the saucepan into a small bowl and allow it to cool down for about 2 minutes.
4. Add one egg at a time to the small bowl of custard and whisk together vigorously.
5. Once all eggs are tempered, pour the egg mixture into the saucepan.
6. Turn custard onto low heat, whisk until it holds marks from the whisk, and the first bubble appears on the surface, about 6 minutes.
7. Pour custard into a heat-proof bowl and allow it to cool to room temperature.
8. Store in mason jars or an airtight container in the fridge for one to two weeks and the freezer for up to three months.

Note

- **If your eggs curdle due to the heat being too high, do not worry! Blend the custard using a handheld emulsifier or a high-speed blender after the custard has cooled down to a warm temperature.**

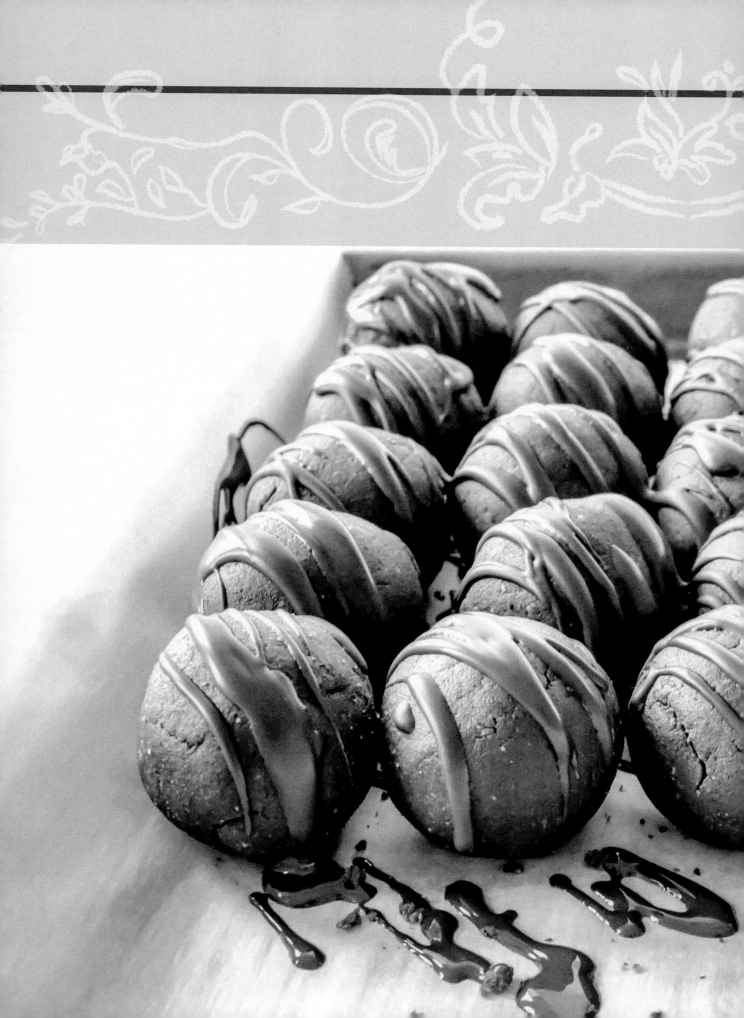

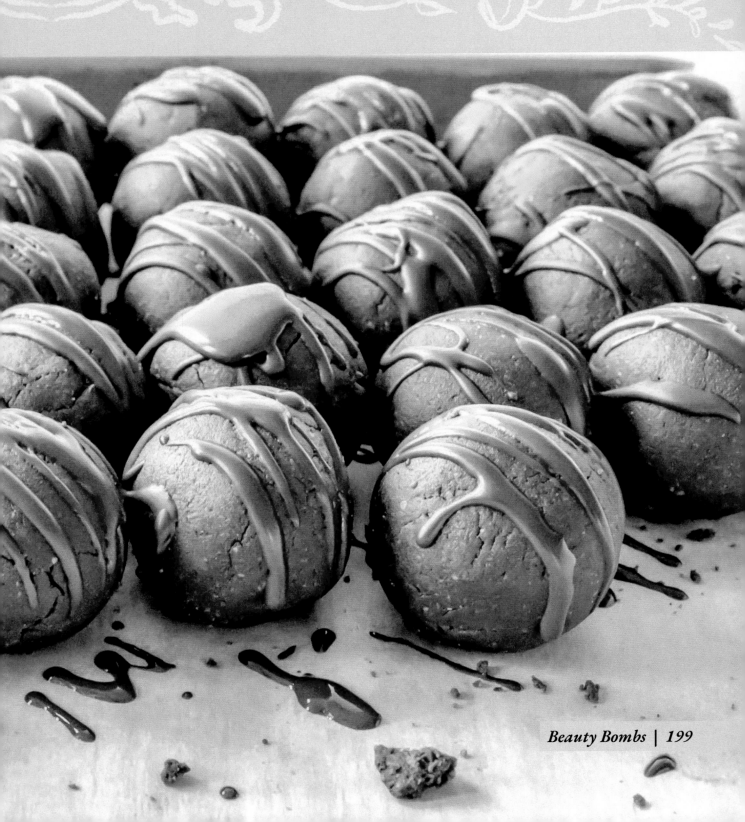

Chapter Ten
BEAUTY BOMBS

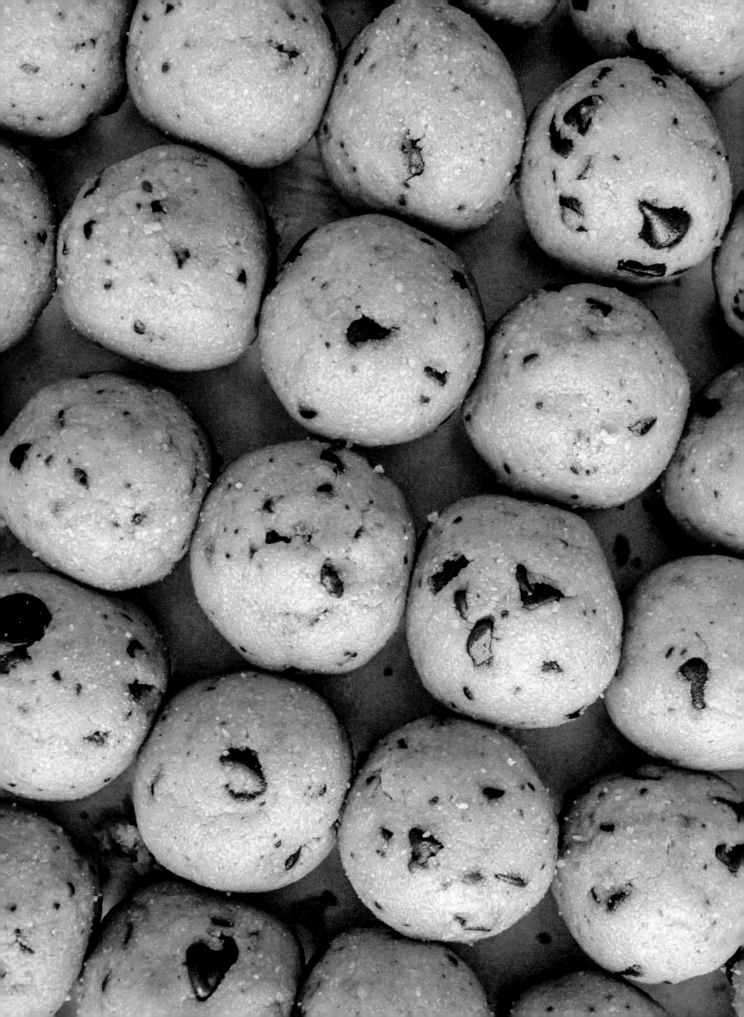

PB Cookie Dough Bombs

prep: *20 min* **cool:** *30 min* **serves:** *15-20 bombs*

These PB Cookie Dough Beauty Bombs were one of the first items in my bakery. They were not only extremely popular because they are incredibly delicious, but these beauties are packed full of beauty-enhancing collagen protein in every bomb. I love to have a stash on me at all times, just in case I get hungry and need to pop one in my mouth, and hunger goes away instantly; they are so satisfying in taste & for crushing cravings!

Dry ingredients

- 168g *(1½ cups)* almond flour
- 68g *(1/2 cup)* coconut flour
- 110g *(1/2 cup)* chocolate chips
  the recipe is found on page 223
- 56g *(1/2 cup)* organic collagen *grass-fed*
- 120g *(1 cup)* powdered sweetener
  monk fruit, erythritol, xylitol
- 1 teaspoon sea salt

Wet ingredients

- 113g *(1/2 cup)* grass-fed butter *room temp*
  sub for palm shortening to make **DF**
- 114g *(1/2 cup)* peanut butter *natural*
- 28g *(1 tablespoon)* coconut oil *extra virgin*
- 14g *(2 teaspoons)* blackstrap molasses
- 10mL *(2 teaspoons)* pure vanilla extract

Instructions

1. Mix all dry ingredients into a medium bowl; whisk until combined, and set aside.
2. In a stand mixer bowl, add all of the wet ingredients. Make sure butter, peanut butter and coconut oil are at room temperature.
3. Pour all dry ingredients on top of the wet ingredients, mix with a paddle attachment, and mix on medium-high speed until incorporated.
4. Prepare a baking sheet with parchment paper, with a small scoop out (*cookie/scoop size: 1.5 Tbsp/ 23 ml/ 0.8 oz)* bombs on a baking sheet with parchment paper. This recipe makes about 15-20 bombs.
5. Roll each bomb in the palm of the hand; A trick to create a perfect ball is to cup your hand slightly.
6. Place bombs in the fridge for 30min to allow them to harden up.
7. Store in an airtight container in the fridge for three to four weeks and freeze for up to three months.

Note

- **You don't need a stand mixer to make these bombs. You can definitely mix them the old fashion way, by hand.**
- **Also, make sure all the wet ingredients are on the warmer side (** *room temp at least* **) to make the rolling & mixing much easier.**

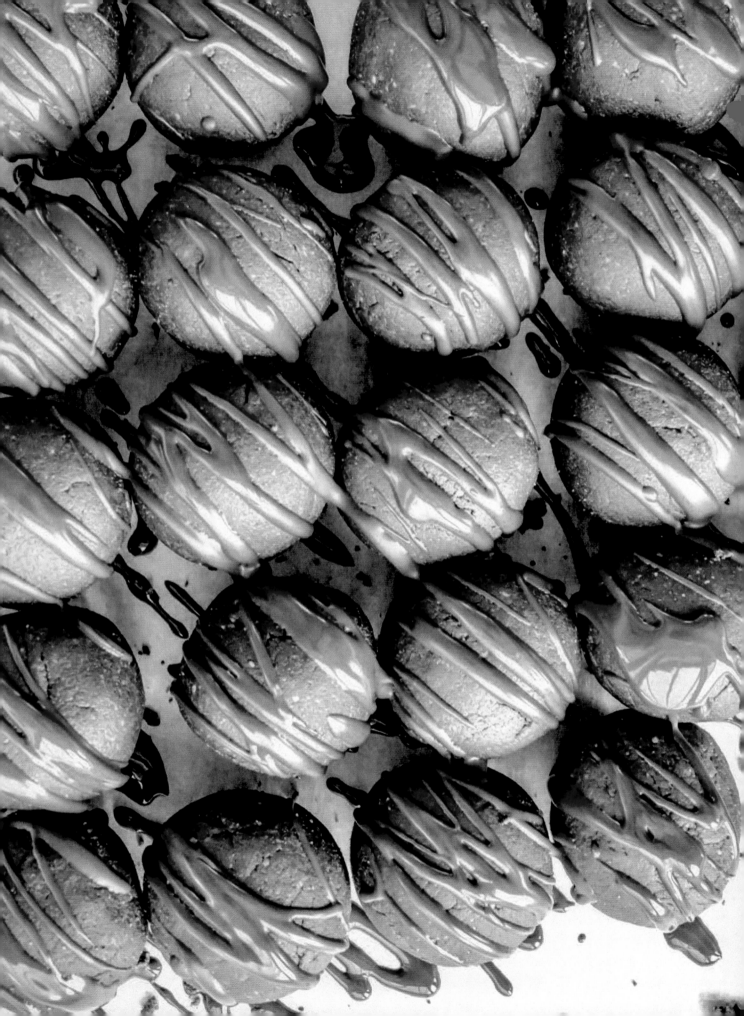

Vegan Truffle Chocolate Bombs

prep: *20 min*   **cool:** *35 min*   **serves:** *15-20 bombs*

Chocolaty goodness that melts in your mouth is exactly what these Vegan Truffle Chocolate Bombs are.

Dry ingredients

- 112g *(1 cup)* almond flour
- 68g *(1/2 cup)* coconut flour
- 56g *(1/2 cup)* cocoa powder
- 28g *(1/4 cup)* vegan collagen *optional*
- 150g *(1¼ cups)* powdered sweetener
  monk fruit, erythritol, xylitol
- 1 teaspoon sea salt

Wet ingredients

- 144g *(3/4 cup)* palm shortening *room temp*
- 57g *(1/4 cup)* peanut butter *natural*
- 56g *(1/4 cup)* coconut oil *extra virgin*
- 14g *(2 teaspoons)* blackstrap molasses
- 10mL *(2 teaspoons)* pure vanilla extract

Chocolate Ganache

- 110g *(1/2 cup)* chocolate chips *melted*
  *the recipe is found on page **223***
- 14g *(1 tablespoon)* coconut oil *extra virgin*

Instructions

1. Mix all dry ingredients into a medium bowl; whisk until combined, and set aside.
2. In a stand mixer bowl, add all of the wet ingredients. Make sure coconut oil, peanut butter and shortening are at room temperature.
3. Pour all dry ingredients on top of the wet ingredients, mix with a paddle attachment, and mix on medium-high speed until incorporated.
4. Prepare a baking sheet with parchment paper, with a small scoop out (***cookie/scoop size: 1.5 Tbsp/ 23 ml/ 0.8 oz***) bombs on a baking sheet with parchment paper. This recipe makes about 15-20 bombs.
5. Roll each bomb in the palm of the hand; A trick to create a perfect ball is to cup your hand slightly.
6. Place bombs in the fridge for 30min to allow them to harden up.
7. **Garnish:** In a small heatproof bowl, melt chocolate chips with coconut oil in the microwave for 10-sec intervals and stir between intervals; repeat 3-5 times until completely melted.
8. Using a small spoon, drizzle chocolate ganache in a zig-zag motion over the bombs.
9. Place bombs in the fridge for 35min to allow them to harden up.
10. Store in an airtight container in the fridge for three to four weeks and freeze for up to three months.

Note

- **You don't need a stand mixer to make these bombs. You can definitely mix them the old fashion way, by hand.**
- **Also, make sure all the wet ingredients are on the warmer side** *(room temp at least)* **to make the rolling much easier.**

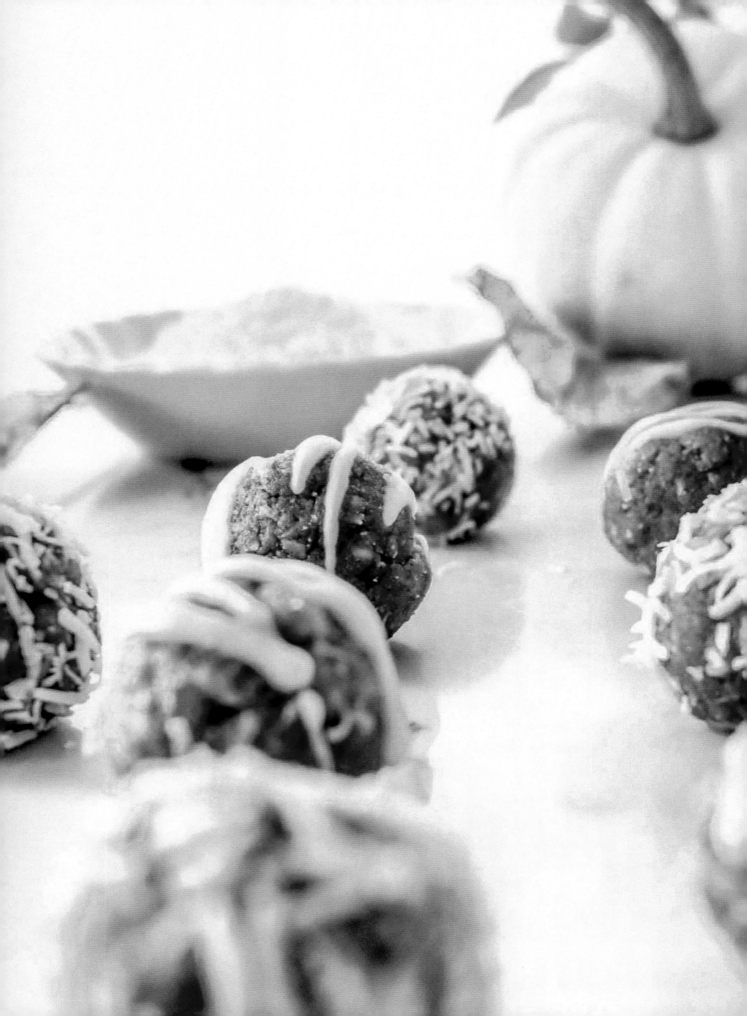

Fall-in-a-Bomb

prep: *20 min*   **cool:** *30 min*   **serves:** *25-30 bombs*

All those warming festive fall flavoures backed into a bomb, that is exactly what these Fall-in-a-Bom simulate!

Dry ingredients

- 168g *(1½ cups)* almond flour
- 46g *(1/3 cup)* coconut flour
- 42g *(1/2 cup)* coconut flakes *unsweetened*
- 55g *(1/2 cup)* pecans *chopped*
- 56g *(1/2 cup)* organic collagen *grass-fed*
- 110g *(1 cup)* carrots *shredded small*
- 120g *(1 cup)* powdered sweetener
    monk fruit, erythritol, xylitol
- 2 teaspoons cinnamon
- 1 teaspoon ginger
- 1/2 teaspoon clove
- 1 teaspoon sea salt

Wet ingredients

- 113g *(1/2 cup)* grass-fed butter *room temp*
    sub for palm shortening to make **DF**
- 114g *(1/2 cup)* almond butter
- 28g *(1 tablespoon)* coconut oil *extra virgin*
- 14g *(2 teaspoons)* blackstrap molasses
- 10mL *(2 teaspoons)* pure vanilla extract

Garnish/Glaze

- 84g *(1 cup)* coconut flakes
- 58mL *(1/4 cup)* coconut milk *full fat*
- 90g *(3/4 cup)* powdered sweetener

Instructions

1. **Preheat oven to 325°F/163°C.** Prep a cookie sheet with two small pieces of parchment paper side by side,
2. Toast coconut flakes for 4-5 minutes, and toast chopped pecans (*1 cup inside the cake & garnish*) for 7 minutes, set aside.
3. With a grater or food processor, grate carrots and set them aside.
4. Mix all dry ingredients into a medium bowl, including toasted nuts and carrots. Make sure carrots are not stuck together, mix until combined, and set aside.
5. In a stand mixer bowl, add all of the wet ingredients. Make sure butter, coconut oil and almond butter are at room temperature.
6. Pour all dry ingredients on top of the wet ingredients, mix with a paddle attachment, and mix on medium-high speed until incorporated.
7. Prepare a baking sheet with parchment paper, with a small scoop out *(cookie/scoop size: 1.5 Tbsp/ 23 ml/ 0.8 oz)* bombs on a baking sheet with parchment paper. This recipe makes about 25-30 bombs.
8. Roll each bomb in the palm of the hand; A trick to create a perfect ball is to cup your hand slightly.
9. **Garnish:** Roll each bomb into coconut flakes, drizzle with glaze, or do half and half; both work beautifully.
10. In a small bowl, mix powdered sweetener and coconut milk. Stir until the mixture becomes light & thin drizzle the glaze over each bomb.
11. Place bombs in the fridge for 30min to allow them to harden up.
12. Store in an airtight container in the fridge for three to four weeks and freeze for up to three months.

Note

- You don't need a stand mixer to make these bombs, You can definitely mix them the old fashion way, by hand.
- Also, make sure all the wet ingredients are on the warmer side *(room temp at least)* to make the rolling much easier.

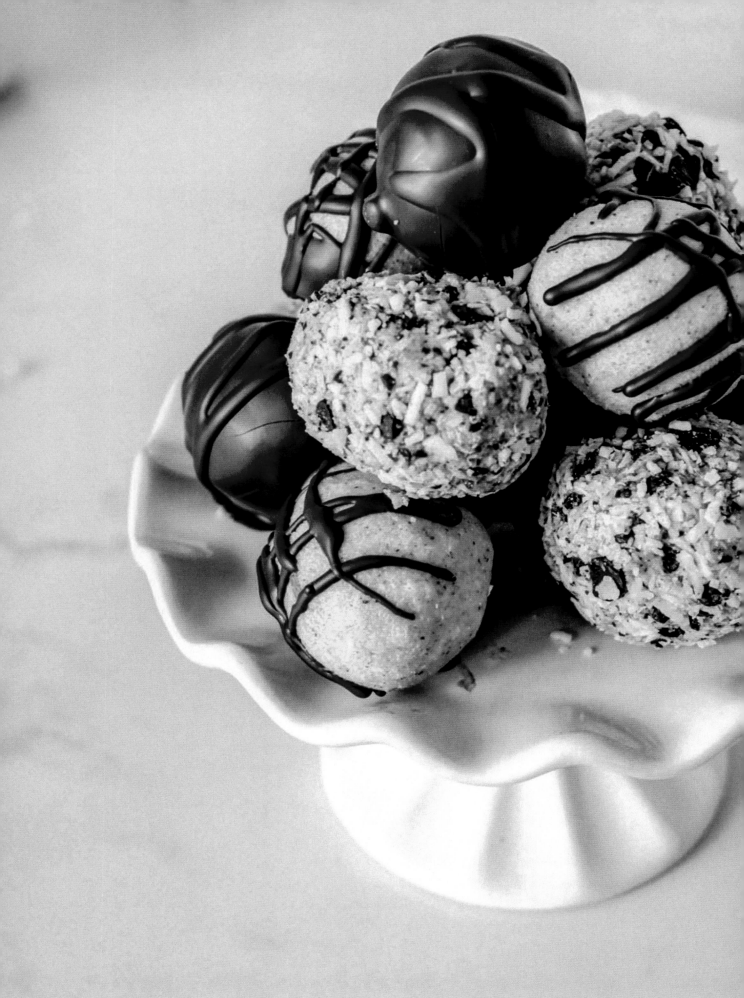

Almond Joy Bombs

prep: *20 min*   **cool:** *35 min*   **serves:** *15-20 bombs*

These almond Joy Bombs truly bring a sweet & satisfying JOY to your taste buds, and there is a little nutty surprise in each bomb.

Dry ingredients

- 168g *(1½ cups)* almond flour
- 46g *(1/3 cup)* coconut flour
- 42g *(1/2 cup)* coconut flakes *unsweetened*
- 56g *(1/2 cup)* organic collagen *grass-fed*
- 120g *(1 cup)* powdered sweetener
  monk fruit, erythritol, xylitol
- 1 teaspoon sea salt
- 15- 20 whole almonds *toasted*

Wet ingredients

- 113g *(1/2 cup)* grass-fed butter *room temp*
  sub for palm shortening to make DF
- 57g *(1/2 cup)* organic almond butter
- 42g *(3 tablespoons)* coconut oil *extra virgin*
- 14g *(2 teaspoons)* blackstrap molasses
- 10mL *(2 teaspoons)* pure vanilla extract
- 2.5mL *(1/2 teaspoon)* pure almond extract

Chocolate Ganache

- 110g *(1/2 cup)* chocolate chips *melted*
  the recipe is found on page 223
- 14g *(1 tablespoon)* coconut oil *extra virgin*
- 42g *(1/2 cup)* coconut flakes *unsweetened*

Instructions

1. Pre-heat oven to 325°F/163°C. Prep a cookie sheet with a piece of parchment paper side.
2. Toast almond whole raw almonds for 7 minutes.
3. Mix all dry ingredients into a medium bowl; *(not including the toasted whole almonds)*, whisk until combined, and set aside.
4. In a stand mixer bowl, add all of the wet ingredients. Make sure butter, peanut butter and coconut oil are at room temperature.
5. Pour all dry ingredients on top of the wet ingredients, mix with a paddle attachment, mix on medium-high speed until incorporated.
6. Prepare a baking sheet with parchment paper, with a small scoop out (***cookie/scoop size: 1.5 Tbsp/ 23 ml/ 0.8 oz***) bombs on a baking sheet with parchment paper. This recipe makes about 15-20 bombs.
7. Push one roasted almond into each center of the bomb.
8. Roll each bomb in the palm of the hand; A trick to create a perfect ball is to cup your hand slightly.
9. **Garnish:** In a small heatproof bowl, melt chocolate chips with coconut oil in the microwave for 10-sec intervals, stirring between intervals; repeat 3-5 times until completely melted.
10. Dunk 1/3 *(6-7 bombs)* of the bombs in the chocolate ganache and scoop out using a fork.
11. Using a small spoon, drizzle chocolate ganache in a zig-zag motion over the other 1/3 of the bombs.
12. Lastly, roll the remaining bombs into coconut flakes.
13. Place bombs in the fridge for 35min to allow them to harden up.
14. Store in an airtight container in the fridge for three to four weeks and freeze for up to three months.

Note

- **You don't need a stand mixer to make these bombs. You can definitely mix them the old fashion way, by hand.**
- **Also, make sure all the wet ingredients are on the warmer side** *(room temp at least)* **to make the rolling much easier.**

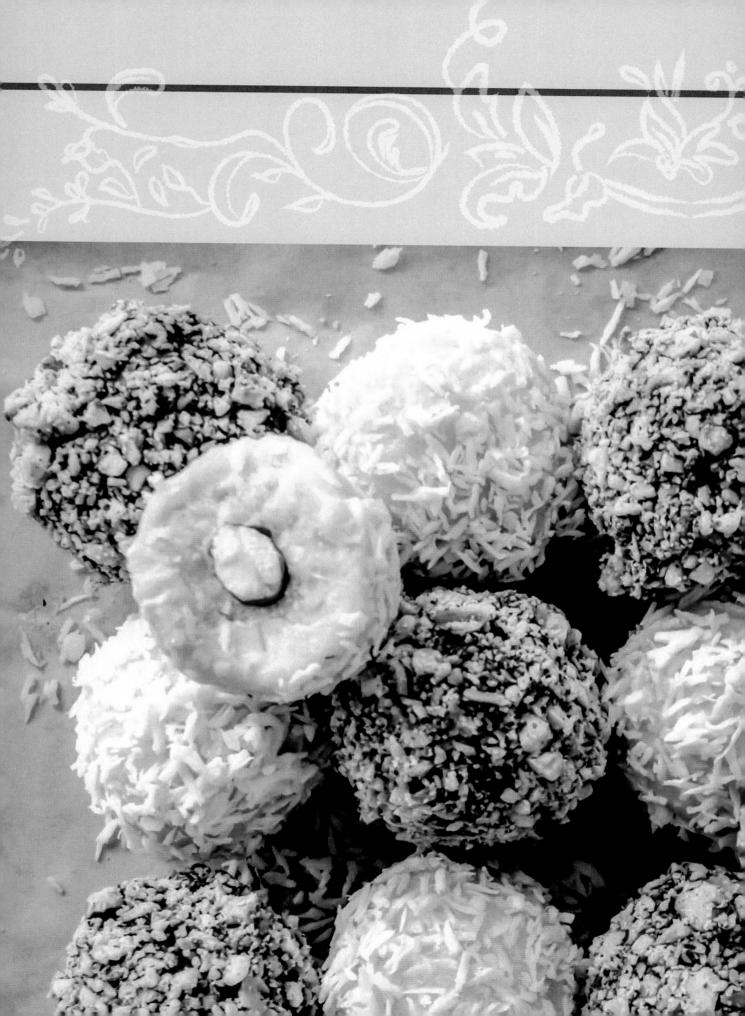

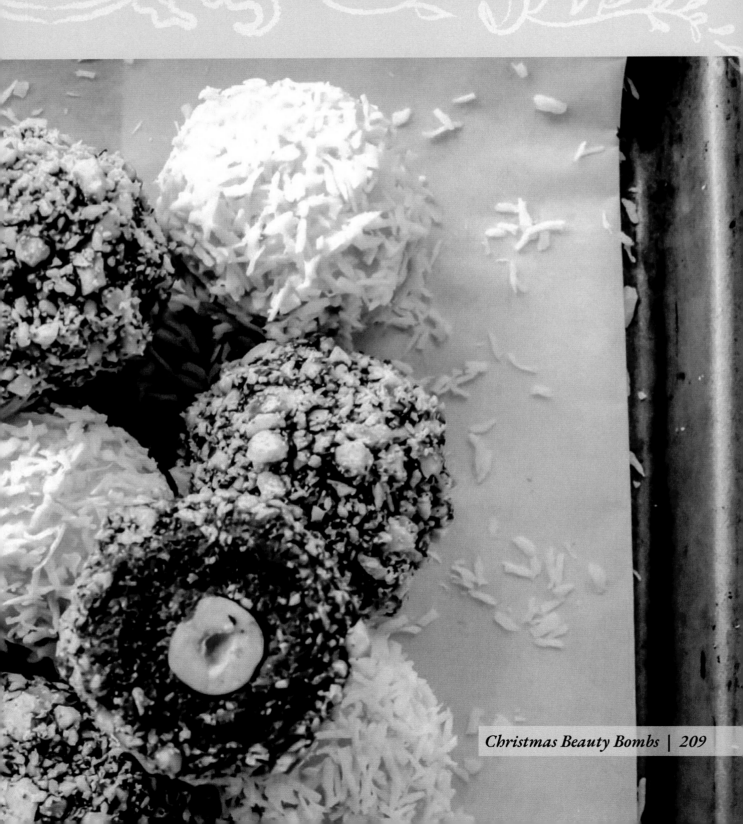

Christmas BEAUTY BOMBS

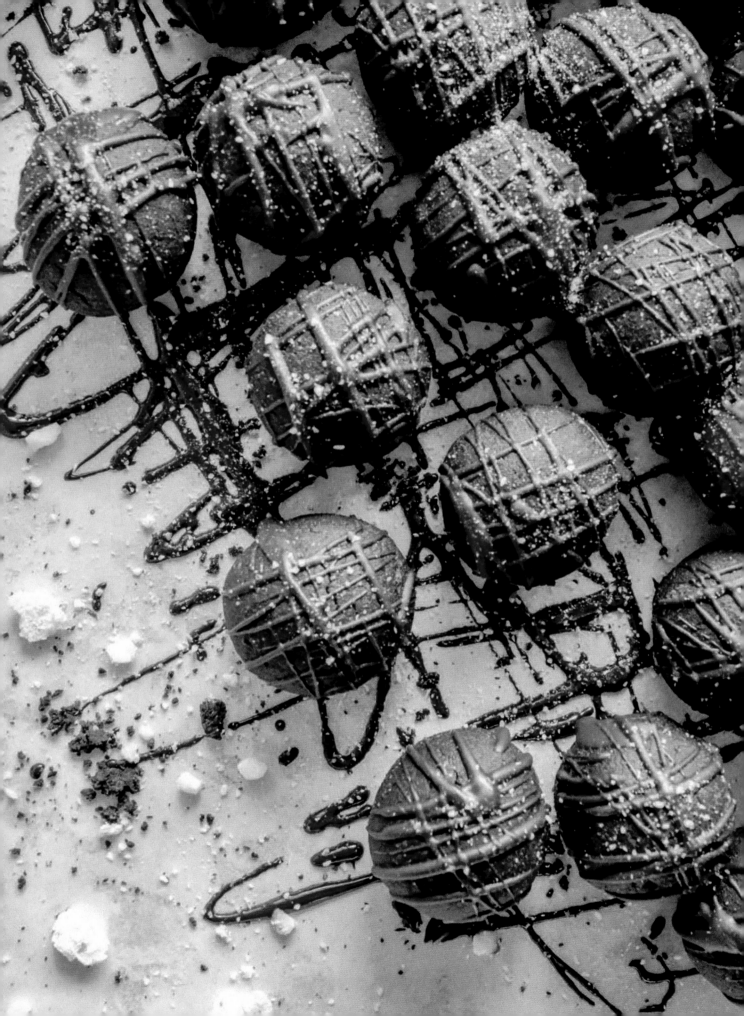

Chocolate Candy Cane Bombs

prep: *20 min*   **cool:** *35 min*   **serves:** *15-20 bombs*

Chocolaty goodness that melts in your mouth is exactly what these Vegan Truffle Chocolate Bombs are.

Dry ingredients

- 140g *(1¼ cups)* almond flour
- 68g *(1/2 cup)* coconut flour
- 56g *(1/2 cup)* cocoa powder
- 28g *(1/4 cup)* organic collagen *grass-fed*
- 150g *(1¼ cups)* powdered sweetener
  monk fruit, erythritol, xylitol
- 1 teaspoon sea salt

Wet ingredients

- 170g *(3/4 cup)* grass-fed butter *room temp*
  sub for palm shortening to make **DF**
- 112g *(1/2 cup)* coconut oil *extra virgin*
- 14g *(2 teaspoons)* blackstrap molasses
- 10mL *(2 teaspoons)* pure peppermint oil
- 5mL *(1 teaspoon)* pure vanilla extract

Chocolate Ganache

- 110g *(1/2 cup)* chocolate chips *melted*
  the recipe is found on page 223
- 14g *(1 tablespoon)* coconut oil *extra virgin*
- 5 starlight mints *sugar-free*

Instructions

1. Mix all dry ingredients into a medium bowl; whisk until combined, and set aside.
2. In a stand mixer bowl, all of the wet ingredients. Make sure the butter and coconut oil are at room temperature.
3. Pour all dry ingredients on top of the wet ingredients, mix with a paddle attachment, and mix on medium-high speed until incorporated.
4. Prepare a baking sheet with parchment paper, with a small scoop out (***cookie/scoop size: 1.5 Tbsp/ 23 ml/ 0.8 oz***) bombs on a baking sheet with parchment paper. This recipe makes about 15-20 bombs.
5. Roll each bomb in the palm of the hand; A trick to create a perfect ball is to cup your hand slightly.
6. **Garnish:** In a small heatproof bowl, melt chocolate chips with coconut oil in the microwave for 10-sec intervals, stirring between intervals; repeat 3-5 times until completely melted.
7. Using a small spoon, drizzle chocolate ganache in a zig-zag motion over the bombs.
8. Chop up starlight mints, and sprinkle over bombs before the chocolate hardens.
9. Place bombs in the fridge for 35min to allow them to harden up.
10. Store in an airtight container in the fridge for three to four weeks and freeze for up to three months.

Note

- You don't need a stand mixer to make these bombs. You can definitely mix them the old fashion way, by hand.
- Also, make sure all the wet ingredients are on the warmer side *(room temp at least)* to make the rolling much easier.

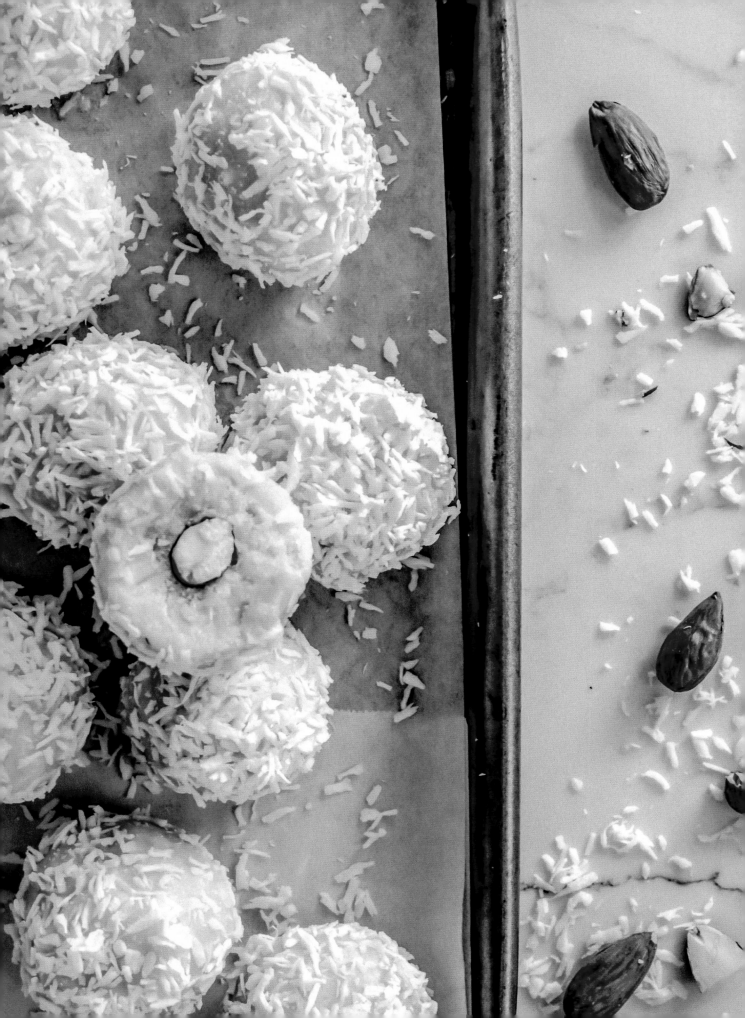

Raffaello Truffles/Bombs

prep: *20 min* **cool:** *35 min* **serves:** *15-20 bombs*

These almond Joy Bombs truly bring a sweet & satisfying JOY to your taste buds, and there is a little nutty surprise in each bomb.

Dry ingredients

- 168g *(1½ cups)* almond flour
- 46g *(1/3 cup)* coconut flour
- 42g *(1/2 cup)* coconut flakes *unsweetened*
- 56g *(1/2 cup)* organic collagen *grass-fed*
- 120g *(1 cup)* powdered sweetener
  monk fruit, erythritol, xylitol
- 1 teaspoon sea salt
- 15- 20 whole almonds *toasted*

Wet ingredients

- *57g (1/4 cup)* organic cacao butter *melted*
- *113g (1/2 cup)* grass-fed butter *room temp*
  sub for palm shortening to make DF
- *56g (1/4 cup)* coconut oil *extra virgin*
- *5mL (1 teaspoon)* coconut extract
- *5mL (1 teaspoon)* pure almond extract
- *10mL (2 teaspoons)* pure vanilla extract

Garnish

- 114g *(1/2 cup)* cacao butter *melted*
- 84g *(1 cup)* coconut flakes *unsweetened*

Instructions

1. **Preheat oven to 325°F/163°C.** Prep a cookie sheet with a piece of parchment paper side.
2. Toast almond whole raw almonds for 7 minutes, and toast almond flour for 4-5 minutes.
3. Mix all dry ingredients into a medium bowl; *(not including the whole toasted almonds)*, whisk until combined, and set aside.
4. In a small heatproof bowl, melt the cacao butter.
5. Add the wet ingredients to a stand mixer bowl, including the melted cacao butter. Make sure that the butter & coconut oil is at room temperature.
6. Pour all dry ingredients on top of the wet ingredients, mix with a paddle attachment, and mix on medium-high speed until incorporated.
7. In a stand mixer bowl, all of the wet ingredients. Make sure coconut oil is at room temperature or melted.
8. Pour all dry ingredients on top of the wet ingredients and mix with the paddle attachment again until incorporated.
9. Prepare a baking sheet with parchment paper, with a small scoop out *(cookie/scoop size: 1.5 Tbsp/ 23 ml/ 0.8 oz)* bombs on a baking sheet with parchment paper. This recipe makes about 15-20 bombs.
10. Push one roasted almond into each center of the bomb.
11. Roll each bomb in the palm of the hand; A trick to create a perfect ball is to cup your hand slightly.
12. Place bombs in the fridge for 20min to allow them to harden up.
13. **Garnish:** For the garnish, in a small heatproof bowl, melt the cacao butter in the microwave for 30-sec or until completely melted.
14. Dunk bombs in the melted cacao butter and scoop out using a fork. And transfer into a small bowl of coconut flakes and roll each bomb completely to cover the outside.
15. Place bombs back into the fridge for 20 min to allow them to harden up.
16. Store in an airtight container in the fridge for three to four weeks and freeze for up to three months.

Note

- **You don't need a stand mixer to make these bombs, you can definitely mix them the old fashion way, by hand.**
- **Also, make sure all the wet ingredients are on the warmer side** *(room temp at least)* **to make the rolling much easier.**

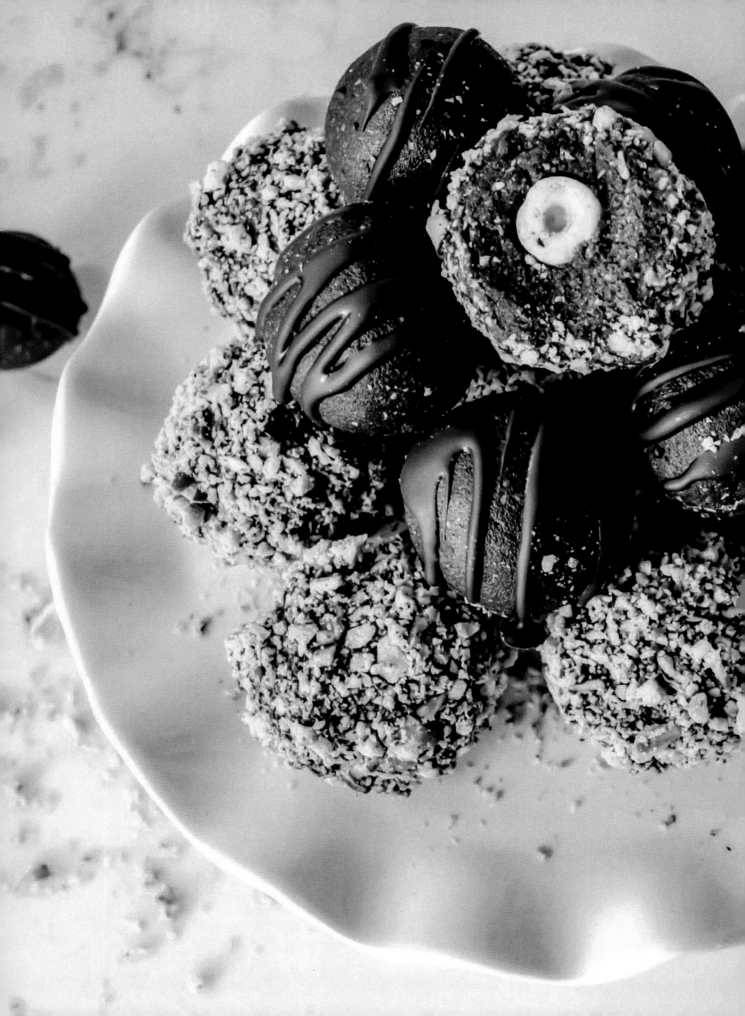

Ferrero Rocher Truffles/Bombs

prep: *20 min*   **cool:** *35 min*   **serves:** *15-20 bombs*

Making these healthy homemade Ferrero Rocher Truffles gifts for friends and family is a beautiful way to express your love through your hands to their bellies. It's a priceless gift.

Dry ingredients

- 140g *(1¼ cups)* hazelnut flour
- 68g *(1/2 cup)* coconut flour
- 56g *(1/2 cup)* cocoa powder
- 28g *(1/4 cup)* organic collagen *grass-fed*
- 150g *(1¼ cups)* powdered sweetener
  monk fruit, erythritol, xylitol
- 1 teaspoon sea salt

Wet ingredients

- 113g *(1/2 cup)* grass-fed butter *room temp*
  sub for palm shortening to make **DF**
- 114g *(1/2 cup)* hazelnut butter
  the recipe is found on page 229
- 56g *(1/4 cup)* coconut oil *extra virgin*
- 10mL *(2 teaspoons)* pure vanilla extract

Garnish & Ganache

- 110g *(1/2 cup)* chocolate chips *melted*
  the recipe is found on page 223
- 14g *(1 tablespoon)* coconut oil *extra virgin*
- 130g *(1 cup) whole* hazelnut
  toasted & chopped fine for rolling

Instructions

1. **Preheat oven to 325°F/163°C.** Prep a cookie sheet with a piece of parchment and toast whole raw hazelnuts for 12 minutes.
2. Transfer hazelnut to a tea towel and rub them inside the tea towel to remove the skin.
3. In a stand mixer bowl, add all of the wet ingredients. Ensure that the butter, hazelnut butter & coconut oil is at room temperature.
4. Pour all dry ingredients on top of the wet ingredients, mix with a paddle attachment, and mix on medium-high speed until incorporated.
5. Prepare a baking sheet with parchment paper, with a small scoop out (*cookie/scoop size: 1.5 Tbsp/ 23 ml/ 0.8 oz*) bombs on a baking sheet with parchment paper. This recipe makes about 15-20 bombs.
6. Push one roasted hazelnut into each center of the bomb.
7. Roll each bomb in the palm of the hand; A trick to create a perfect ball is to cup your hand slightly.
8. Place bombs in the fridge for 20min to allow them to harden up.
9. **Garnish:** Finely chop toasted hazelnuts and place them in a small bowl.
10. In a small heatproof bowl, melt chocolate chips with coconut oil in the microwave for 10-sec intervals and stir between intervals; repeat 3-5 times until completely melted.
11. Dunk the bombs in the chocolate ganache, and scoop them out using a fork. And transfer into the small bowl of finely chopped hazelnuts, and roll each bomb completely to cover the outside in hazelnuts.
12. Place bombs back in the fridge for 30min to allow them to harden up.
13. Store in an airtight container in the fridge for three to four weeks and freeze for up to three months.

Note

- You don't need a stand mixer to make these bombs. You can definitely mix them the old fashion way, by hand.
- Also, make sure all the wet ingredients are on the warmer side *(room temp at least)* to make the rolling much easier.

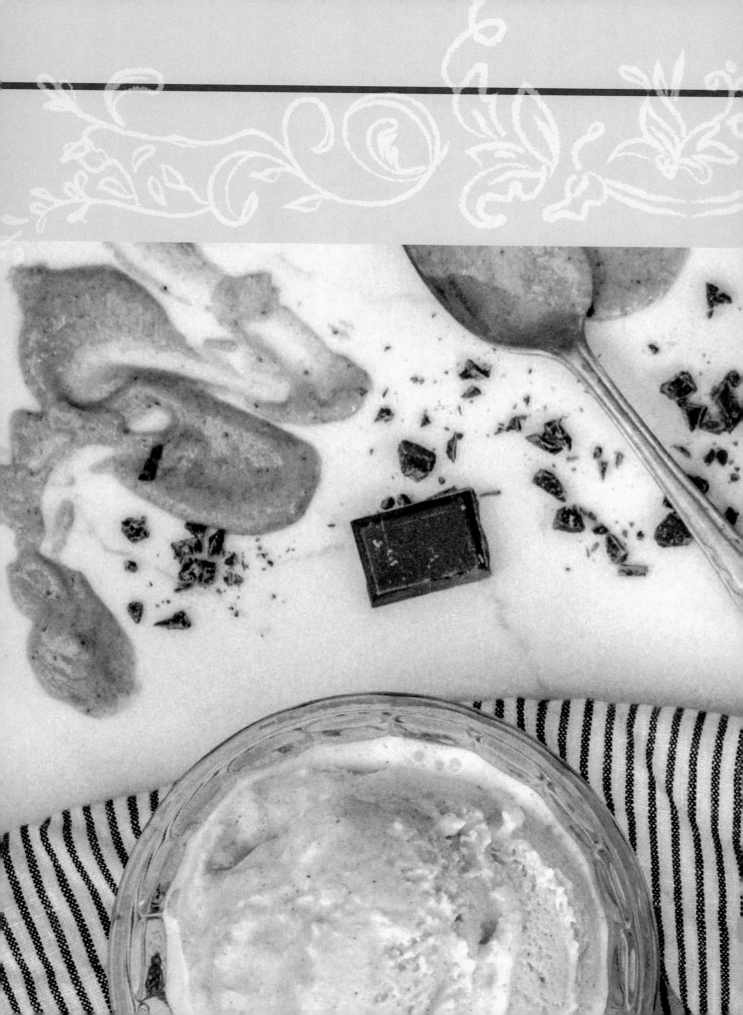

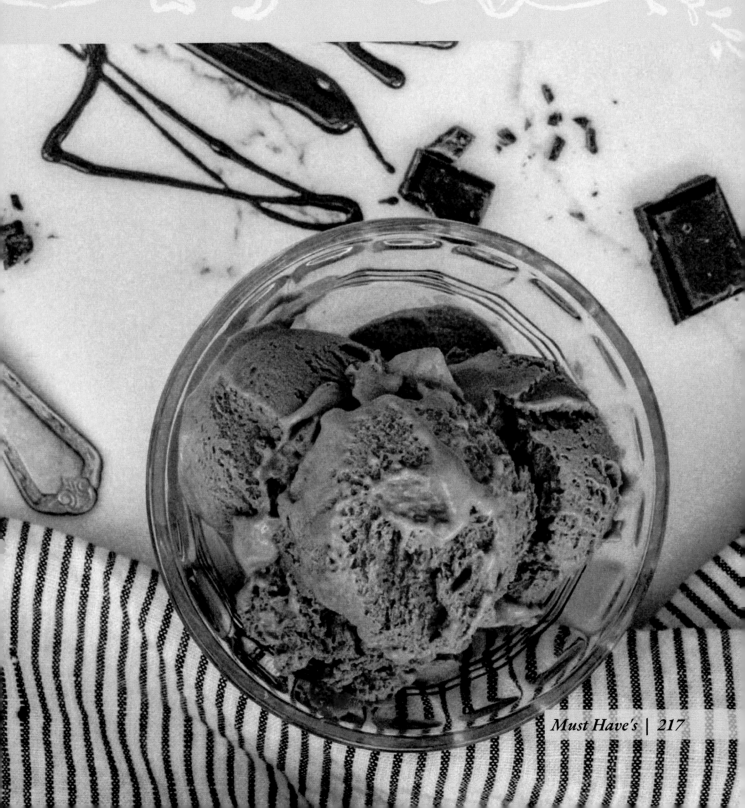

Chapter Eleven

MUST HAVE'S

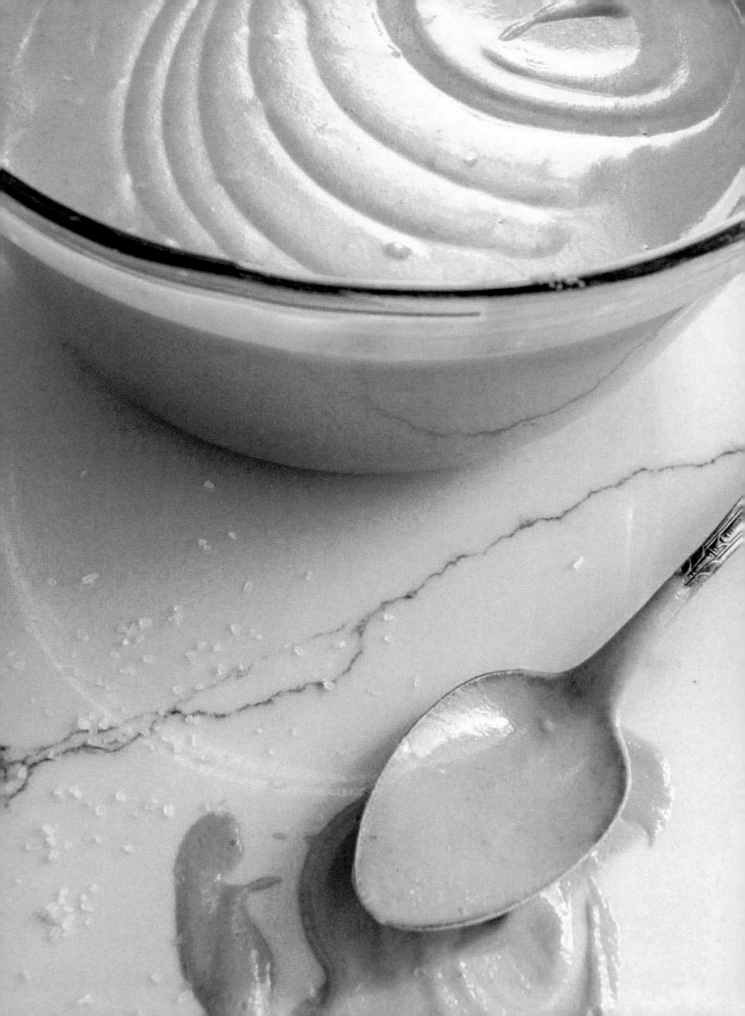

Salted Raw Caramel Sauce

prep: *20 min*   **cool:** *35 min*   **serves:** *3 cups*

This Salted Raw Caramel Sauce is a must-have for so many Bakerlita recipes. This caramel sauce is creamier than traditional caramel sauce, making it a wonderful garnish, donut glaze, and filling!

Dry ingredients

- 280g *(2 cups)* raw cashews soaked *overnight*
- 120g *(1 cup)* powdered sweetener
  monk fruit, erythritol, xylitol
- 90g *(4-5)* Medjool date
- 56g *(1/2 cup)* collagen *grass-fed*
- 15g *(1 tablespoon)* maca powder
- 2 teaspoons sea salt

Wet ingredients

- 118mL *(1/2 cup)* coconut oil *melted*
- 118mL *(1/2 cup)* coconut milk *in can*
  monk fruit, erythritol, xylitol
- 45g *(3 tablespoons)* blackstrap molasses
- 1 teaspoon pure vanilla extract
- 2 teaspoon caramel extract extract

Instructions

1. To make the caramel sauce, you must soak cashews for at least 6 hours in warm water or overnight for best results.
2. In a medium heatproof bowl, weigh/measure wet ingredients.
3. Warm up in the microwave or double broiled to melt all wet ingredients until fully melted and on the hot/warm side. *(you may also use a microwave)*
4. In a high-powered blender, combine all the ingredients, starting with the soaked cashews, the warm wet ingredients, and the dry ingredients.
5. Blend for 5-10 minutes, in 2-3 intervals crapping the sides of the blender if necessary. Blend until the mixture is silky smooth, and creamy.
6. You may need to add a bit more coconut milk or coconut oil to get it to blend smoothly if your blender isn't super high-powered.
7. Once it's smooth, taste the mixture and adjust the sweetness and saltiness to your desired taste,
8. Pour into an airtight container and store in the fridge for one month or in the freezer for four months.

Note

- **The added dates and maca root create such a lovely natural caramel flavour with many minerals, vitamins and energy-boosting properties.**

White Chocolate DF

prep: *15 min*   **cool:** *35 min*   **serves:** *2 large chocolate bars*

Finding a dairy-free, sugar-free and delicious white chocolate bar is basically impossible, and that is precisely why I had to make my own white chocolate recipe. Follow the instructions carefully, and enjoy the most robust flavoured white chocolate bar ever.

Ingredients

- 76g *(1/3 cup)* cocoa butter
- 14g *(1 tablespoon)* coconut oil *melted*
- 45g *(1/3 cup)* coconut cream powder
  you can also use MCT oil powder
- 40g *(1/3 cup)* powdered sweetener
  monk fruit, erythritol, xylitol
- 1/4 teaspoon sunflower lecithin
- 1/4 teaspoon sea salt
- 1/8 teaspoon vanilla bean powder

Instructions

1. It's best to use indirect heat to melt the cocoa butter by using a double boiler with a glass heat-proof or a metal bowl on top of low heat.
2. Before adding the cocoa butter, be sure that the simmering water isn't touching the bottom of the bowl. Also, make sure that no water or steam will reach the white chocolate mixture.
3. Add the cocoa butter to the double boiler bowl and whisk/stir until melted.
4. At this time, you may use a thermometer if you have one. The melted cocoa butter should be around 120°F.
5. Whisk in the sunflower lecithin, vanilla bean powder, salt and powdered sweetener a few tablespoons at a time.
6. Once the melted chocolate appears smooth, add in the coconut cream powder a few tablespoons at a time. Make sure you whisk very vigorously to ensure a smooth texture. Adding in the coconut milk powder too quickly can cause it to split and become grainy.
7. The white chocolate mixture will begin to turn into a thick paste texture. Add in one tablespoon of coconut oil *(14g)*, and whisk until smooth. If the consistency is still too thick, add one more tablespoon of coconut oil if needed until the mixture smooths out once again.
8. If the white chocolate mixture becomes grainy, don't worry! Pour the melted white chocolate into a high-speed blender, and blend until smooth.
9. Pour into chocolate bar silicone moulds.
10. Leave chocolate bars out to cool to room temperature *(15-20 minutes)* and place them in the fridge until the chocolate bar has set.
11. Store in an airtight container in the fridge for three to four weeks and freeze for up to three months.

Note

- **Sunflower lecithin is a natural emulsifier to help improve the moulding processes when making a chocolate bar.**

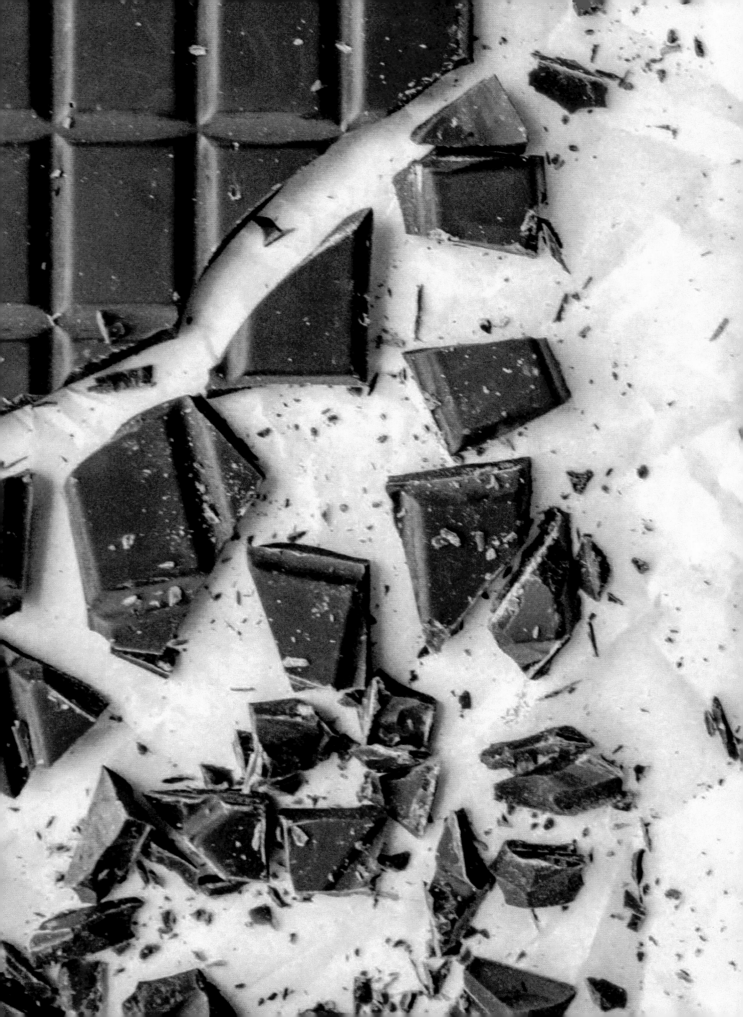

Dark Chocolate Bar/Chips

prep: *15 min*   **cool:** *35 min*   **serves:** *2 large chocolate bars*

Unlike white chocolate, finding a high-quality keto & paleo-approved chocolate bar and chips is relatively easy. My two favourite brands are Lakanto and Lily's. Making your chocolate is simple and much more affordable. Dark chocolate is much easier to make than white chocolate, so load up on a few batches!

Ingredients

- 30g *(2 tablespoons)* cocoa butter
- 120g *(3/4 cup)* baker's chocolate *unsweet*
- 60g *(1/2 cup)* powdered sweetener
  monk fruit, erythritol, xylitol
- 1/4 teaspoon sunflower lecithin
- 1/4 teaspoon sea salt
- 1 teaspoon vanilla extract

Instructions

1. To melt the cocoa butter and baker's chocolate, it's best to use indirect heat by using a double boiler with a glass heat-proof or a metal bowl on top on low heat.
2. Before adding the cocoa butter and baker's chocolate, be sure that the simmering water isn't touching the bottom of the bowl. Also, make sure that no water or steam will reach the white chocolate mixture.
3. Add the cocoa butter and baker's chocolate to the double boiler bowl and whisk/stir until melted.
4. At this time, you may use a thermometer if you have one. The melted cocoa butter should be around 120°F.
5. Whisk in the sunflower lecithin, vanilla extract, sea salt and powdered sweetener, a few tablespoons at a time.
6. Pour into chocolate bar silicone moulds.
7. Leave chocolate bars out to cool to room temperature *(15-20 minutes)* and place them in the fridge until the chocolate bar has set.
8. Store in an airtight container in the fridge for three to four weeks and freeze for up to three months.

Note

- **Sunflower lecithin is a natural emulsifier to help improve the moulding processes when making a chocolate bar.**
- **Chop chocolate bar into small pieces and use in place of chocolate chips!**

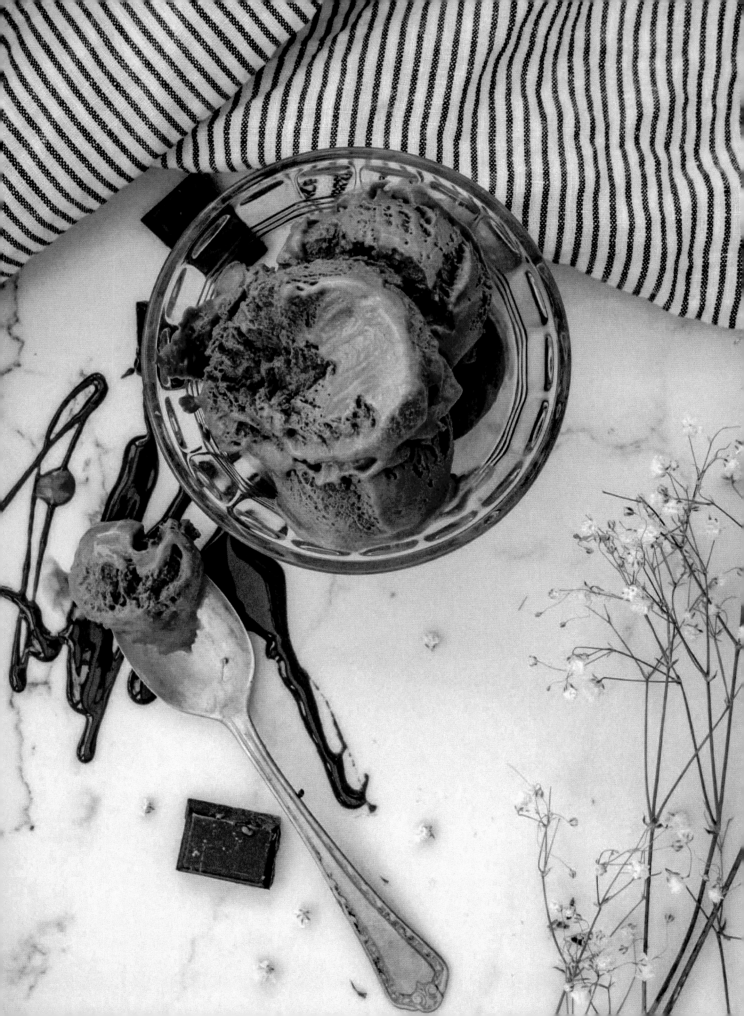

Chocolate Ice Cream DF

prep: *15 min*   **cook:** *15 min*   **freeze:** *4-6 hours*   **serves:** *10-12 scoops*

Making a creamy, fluffy, scoopable sugar-free ice cream can be tricky; however, I have mastered the perfect ice-cream recipe that you will be creaming for another spoon full! Please read the instructions and notes fervently.

Ingredients

- 400mL *(1 can)* coconut milk *full-fat*
- 120g *(1 cup)* xylitol sweetener
  56g *(1/2 cup)* cocoa powder
  use more if you like dark chocolate
- 1 teaspoon arrowroot flour *to thicken*
- 30mL *(2 tablespoons)* alcohol
  using any type of alcohol helps the ice cream become scoopable without the added sugars
- 1/4 teaspoon sea salt
- 1 teaspoon pure vanilla extract

Whipped Cream

- 1 batch of coconut whipped cream
  the recipe is found on page 189

Instructions

1. Add full-fat coconut milk, sweetener, cocoa and sea salt to a medium/small saucepan over medium heat.
2. Mix using a handheld immersion blender for best results. You may also use a whisk until all the solids from the coconut milk have dissolved and the mixture is completely smooth.
3. Next, sprinkle the arrowroot flour and whisk/blend until thoroughly combined.
4. **NOTE:** Arrowroot can clump up. To be safe, quickly run the mixture through a high-speed blender if needed.
5. Remove the chocolate mixture from the heat and allow the mixture to cool completely.
6. **Whipped cream:** Add chilled coconut cream to a large chilled bowl and whip with a handheld electric mixer or a stand mixer until soft peaks form. *See page 189 for the recipe and instructions.*
7. Once whipped coconut cream is finished, add the cooled chocolate mixture and whisk until well incorporated.
8. Add in the alcohol of choice *(this is optional)*. The mixture should be thick and creamy.
9. Transfer the chocolate ice cream to an airtight container and place the ice cream in the freezer until frozen *(4-6 hours to overnight)*.
10. If you store ice cream overnight in the freezer, take it out 15-20 minutes before serving, depending on your room temperature.
11. Store ice cream in an airtight container for two months in the freezer.

Note

- **Using xylitol for your sweetener works the best in homemade ice creams because it ensures a more scoopable/soft result. The added alcohol does the trick as well *(optional)*.**

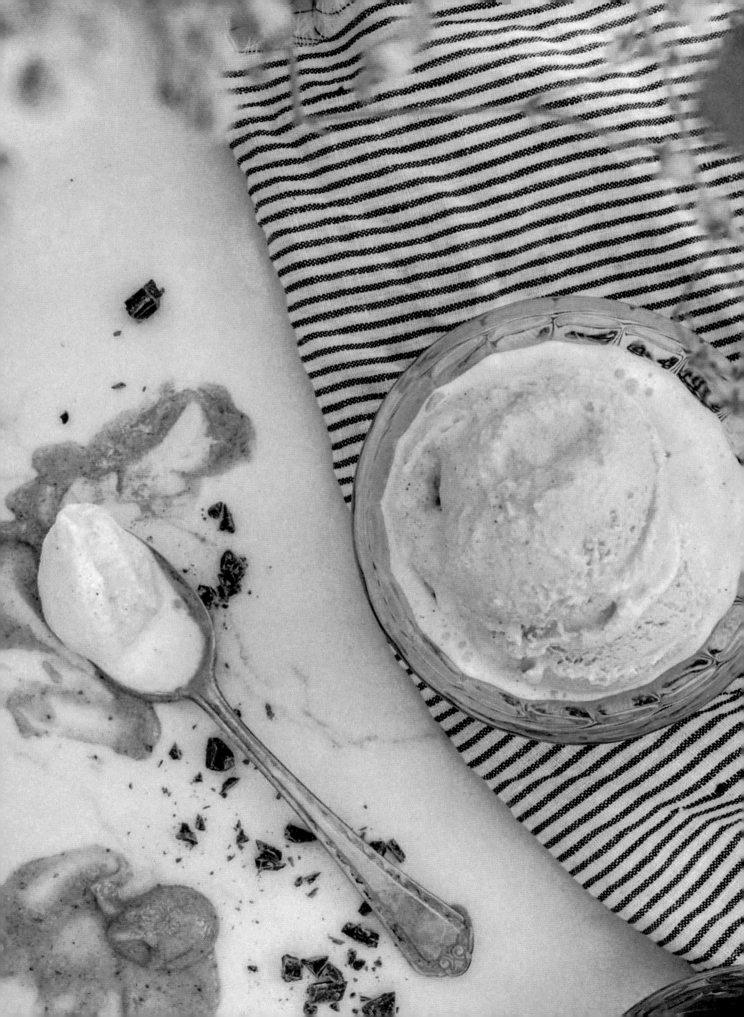

Vanilla Ice Cream DF

prep: *15 min*   **cook:** *15 min*   **freeze:** *4-6 hours*   **serves:** *10-12 scoops*

Making a creamy, fluffy, scoopable sugar-free ice cream can be tricky; however, I have mastered the perfect ice-cream recipe that you will be creaming for another spoon full! Please read the instructions and notes fervently.

Ingredients

- 400mL *(1 can)* coconut milk *full-fat*
- 120g *(1 cup)* xylitol sweetener
- 2 teaspoons arrowroot flour *to thicken*
- 30mL *(2 tablespoons)* alcohol

using any type of alcohol helps the ice cream become scoopable without the added sugars

- 1/4 teaspoon sea salt
- 1/2 teaspoon vanilla bean powder
- 2 teaspoons pure vanilla extract

Whipped Cream

- 1 batch of coconut whipped cream

the recipe is found on page 189

Instructions

1. Add full-fat coconut milk, sweetener and sea salt to a medium/small saucepan over medium heat.
2. Mix using a handheld immersion blender for best results. You may also use a whisk until all the solids from the coconut milk have dissolved and the mixture is completely smooth.
3. Next, sprinkle the arrowroot flour and whisk/blend until thoroughly combined.
4. **NOTE:** Arrowroot can clump up. To be safe, quickly run the mixture through a high-speed blender if needed.
5. Remove the creamy vanilla mixture from the heat and allow the mixture to cool completely.
6. **Whipped cream:** Add chilled coconut cream to a large chilled bowl and whip with a handheld electric mixer or a stand mixer until soft peaks form. ***See page 1829 for the recipe and instructions.***
7. Once whipped coconut cream is finished, add the cooled chocolate mixture and whisk until well incorporated.
8. Add in the alcohol of choice *(this is optional)*. The mixture should be thick and creamy.
9. Transfer the chocolate ice cream to an airtight container and place the ice cream in the freezer until frozen *(4-6 hours to overnight)*.
10. If you store ice cream overnight in the freezer, take it out 15-20 minutes before serving, depending on your room temperature.
11. Store ice cream in an airtight container for two months in the freezer.

Note

- **Using xylitol for your sweetener works the best in homemade ice creams because it ensures a more scoopable/soft result. The added alcohol does the trick as well *(optional)*.**

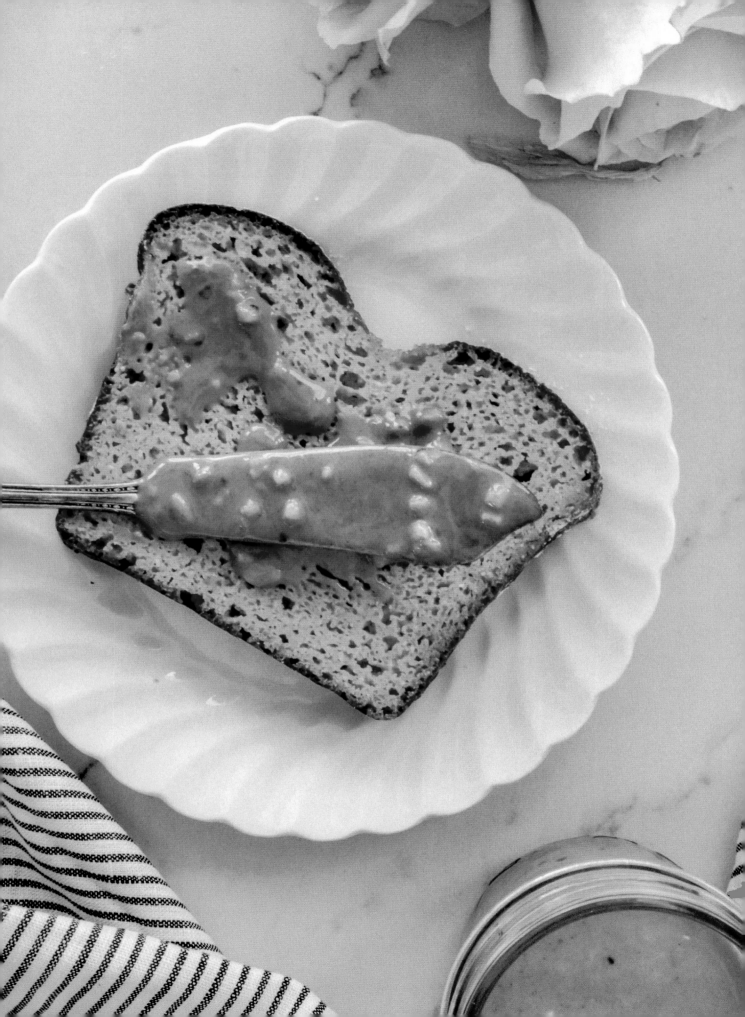

Homemade Nut Butters

prep: *10 min*   **cook:** *15 min*   **cool:** *10-12 min*   **serves:** *20*

Making your organic nut butter is very simple and much more affordable. Use any nut you desire, or make all of them! My favourite is pecan butter, yum! I love having a variety of nut butter stocked in my pantry.

Ingredients

- 420g *(3 cups)* raw nuts *organic*
  almonds
  pecans
  walnuts
  cashews
  macadamia
  hazelnuts
  peanuts
- 30mL *(2 tablespoons)* MCT oil
- 1 teaspoon sea salt

Instructions

1. **Preheat the oven to 325°F/163°C.** Spread the nut of choice *(almonds, walnuts, hazelnuts, macadamias, cashews or pecans)* on a large cookie/baking sheet and toast the nuts for about 12-15 minutes, mixing halfway.
2. **NOTE:** Don't bake the nuts too long because it will wreck the flavour.
3. Let the nuts cool for about 10-12 minutes until they become warm, not cool.
4. Transfer the toasted nuts, MCT oil and sea salt to a high-speed blender or food processor. Using a rubber spatula, scrape down the sides as necessary. Blend nuts, and be patient.
5. Keep blending until the nut butter becomes smooth and creamy.
6. Using a food processor may take a while for the nuts to transform into nut butter *(it may turn into a ball before smooth nut butter)*. Continue to scrape down the sides.
7. Once the nut butter is very creamy, add more salt if needed.
8. Transfer the homemade nut butter into an air-tight container/glass jar. Store in the refrigerator for up to four weeks.

Note

- **Hazelnuts will need an additional 1-2 minutes in the oven to allow the skin to loosen. While the hazelnuts are still warm, use a tea towel and wrap hazelnuts inside and rub them together to remove the skins.**

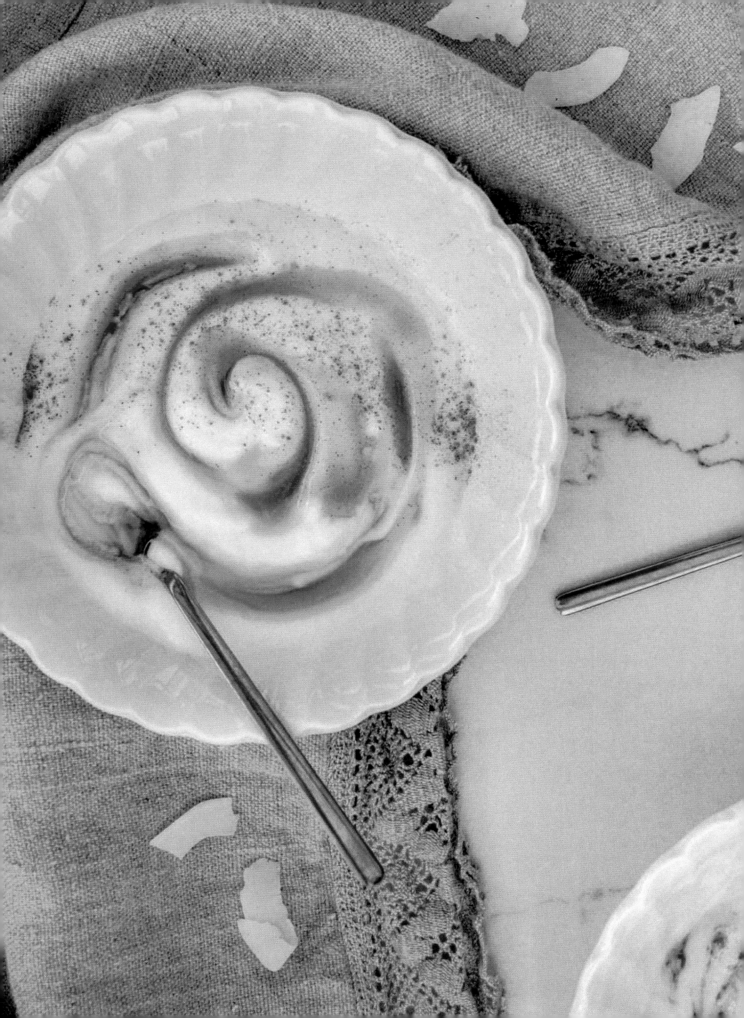

Coconut Collagen Yogurt

prep: *15 min*   **cook:** *15 min*   **freeze:** *4-6 hours*   **serves:** *10-12 scoops*

I always loved Greek yogurt due to its super creamy thick texture, tanginess & tremendous amounts of protein. I enjoyed it when I first made coconut yogurt; yet, I needed to add the missing protein as Greek yogurt had. And that's how I came up with my own **Coconut Collagen Yogurt** *creation!*

Ingredients

- 800mL *(2 cans)* coconut milk *full-fat*
- 112g *(1 cup)* organic collagen *grass-fed*
- 4 capsules of probiotics
  capsules can be easily opened and emptied

Add-ins

- 60g *(1/2 cup)* powdered sweetener
  monk fruit, erythritol, xylitol
- 1 teaspoon cinnamon
- 1 teaspoon vanilla extract

Fruity Add-ins

- 280g *(2 cups)* berry jams *recipe page 193*

Instructions

1. Make sure you buy high-quality, full-fat organic BPA-free coconut milk in the can.
2. Shake the cans of full-fat coconut milk extremely well. Open cans and pour them into a clean, sterilized glass jar or bowl.
3. Add 1 cup of coconut milk and collagen to a small bowl and empty the probiotic capsules. Stir using a wooden or plastic spoon to stir *(not metal, as a metal spoon can react negatively with the probiotics)* Stir until it creates a smooth paste.
4. Cover the yogurt with a cheesecloth or a very thin, clean tea towel and secure it with a rubber band.
5. Place the jar in a warmer spot in your house. Let the coconut yogurt activate for at least 24 hours and up to +48 hours.
6. The longer the yogurt rests, the tangier/tart the yogurt will become.
7. Taste test with a wooden spoon, and once the coconut yogurt has reached the desired amount of tanginess and thickness for your liking, place an air-tight lid over the yogurt and refrigerate until cold.
8. Once your yogurt has been refrigerated for a couple of hours, it will thicken even more, almost to that desirable Greek yogurt consistency.
9. Transfer the homemade yogurt into an air-tight container/glass jar. Store in the refrigerator for up to four weeks.

Note

- To make a delicious tangy yogurt, it must be activated at a warm temperature. If your house is on the cooler side, place the yogurt in the oven with the light on *(do not turn on the oven, just the oven light)*. **This** should provide the perfect amount of heat to activate the yogurt.

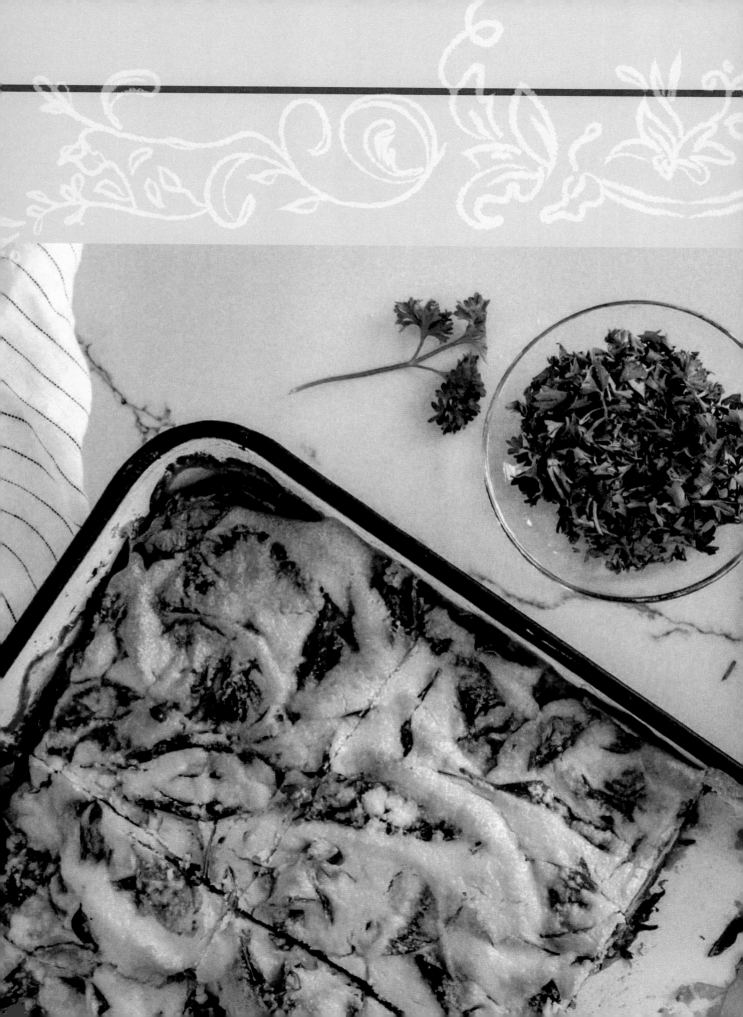

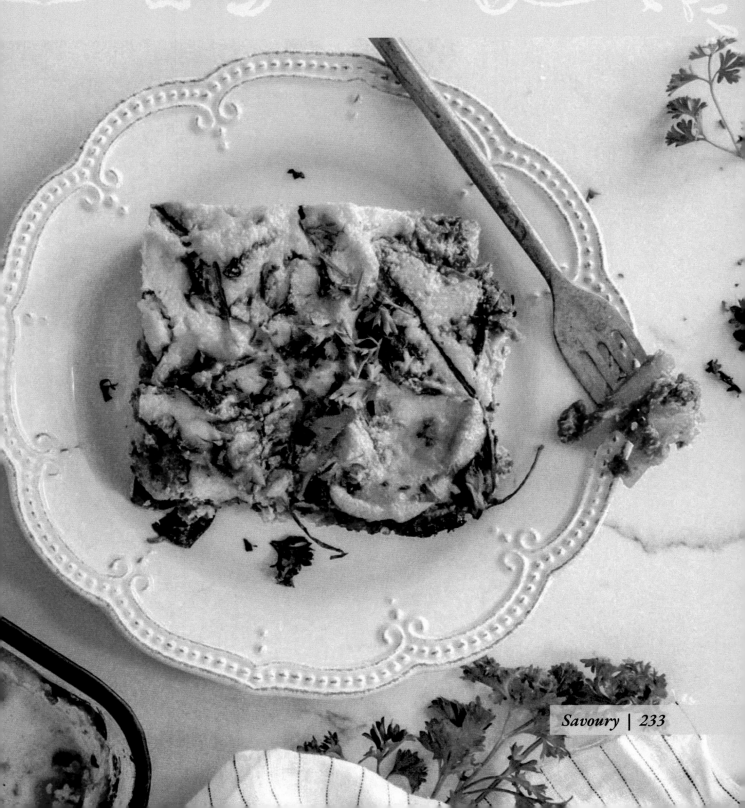

Chapter Twelve

SAVOURY

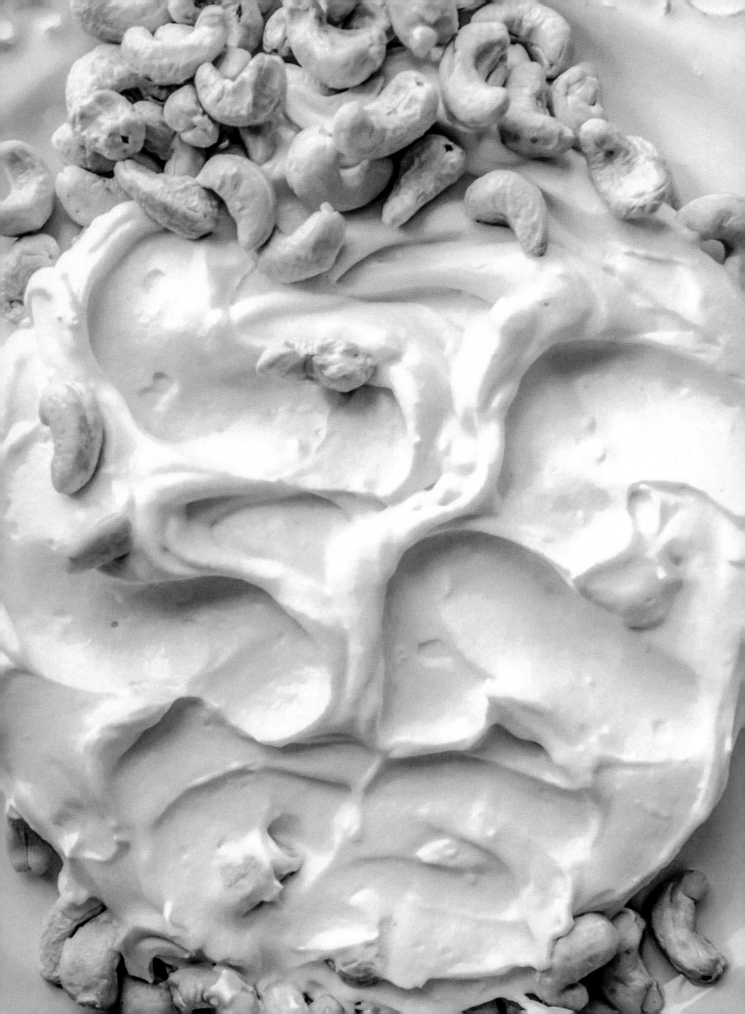

Cashew Cream Cheese & Sauce

prep: *20 min* **cool:** *35 min* **serves:** *3 cups*

Making your own homemade cashew cream cheese and cheese sauce is defiantly a win, win for your tummy since they are both 100% dairy-free and your wallet. Buying pre-made cashew cream cheese from your local grocery store can be highly pricy per the quantity you will get.

Cream cheese ingredients

- 280g *(2 cups)* raw cashews *soaked overnight*
- 118g *(1/2 cup)* plain coconut yogurt
  the recipe is found on page 220
  OR *you can buy it at a local health food store*
- 2 teaspoons sea salt
- +15mL *(1-2 tablespoons)* warm water
  if needed to help with blending

Cheese sauce ingredients

- 280g *(2 cups)* raw cashews *soaked overnight*
- 45g *(1/2 cup)* nutritional yeast
- 177mL *(3/4 cup)* warm water
- 56mL *(1/4 cup)* lemon juice
- 2 teaspoons sea salt

Cream cheese instructions

1. Soak cashews overnight in filters water.
2. Strain water from the cashews and place them into a food processor or a high-speed blender.
3. Add coconut yogurt and sea salt. Blend until creamy, thick and smooth.
4. Scrape down sipes with a rubber spatula every few minutes to ensure no chucks get stuck to the bottom and sides of the blender/food processor.
5. Add warm water to help cashew cream cheese reach its perfect consistency.
6. Store this delicious cashew cream cheese in an air-tight container in the fridge for up to two weeks, or freeze it for three months.

Cheese Sauce instructions

1. Soak cashews overnight in filters water.
2. Strain water from the cashews and place them into a high-speed blender.
3. Add all the rest of the ingredients and blend until creamy and smooth.
4. Scrape down sipes with a rubber spatula every few minutes to ensure no chucks get stuck to the bottom and sides of the blender/food processor.
5. Add warm water to help cashew cream cheese reach its perfect consistency. You don't want cashew cheese sauce to be too thick or runny.
6. Store this cheesy cashew cheese sauce in an air-tight container in the fridge for up to two weeks, or freeze for three months.

Note

- **These two recipes are very straightforward to make. However, they work the best when the cashews are well soaked** *(at least 6 hours in warm water).*

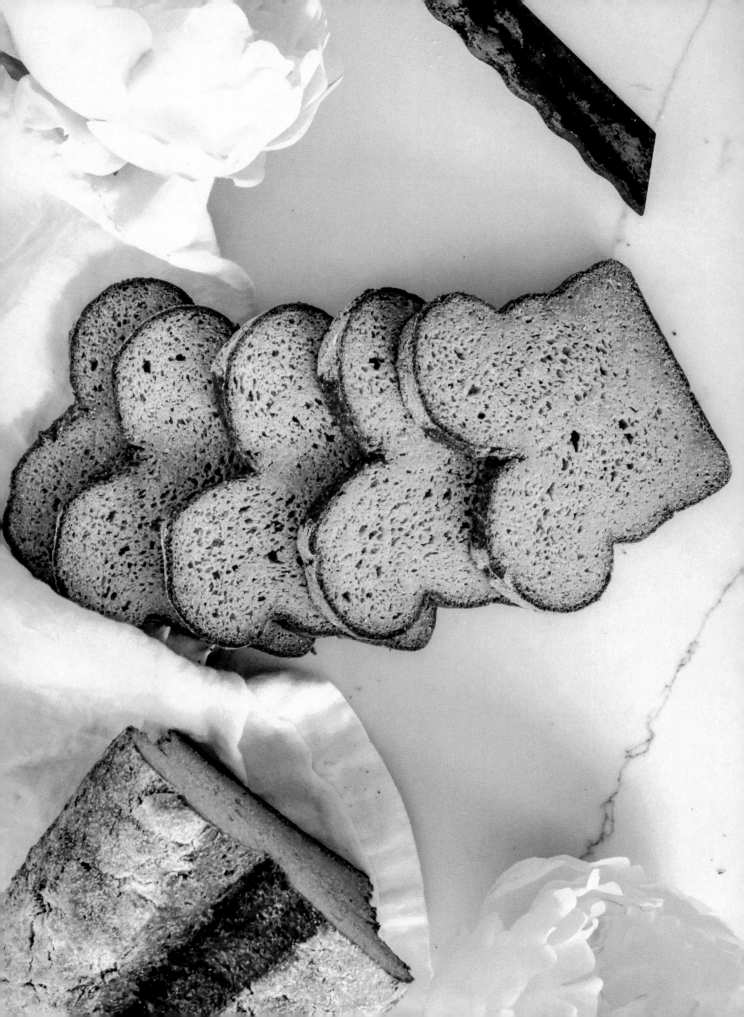

Artisan Sandwich Bread

prep: *15 min*   **bake:** *45-55 min*   **cool:** *50 min*   **serves:** *1 loaf / 20 slices*

*Bread was one of the hardest things to give up when I went on a keto/paleo diet. It became a quest I wouldn't give up until I created a bread that I loved! My **Artisan Sandwich Bread** reminds me of a heavier rye sourdough bread. My favourite way to eat this bread is making avocado toast on-page.*

Dry ingredients
- 140g *(1¼ cups)* almond flour
- 68g *(1/2 cup)* coconut flour
- 44g *(1/4 cup)* psyllium husk powder
- 56g *(1/2 cup)* organic collagen *grass-fed*
- 20g *(2 tablespoons)* flaxseed meal
- 1 teaspoon baking soda
- 1 teaspoon baking powder
- 2 teaspoons instant yeast
- 2 teaspoons sea salt

Wet ingredients:
- 4 free-run eggs *room temp*
- 3 egg whites *room temp*
- 177mL *(3/4 cup)* warm water
- 15mL *(1 tablespoon)* honey *activates yeast*
- 118mL *(1/2 cup)* apple cider vinegar

Garnish:
- 1 tablespoon of arrowroot flour *optional*

Instructions
1. **Preheat oven to 350°F/180°C.** Prep an 8x4 inch bread/loaf pan with parchment paper.
2. In a medium bowl, measure all dry ingredients, whisk together and set aside.
3. In a separate medium bowl, add all wet ingredients, whisk together, and pour the entire wet ingredients onto the dry ingredients in a separate medium bowl.
4. . Using a rubber spatula, mix until well incorporated.
5. The dough should form a ball of dough.
6. **Garnish:** Place bread dough in the repaired loaf pan and dust with arrowroot flour to give it that artisan look.
7. Using a knife, make a slice/slash down the length of the loaf.
8. Bake the bread for 45-55 minutes or until lightly golden brown on top.
9. Cool bread in the loaf pan for about 15min, then remove the bread and let it completely cool on a cooling rack for 45minutes.
10. Slice the bread into 20-18 slices.
11. Store bread in a durable zip-lock bag in the fridge for up to two weeks or in the freezer for two months.

Note

- **Dusting the top with a small amount of arrowroot flour truly makes this bread look beautiful and gives it that iconic artisan look.**

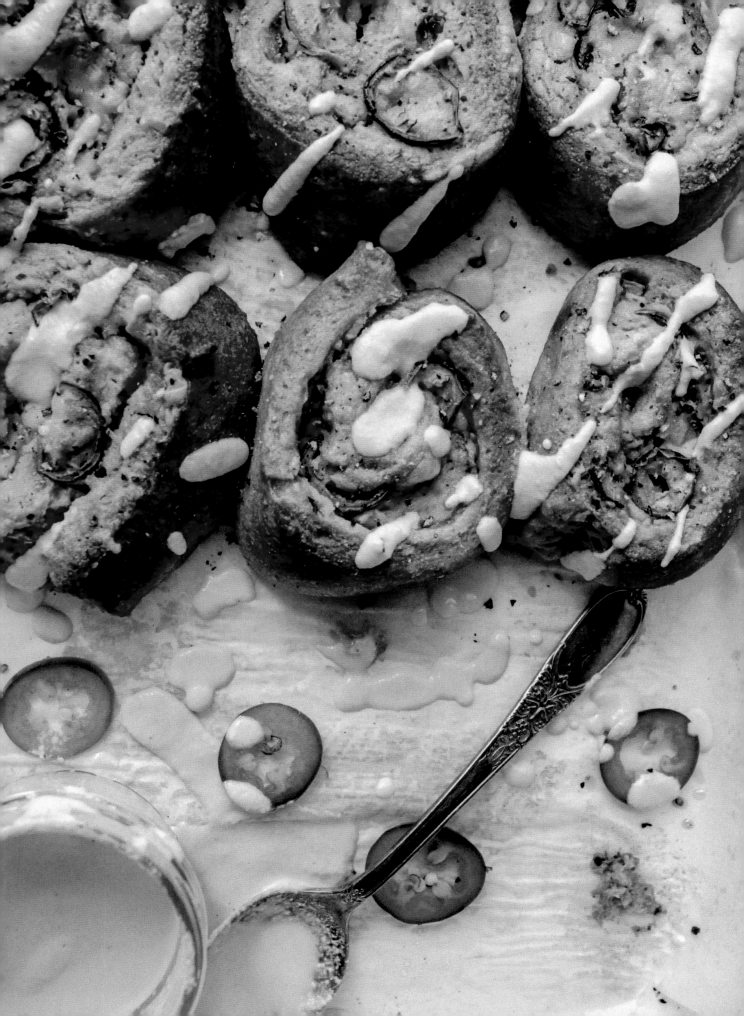

Cheesy Jalapeño Rolls

prep: *25 min*   **bake:** *30-35 min*   **cool:** *20 min*   **serves:** *8 large rolls*

Dough dry ingredients

- 168g *(1½ cups)* almond flour
- 34g *(1/4 cup)* coconut flour
- 44g *(1/4 cup)* psyllium husk powder
- 1 teaspoon baking soda
- 1 teaspoon baking powder
- 2 teaspoons instant yeast
- 2 teaspoons sea salt

Dough wet ingredients:

- 2 free-run eggs *room temp*
- 3 egg whites *room temp*
- 118mL *(1/2 cup)* warm water
- 15mL *(1 tablespoon)* honey *activates yeast*
- 60mL *(1/4 cup)* apple cider vinegar

Filling ingredients:

- 120mL *(1/2 cup)* cashew cheese sauce
  the recipe is found on page 235
- 60mL *(1/4 cup)* tomato sauce
- 1 fresh jalapeño *chopped*
  remove seeds to make it less spicy
- 140g *(1/2 cup)* pickled jalapeño *chopped*
- 1 clove fresh garlic
- 1 teaspoon sea salt & black pepper.

Garnish ingredients:

- 60mL *(1/4 cup)* cashew cheese sauce
- 1 fresh jalapeño *sliced thin*
- freshly cracked black pepper.

Instructions

1. **Preheat oven to 350°F/180°C,** and prep an 8x8 inch pan with parchment paper.
2. In a medium bowl, measure all dry ingredients, whisk together and set aside.
3. In a separate medium bowl, add all wet ingredients, whisk together, and pour the entire wet ingredients onto the dry ingredients in a separate medium bowl. Using a rubber spatula, mix until well incorporated.
4. Place a piece of saran wrap to cover the bowl, and place in the dough fridge for about 10 minutes to firm up.
5. **Filling:** Mix the tomato sauce, fresh garlic *(pressed or chopped fine),* and sea salt in a small bowl.
6. Chop up fresh and pickled jalapeños, and set them aside.
7. Have cheese sauce pre-made. **See page 235.**
8. Place a large piece of saran wrap onto the surface of your countertop.
9. Place the chilled dough onto the saran wrap surface. Take another piece of saran wrap, place it on top of the dough and press down.
10. Using a rolling pin, roll the dough out into a 16x8-inch rectangle.
11. First, spread tomato sauce evenly over the whole surface of the dough, then drizzle cashew cheeses sauce, and sprinkle chopped jalapeños over the entire surface.
12. Roll the dough by folding the saran wrap under the dough, the side closest to yourself, rolling it up until it rolls into a big log roll.
13. Using a sharp knife, cut the roll in half, then cut each half into 3-4 pieces, leaving you with 6-8 rolls, and place a greased 8x8 baking/casserole pan.
14. **Garnish:** Place thinly sliced jalapeños on top of the roll.s
15. Bake the rolls for 30-35 minutes or until lightly golden brown on top.
16. Let rolls cool down for about 20 min.
17. Once rolls are cooled, drizzle extra cashew cheese on top & enjoy!
18. Store in an air-tight container in the fridge for one week or in the freezer for two months.

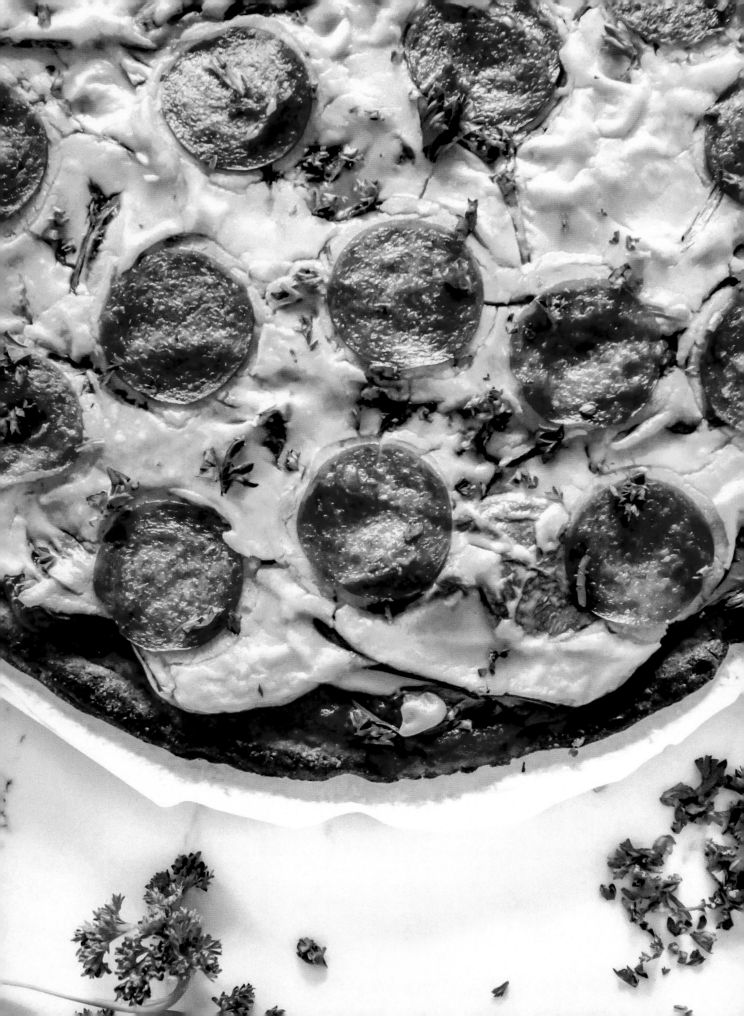

Andrea's Pepperoni Pizza

prep: *25 min*   **bake:** *30-35 min*   **cool:** *20 min*   **serves:** *2 medium pizzas*

Who doesn't crave pizza once in a while? Now you can enjoy pizza again without loads of carbs & dairy, which means you will have a happy tummy, and a satisfied soul!

Dough dry ingredients
- 168g *(1½ cups)* almond flour
- 34g *(1/4 cup)* coconut flour
- 33g *(3 tablespoons)* psyllium husk powder
- 1 teaspoon baking soda
- 1 teaspoon baking powder
- 2 teaspoons instant yeast
- 2 teaspoons sea salt

Dough wet ingredients:
- 2 free-run eggs *room temp*
- 3 egg whites *room temp*
- 118mL *(1/2 cup)* warm water
- 15mL *(1 tablespoon)* honey *activates yeast*
- 60mL *(1/4 cup)* apple cider vinegar

Topping ingredients:
- 240mL *(1 cup)* pizza sauce
- 1 clove fresh garlic *minced*
- 35g *(1 cup)* baby spinach *packed*
- 240mL *(1 cup)* cashew cheese sauce
  the recipe is founf on page 235
- 150g *(1 cup)* pepperoni *grass-fed*
- 1 teaspoon sea salt & black pepper.

Garnish ingredients:
- fresh parsley *chopped*

Instructions

1. Preheat oven to 350°F/180°C.
2. In a medium bowl, measure all dry ingredients, whisk together and set aside.
3. In a separate medium bowl, add all wet ingredients, whisk together, and pour the entire wet ingredients onto the dry ingredients in a separate medium bowl. Using a rubber spatula, mix until well incorporated.
4. Using two medium 12-inch pizza pans, cut out two pieces of parchment paper for the bottom of each pizza pan.
5. Split the dough in half, and place each piece of the dough on the prepared parchment paper on a flat surface. With your hands, slightly press down the dough.
6. Using a rolling pin and plastic wrap, place plastic wrap over the dough, start rolling the dough only where the plastic wrap is, and roll to the edges on the cut parchment paper.
7. Once the dough is rolled out, transfer the dough to pizza pans, poke a few holes in the top of the dough, using a fork for a more even bake.
8. Par-bake the pizza crust for 10 min at 350°F/180°C.
9. Once the pizza dough is par-baked, it is time to build the pizzas.
10. **Topping:** First, spread pizza sauce and minced garlic evenly over each surface of the dough, add spinach, then drizzle with cashew cheeses sauce. Using a back of a spoon, spread cheese sauce to the edges evenly.
11. Add pepperoni on top of the cashew cheese *(or any toppings you desire)*
12. Bake the pizzas for 30-35 minutes or until the cheese becomes lightly golden.
13. **Garnish:** Let the pizzas cool down for about 10 min. Once pizzas are cooled, garnish with fresh parsley, slice & enjoy!
14. Store in an air-tight container in the fridge for one week or in the freezer for two months.

Note

- **Be creative, use any topping you desire to make your dream pizza!**

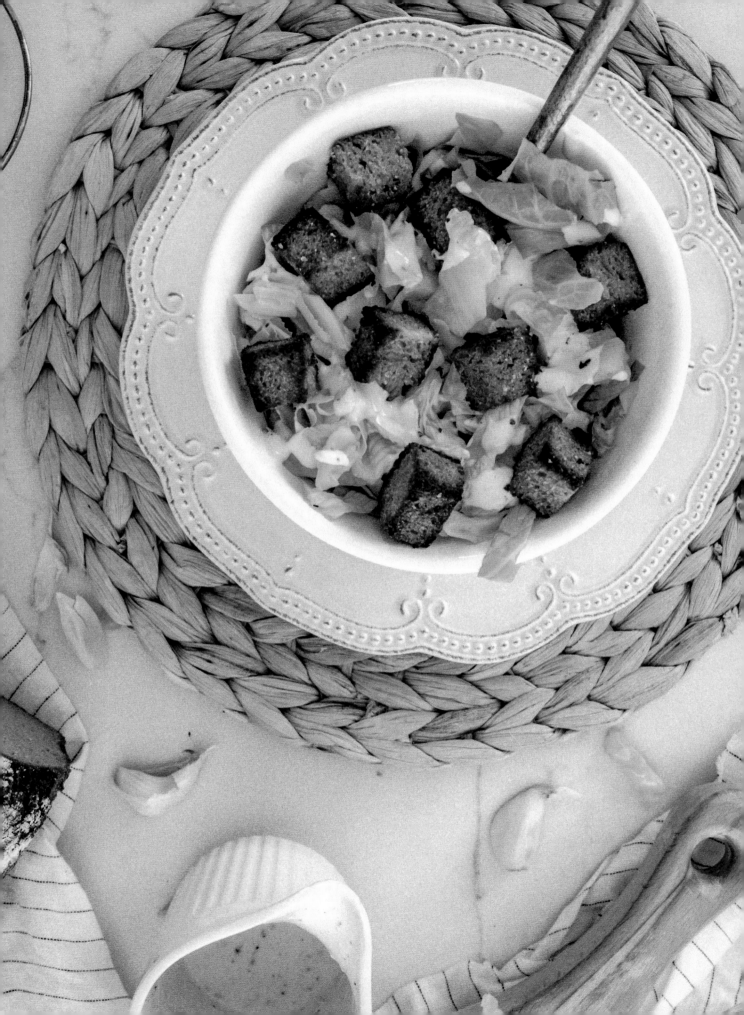

Crouton Heaven Caesar Salad

prep: *25 min*   **bake:** *10 min*   **cool:** *5 min*   **serves:** *4 large salads*

As weird, but as true as it is, salads are one of my most loved meals for lunch and dinner. This Crouton Heaven Caesar Salad is next level, with the crunchy Romain lettuce, the most delicious crustons ever, and the Caesar Aoöli that should be ilegal.

Crouton Ingredients

- 1/2 loaf of artisan sandwich bread *cubbed*
  The recipe is found on page 237
- 30mL *(2 tablespoons)* avocado oil
- 1 teaspoon garlic powder
- 1/2 teaspoon sea salt
- 1/2 teaspoon black pepper

Caesar Aioli ingredients:

- 1 egg *room temp*
- 240mL *(1 cup)* avocado oil
- 15mL *(1 tablespoon* Dijon mustard
- 15mL *(1 tablespoon)* lemon juice
- 45g *(1/2 cup)* nutritional yeast
- 2 small garlic cloves *minced*
- 1 teaspoon anchovy paste *in a can*
- 1/2 teaspoon sea salt
- 1/2 teaspoon black pepper

Salad ingredients:

- 3 heads of organic Romaine lettuce *chopped*

Instructions

1. Preheat oven to 350°F/180°C. Prep a small pan with parchment paper.
2. **Croutons:** In a medium bowl, measure all crouton ingredients and stir the croutons covered in oil, garlic, sea salt and pepper.
3. Bake the croutons for 10-min or until they become lightly golden on top.
4. **Caesar aioli:** Crack one whole egg into the bottom of a tall large glass jar with a wide-mouth glass jar. *(Use anything that will be big enough for an immersion blender to fit. But do not use a bowl.)*
5. Add the rest of the Caesar aioli dressing on top of the egg, trying not to break the egg, and make sure you don't whisk or stir either.
6. Pour the avocado oil on top.
7. Carefully submerge the immersion blender into the bottom of the jar/glass, and place it right where the egg is. Blend on low power for about 15-20 seconds without moving from where the egg was.
8. Blend until you see most of the aioli has turned white and pail.
9. Next, slowly move the blender while blending upward without lifting the blender out into the air. Once you reach the top of the oil, slowly roll back down to the bottom.
10. Repeat this motion in step 9 until the mayonnaise forms a rich, creamy texture.
11. **Salad:** Chop Romaine lettuce into a large brown, add 1/2 cup of Caesar Aioli Dressing and the baked croutons, toast the salad and serve!
12. Store the homemade aioli avocado mayonnaise right in the jar in the refrigerator for two months.

Note

- **Be creative, add chicken or wild boar bacon to make it a full meal.**

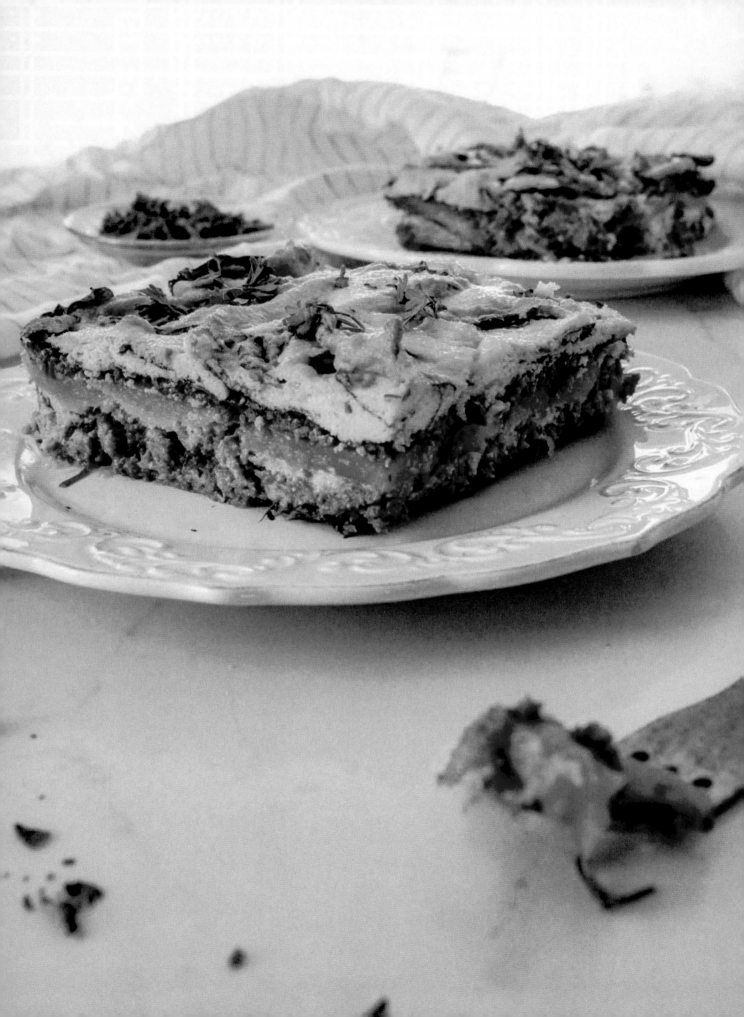

Creamy Butternut Lasagna

prep: *35 min*   **bake:** *50-65 min*   **cool:** *15 min*   **serves:** *6 large pieces*

Who doesn't crave pizza once in a while? Now you can enjoy pizza again without loads of carbs & dairy, which means you will have a happy tummy, and a satisfied soul!

Meat sauce ingredients
- 2 pounds *(910g)* beef *organic grass-fed*
- 240mL *(1 cup)* tomato sauce *organic*
- 118mL *(1 cup)* tomato paste *organic*
- 2 small garlic cloves *minced*
- 1 teaspoon dried basil
- 1 teaspoon dried oregano
- 2 teaspoons red chilli flakes
- 2 teaspoons sea salt

Layer ingredients:
- 1 extra-large butternut squash
- 480mL *(2 cups)* cashew cheese sauce
  the recipe is found on page 235
- 125g *(4 cups)* baby spinach *packed*

Garnish ingredients:
- fresh parsley *chopped*

Assembly

- **BUTTERNUT**
- **MEAT SAUCE**
- **SPINACH**
- **CASHEW CHEESE**
-
- **BUTTERNUT**
- **MEAT SAUCE**
- **SPINACH**
- **CASHEW CHEESE**

Instructions

1. **Preheat oven to 375°F/190°C.**
2. **Meat sauce:** In a large saucepan, add beef, tomatoes, sauce & paste, and herbs and spices. Place a lid on the pot, and turn the heat to medium.
3. Allow the beef to soften/warm up and break it down with a large spoon.
4. Stir and break down the meat sauce until thoroughly cooked.
5. **Layer:** Peel and sliced butternut squash in 1/4 inch, and if using the bulb of butternut squash, peel and de-seed. Cut the bulb into a moon shape. *(best to use these pieces for the top layer)*
6. Make sure the cashew cheese sauce is already pre-made. ***The recipe is on page 235.***
7. In a 10x 13-inch casserole dish *(or any deep dish baking pan close to that measurement)*, layer the thin butternut slices to completely cover the bottom of the casserole dish.
8. Add 1/2 the meat sauce on top of the butternut layer, then add 2 cups of spinach and 1 cup of cashew cheese. Spread cashew sauce evenly over the spinach using the back of a spoon.
9. Repeat instructions 7-8 to create another layer. Start with the leftover butternut slices and end with the cashew cheese sauce on top.
10. Bake the lasagna for 50-65 minutes or until you, test the butternut by poking the lasagna with a knife to see if the butternut is soft.
11. **Garnish:** Let the lasagna cool down for about 15 min. Once it's cooled, garnish with fresh parsley, serve & enjoy!
12. Store in an air-tight container in the fridge for up to three to four days or in the freezer for two months.

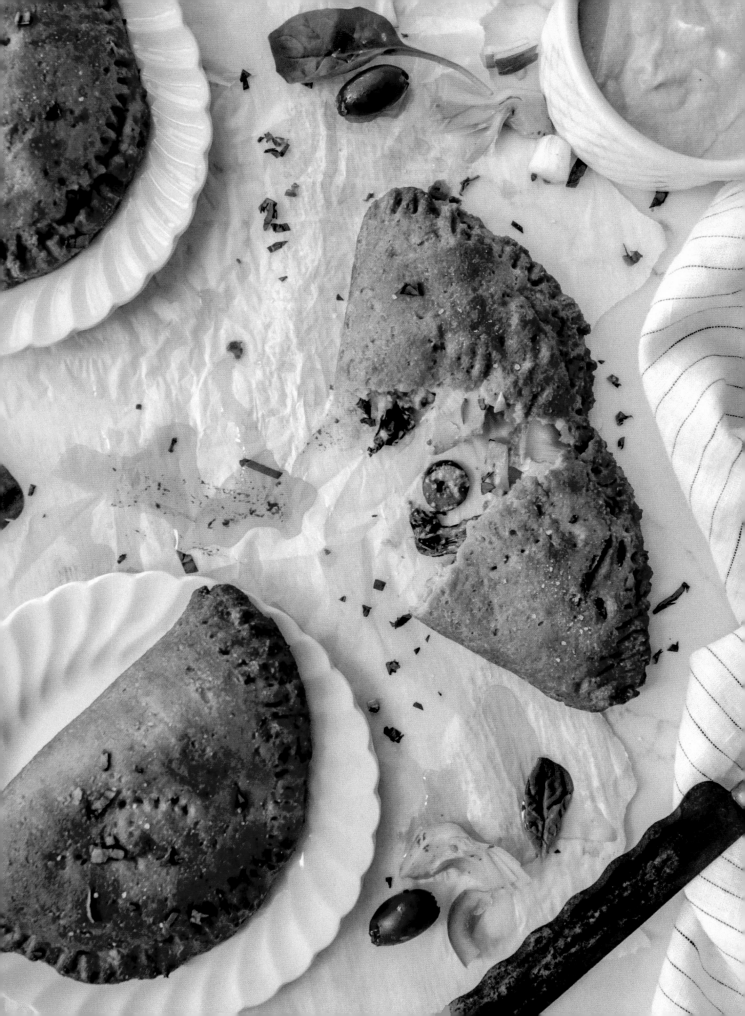

Mediterranean Clazones

prep: *25 min*   **bake:** *30-35 min*   **cool:** *20 min*   **serves:** *5 medium calzones*

Dough dry ingredients
- 168g *(1½ cups)* almond flour
- 34g *(1/4 cup)* coconut flour
- 44g *(1/4 cup)* psyllium husk powder
- 1 teaspoon baking soda
- 1 teaspoon baking powder
- 2 teaspoons instant yeast
- 2 teaspoons sea salt

Dough wet ingredients:
- 2 free-run eggs *room temp*
- 3 egg whites *room temp*
- 118mL *(1/2 cup)* warm water
- 15mL *(1 tablespoon)* honey *activates yeast*
- 30mL *(2 tablespoons)* olive oil
- 30mL *(2 tablespoons)* apple cider vinegar

Filling ingredients:
- 80mL *(1/3 cup)* tomato sauce *organic*
- 175mL *(3/4 cup)* cashew cheese sauce
  the recipe is found on page 235
- 56g *(1/3 cup)* artichokes *chopped*
- 55g *(1/3 cup)* kalamata olives *sliced*
- 50g *(1/3 cup)* red onion *sliced*
- 55g *(1/3 cup)* green bell pepper *chopped*
- 1 garlic clove *minced*
- 1 teaspoon dried basil
- 1 teaspoon dried oregano
- 1/2 teaspoon cayenne pepper

Instructions
1. **Preheat oven to 350°F/180°C.** Prep a baking sheet with parchment paper and set it aside.
2. In a medium bowl, measure all dry ingredients, whisk together and set aside.
3. In a separate medium bowl, add all wet ingredients, whisk together, and pour the entire wet ingredients onto the dry ingredients in a separate medium bowl. Using a rubber spatula, mix until well incorporated.
4. Split the dough into five pieces *(you can weigh it on a food scale to ensure the same size, or you can eye it).*
5. *Roll the dough in your hand,* and place each piece of the dough on the prepared parchment paper on a flat surface. With your hands, slightly press down the dough.
6. Using a rolling pin and plastic wrap, place plastic wrap over the dough, and start rolling the dough to make a flat, even circle, about 8-inches.
7. Once each dough round is rolled out, carefully transfer the dough to prepped pans.
8. **Filling:** Add tomato sauce and mix fresh herbs, spices, garlic, salt, and pepper in a small bowl.
9. Add all the ingredients to one side of the dough to assemble the calzone.
10. Chop artichokes, olives, red onion, and bell peppers.
11. Add 2 tablespoons of cashew on one side, spreading the centre, adding 1 tablespoon of tomato sauce, and 1 tablespoon of each chopped veggie.
12. Gently fold the top half *(the half with nothing)* on top of the filled half. Using your fingers, pinch Calzone closed. Slash the top with two small holes to allow airflow inside.
13. **Bake calzones for 25-35min at 350°F/180°C.**
14. Let them cool down for about 10-min. Once calzones are cooled, enjoy them right away!
15. Store in an air-tight container in the fridge for up to four to five days or in the freezer for two months.

Note

- **Add/sub anything you desire in this recipe. You can even fill it with your favourite meat to make it a complete meal.**

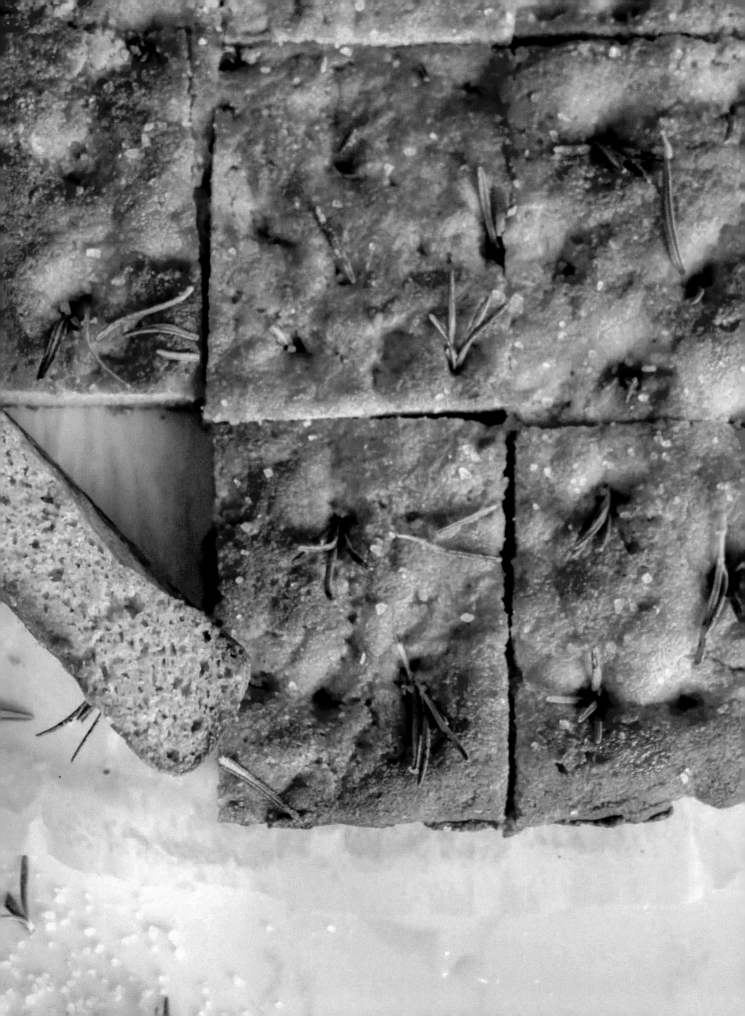

Garlic Focaccia Bread

prep: *15 min*   **bake:** *25-25 min*   **cool:** *30 min*   **serves:** *9 large pieces*

Focaccia bread makes an excellent side for dinner, or even toast is and makes an Italian salami sandwich, YUM!

Dry ingredients
- 168g *(1½ cups)* almond flour
- 68g *(1/2 cup)* coconut flour
- 44g *(1/4 cup)* psyllium husk powder
- 56g *(1/2 cup)* organic collagen *grass-fed*
- 2 garlic cloves *minced*
- 1 teaspoon baking soda
- 1 teaspoon baking powder
- 2 teaspoons instant yeast
- 2 teaspoons sea salt

Wet ingredients:
- 4 free-run eggs *room temp*
- 3 egg whites *room temp*
- 118mL *(1/2 cup)* warm water
- 56mL *(1/4 cup)* olive oil *extra virgin*
- 15mL *(1 tablespoon)* honey *activates yeast*
- 118mL *(1/2 cup)* apple cider vinegar

Garnish:
- 1-2 stems of fresh rosemary
- 30mL *(2 tablespoons)* olive oil *extra virgin*
- flaky sea salt

Instructions

1. Preheat oven to 350°F/180°C, and prep an 8x8-inch pan with parchment paper.
2. In a medium bowl, measure all dry ingredients, whisk together and set aside.
3. In a separate medium bowl, add all wet ingredients, whisk together, and pour the entire wet ingredients onto the dry ingredients in a separate medium bowl. Using a rubber spatula, mix until well incorporated.
4. The dough should form a ball of dough.
5. Place focaccia dough in the repaired pan, and flatten/shape the dough to evenly fill the pan.
6. **Garnish:** Using your fingertips, poke holes over the entire surface of the dough. Drizzle with olive oil, cut rosemary stems into small pieces and insert them into the holes.
7. Bake the focaccia bread for 25-35 minutes or until lightly golden brown on top.
8. Cool focaccia bread in the pan for about 10min, and then remove the focaccia and let it completely cool on a cooling rack for 35minutes.
9. Sprinkle flaky sea salt on top, and slice the focaccia bread into 9 large squares.
10. Store in a durable zip-lock bag in the fridge for up to two weeks or in the freezer for two months.

Note

- **Try to serve this focaccia bread with balsamic vinegar and olive oil for dipping on a small side plate.**

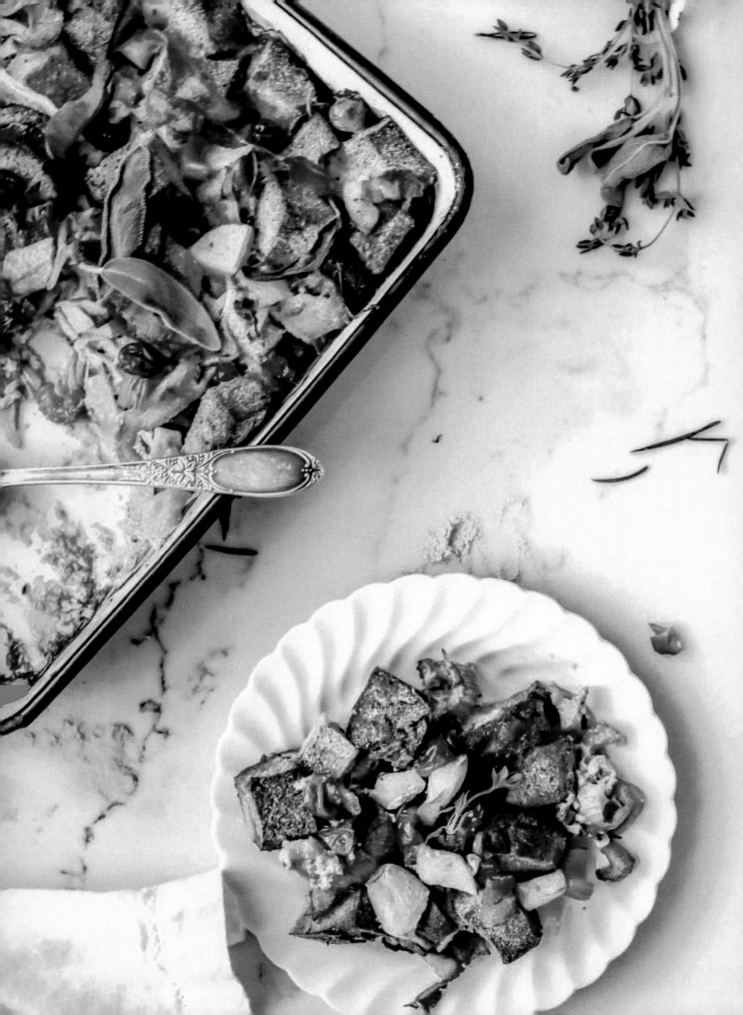

Apple Cranberry Bacon Stuffing

prep: *25 min*   **bake:** *45-50 min*   **cool:** *10 min*   **serves:** *9-12 servings*

Christmas and Thanksgiving cannot be celebrated without the tradition of stuffing served around the table. This Apple Cranberry Bacon Stuffing is packed with endless flavours, from tart, rich, savoury and sweet.

Stuffing Ingredients

- 1 loaf of artisan sandwich bread *cubbed*
  the recipe is found on page 237
- 375mL *(1½ cups)* chicken bone broth *organic*
- 1 granny smith apple *chopped*
- 118g *(1/2 cup)* grass-fed butter
  sub for avocado oil to make it **DF**
- 2 free-run eggs
- 5 slices of wild boar bacon
- 1 cup fresh cranberries
- 1 medium white onion *chopped*
- 4 stalks of celery *organic*
- 2 tablespoons fresh parsley
- 1 tablespoon fresh rosemary
- 1 tablespoon fresh sage
- 1 tablespoon fresh thyme
- 2 teaspoons sea salt
- 1 teaspoon black pepper

Instructions

1. Preheat oven to 375°F/190°C.
2. In a large skillet, turn on the stove element to medium heat, add the grass-fed butter and allow it to melt; add the onions and celery along with a pinch of salt and sauté for about 5 to 7 minutes or starts to become translucent.
3. In a large bowl, mix bread cubes, peeled & chopped apples, cranberries, fresh herbs and seasonings *(salt & pepper)*, along with the cooked onions & celery.
4. Next, mix the chicken bone broth in the large bowl with the stuffing until combined.
5. Pour the stuffing into a medium/large casserole baking dish.
6. Chop up six slices of wild boar bacon & spread chopped bacon all over the top of the stuffing so the fat melts down into the stuffing to create a fantastic flavour!
7. Cover with foil and bake for 20 minutes; remove foil and bake for another 30 minutes or until the top is lightly golden brown and the bacon is nice and crispy!
8. Serve at Christmas dinner or Thanksgiving dinner!
9. Store in an air-tight container in the fridge for up to four to five days or in the freezer for two months.

Note

- There are no fundamental rules when it comes to stuffing, so add anything you love. I love adding pecans in this recipe as they add an extra crunch.

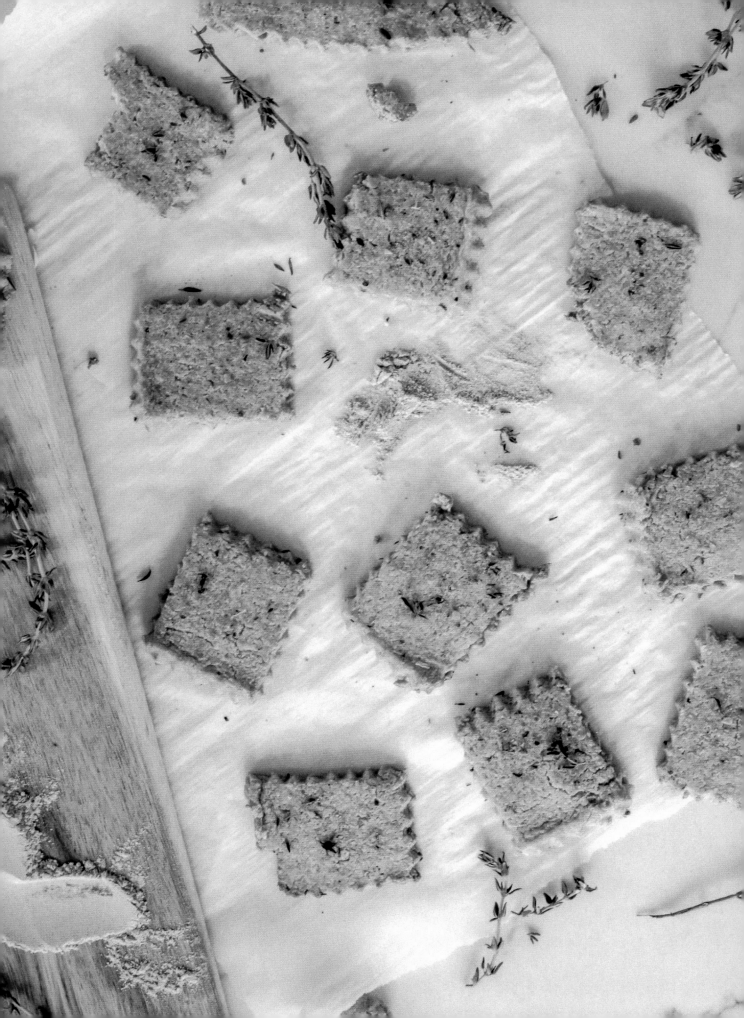

Veggie & Herb Crackers

prep: *25 min*   **bake:** *8-10 min*   **cool:** *15 min*   **serves:** *2-3 dozen*

Crackers are very simple to make, and they taste absolutely amazing! Impress your guest and have these Veggie & Herb Crackers out as an API with come homemade cashew cheese; I am sure their won't be any leftovers.

Dry ingredients
- 224g *(2 cups)* almond flour
- 2 tablespoons veggie broth powder *organic*
- 45g *(1/2 cup)* nutritional yeast
- 1 teaspoon garlic powder
- 1 teaspoon dried parsley
- 1 teaspoon dried rosemary
- 1 teaspoon dried sage
- 1 teaspoon dried thyme
- 2 teaspoons sea salt
- 1 teaspoon black pepper

Wet ingredients:
- 2 free-run eggs *room temp*
- 82g *(1/3 cup)* grass-fed butter *melted sub for palm shortening to make* **DF**
- 15mL *(1 tablespoon)* apple cider vinegar

Garnish:
- flaky sea salt

Instructions

1. **Preheat oven to 350°F/180°C.** Prep a baking/cookie sheet with parchment paper.
2. Melt butter in a small pot on low heat; let it simmer, add the veggie broth, mix it until well incorporated, and then turn off the heat. Set aside to cool while you mix the flour.
3. In a small bowl, whisk the eggs.
4. Add all the dry ingredients to a medium bowl and whisk thoroughly. Pour in the butter/veggie broth mixture and mix until evenly distributed *(I use my hands!)*.
5. Add in the whisked eggs and continue to knead until it forms into a ball. Cover in cling film and place in the freezer for 5 minutes to solidify the butter.
6. Roll out the dough between two sheets of parchment paper.
7. Trim to desired cracker size and separate gently. The dough is fragile, so I split the pieces by running a knife underneath and place on the baking sheet.
8. **Garnish:** Sprinkle the flaky sea salt.
9. Bake the veggie herb crackers for 8-12 minutes in the oven at 350°F/180°C or until lightly golden *(time will depend on size and thickness)*. And to make them extra crisp!
10. Cool the crackers for about 15min before serving.
11. Enjoy these with some creamy **cashew cheese on page 235.**
12. Store in an air-tight container for up to three weeks.

Note
- **Try any flavour cracker you like. One of my favourites is adding sesame oil, garlic, and sesame seeds on top.**

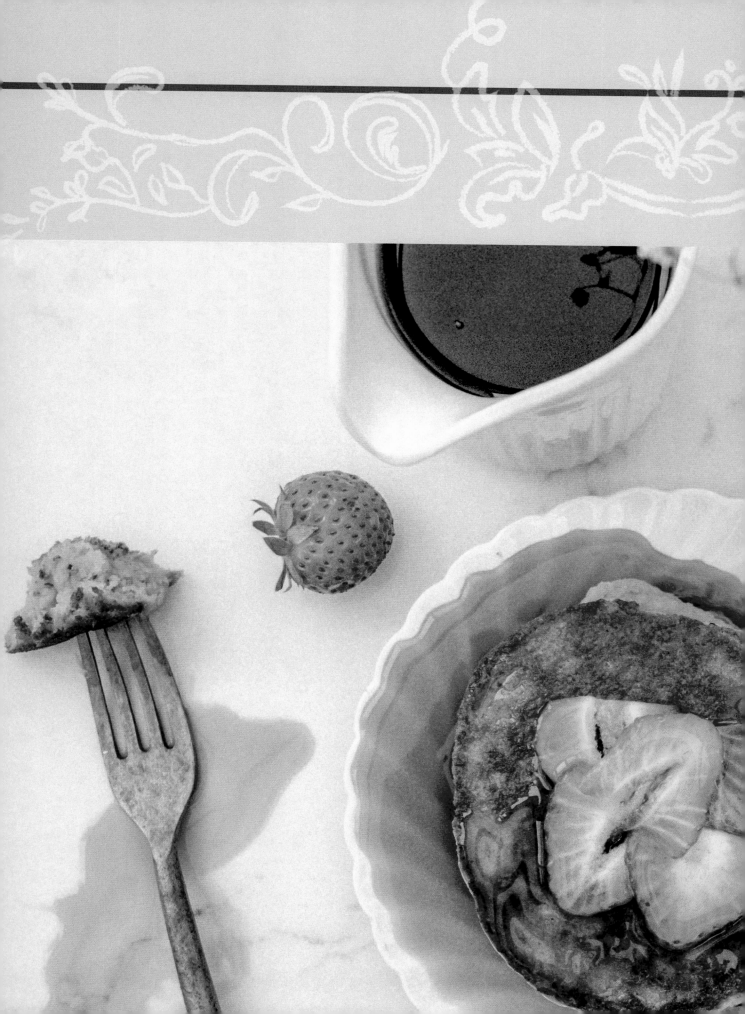

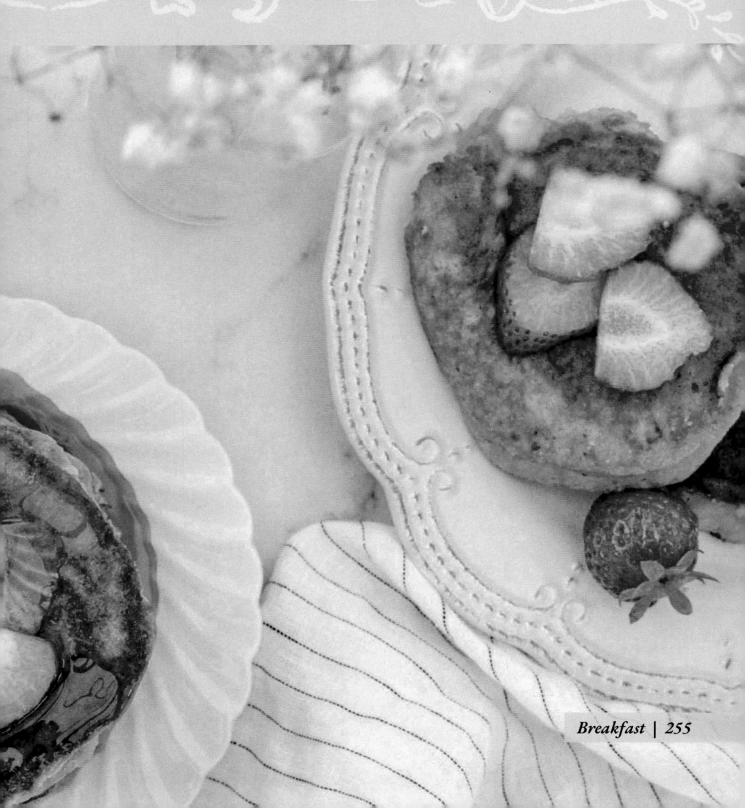

Chapter Thirteen
BREAKFAST

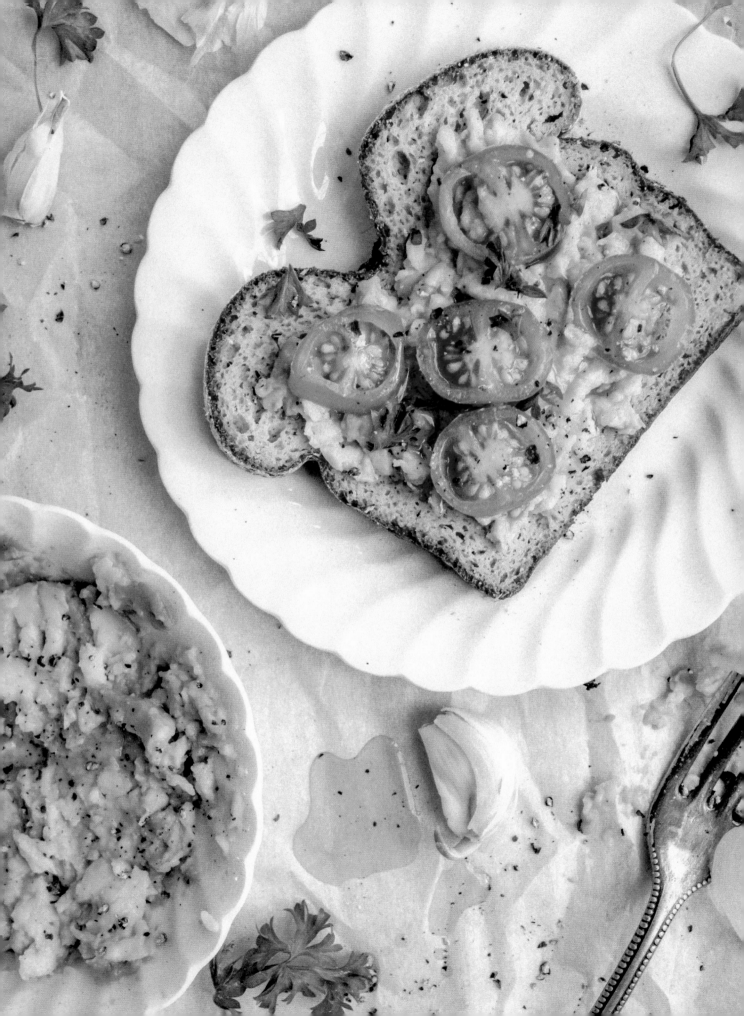

Avocado Toast - *the right way*

prep: *15 min*   **cook:** *8 min*   **cool:** *10 min*   **serves:** *2 toasts*

*Avocado is defiantly the new radge, and I totally understand why! It's because it's simple, delicious and satisfying. Yet, my avocado toast is called **"the right way"** because having this for breakfast will carry you along to lunchtime without the crash/ cravings and hunger pains due to using my **Artisan Sandwich Bread** due to its high amounts of collagen proteins, high fibre and healthy fats.*

Ingredients

- 2 slices artisan sandwich bread
  the recipe is found on page 237
- 1 whole ripe avocado *mashed*
- 6 cherry tomatoes *sliced thin*
- 1 fresh parsley *chopped fine*
- 1 clove garlic *minced*
- 2 teaspoons Dijon mustard *optional*
- 1/8 teaspoon sea salt
- 1/2 teaspoon black pepper

Instructions

1. Add ripe avocado, Dijon mustard, minced garlic, sea salt and pepper in a small bowl.
2. Using a large fork, mash as much as you like to create a smooth mash or a chunky mash.
3. Toast bread to your liking.
4. Slice cherry tomatoes thinly, chop fresh parsley finely and set aside.
5. Add mashed avocado mash to the toast, and spread evenly to the edges.
6. Top with tomatoes and parsley, and add extra salt and pepper if needed.
7. Enjoy this simple *Avocado Toast the right way* to satisfy and fuel yourself for a fruitful day!

Note

- **Of course, you can add anything you dearly love to your avocado toast. Cucumbers, jalapenös, sprouts, banana peppers, you name it!**

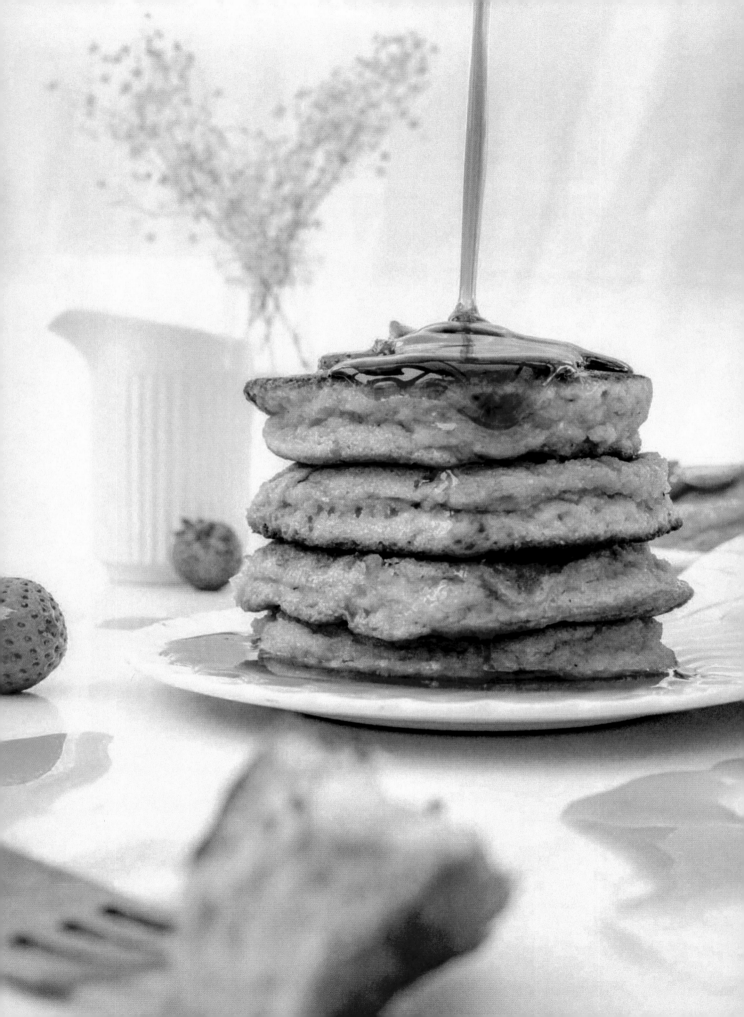

Fluffy Perfect Pancakes

prep: *10 min*　**cook:** *15 min*　**cool:** *5 min*　**serves:** *8 medium pancakes*

*Make these delicious **Fluffy Perfect Pancakes** in a pinch, and have yourself a perfectly balanced breakfast! Saturday morning, my hubby and I have a tradition to make these pancakes while enjoying a coffee in the presence of each other, and we can't wait to carry on this enjoyable little tradition as our family grows.*

Dry ingredients

- 112g *(1 cup)* almond flour
- 34g *(1/4 cup)* coconut flour
- 11g *(1 tablespoon)* psyllium husk powder
- 56g *(1/2 cup)* organic collagen *grass-fed*
- 51g *(1/4 cup)* sweetener
  monk fruit, erythritol, xylitol
- 1 teaspoon baking soda
- 1 teaspoon baking powder
- 1/2 teaspoon sea salt

Wet ingredients:

- 2 free-run eggs *room temp*
- 177mL *(3/4 cup)* coconut milk *full fat*
- 30mL *(2 tablespoons)* apple cider vinegar

Toppings:

- fresh berries of choice
- maple syrup *keto & paleo approved*
- nut butter of choice
  the recipe is found on page 229
- coconut whipped cream
  the recipe is found on page 189

Instructions

1. In a medium bowl, measure all dry ingredients, whisk together and set aside.
2. Add coconut milk *(full-fat from a can) in a small bowl* and slightly heat up in the microwave for 20-30sec.
3. Add the remainder of the wet ingredients, whisk together, and pour onto the dry ingredients.
4. Using a whisk, mix until well incorporated.
5. The pancake batter should be on the more liquid side.
6. In a non-stick large frying pan, on medium/high heat, add grass-fed butter *(or avocado oil if dairy-free)* to grease the pan.
7. Using a large cookie scoop *(5.4 Tbsp/ 81 ml/ 2.7 oz)*, spoon 3-4 heaping *(making 3-4 pancakes at a time)* scoops on the hot frying pan.
8. Once you see tiny bubbles form on the top of the pancakes, flip them imminently.
9. Cook the other side for about 2 minutes and transfer it onto a plate.
10. Add butter or oil to the pan, and repeat until you have no more pancake batter left.
11. **Topping:** Serve with any toppings you desire. I love fresh berries, almond butter and coconut whipped cream. YUM!
12. Store leftover pancakes in an air-tight container in the fridge for four to five days.

Note

- **Make sure coconut milk is full fat and warmed up for creating the perfect fluffy pancakes.**

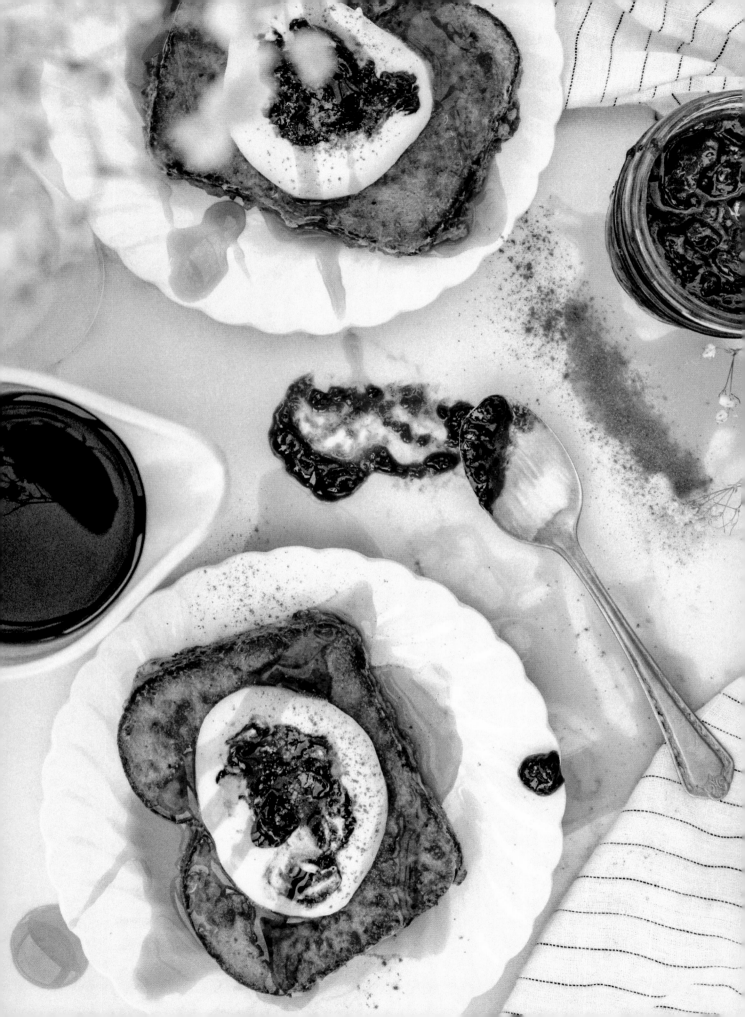

Cinnamon French Toast

prep: *10 min* **cook:** *15 min* **cool:** *5 min* **serves:** *6 slices*

*This recipe works so well with my **Artisan Sandwhich Bread** since it it a denser bread, and is able to soak up all that creamy goodness to create a fabulous french toast breakfast.*

French toast ingredients

- 1/2 loaf of artisan sandwich bread *sliced thick* *the recipe is found on page 237*
- 118mL *(1/2 cup)* coconut milk *full fat*
- 3 free-run eggs *room temp*
- 103g *(1/2 cup)* sweetener
  monk fruit, erythritol, xylitol
- 1 teaspoon cinnamon
- 1/2 teaspoon sea salt

Toppings:

- berry jams
  the recipe is found on page 193
- maple syrup *keto & paleo approved*
- nut butter of choice
  the recipe is found on page 229
- coconut whipped cream
  the recipe is found on page 189

Instructions

1. Cut bread about 1 inch thick.
2. Add coconut milk *(full-fat from a can) in a small bowl* and slightly heat up in the microwave for 20-30sec.
3. Add the eggs, sweetener, vanilla, cinnamon and sea salt; mix until well incorporated using a whisk.
4. Pour the liquid into an 8x8-inch pan, and place the thick-cut bread into the creamy egg mixture. Use your finger to press the creamy liquid into the bread.
5. Let it soak on each side in the creamy liquid for at least 5 minutes.
6. As the french toast is soaking, turn a non-stick large frying pan on medium heat. Add grass-fed butter *(or avocado oil if dairy-free)* to grease the pan.
7. As the soaked french toast into the hot greased pan, let the first side cook for about 4 minutes, and once you flip the french toast, cook the other side for an additional 2-3 minutes.
8. Transfer the french toast onto a plate, add more butter or oil to the pan, and repeat until all your soaked bread has been fried.
9. Topping: Serve with any toppings you desire. I love blueberry jam and coconut whipped cream. YUM!
10. Store leftover french toast in an air-tight container in the fridge for three to four days.

Note

- **Make sure coconut milk is full fat and warmed up so that it can be easily absorbed into the bread.**

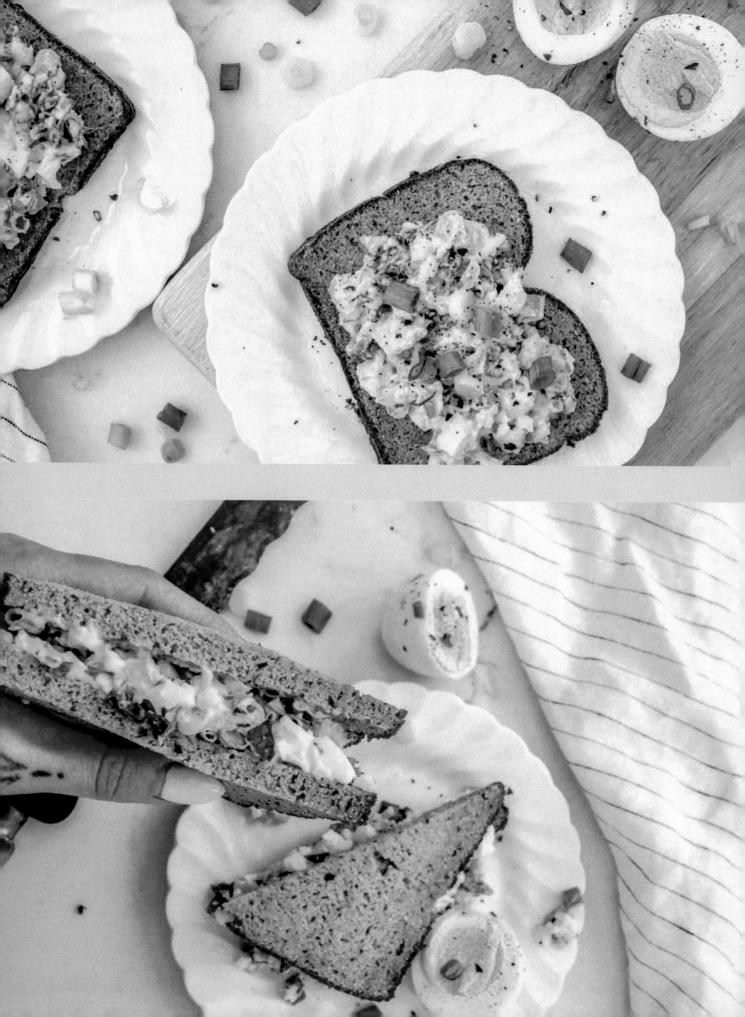

Chive Egg Salad Sandwich

prep: *15 min*   **cook:** *8 min*   **cool:** *10 min*   **serves:** *2 sandwiches*

*This recipe works so well with my **Artisan Sandwich Bread** since it it a denser bread, and is able to soak up all that creamy goodness to create a fabulous french toast breakfast.*

Dry Ingredients

- 4 slices artisan sandwich bread
  the recipe is found on page 237
- 4 free-run eggs *soft boiled*
- 2 green chives/onions *chopped fine*
- 1/2 English cucumber *chopped fine*
- 1 teaspoon garlic powder
- 1/2 teaspoon sea salt
- 1/2 teaspoon black pepper

Mayo ingredients:

- 1 free-run egg *room temp*
- 240mL *(1 cup)* avocado oil
- 15mL *(1 tablespoon)* Dijon mustard
- 15mL *(1 tablespoon)* apple cider vinager
- 1/2 teaspoon sea salt
- 1/2 teaspoon black pepper

Instructions

1. In a small pot, bring to a boil.
2. Add 4 eggs *(best to use room temperature)* to the boiling water, and boil for 7-8 minutes.
3. Immediately, add the boiled eggs into a small bowl with cold water and ice cubes.
4. As the eggs are cooling, prep the avocado mayo.
5. **Mayo:** Crack one whole egg into the bottom of a tall large glass jar with a wide-mouth glass jar. *(Use anything that will be big enough for an immersion blender to fit. But do not use a bowl.)*
6. Add the rest of the mayo ingredients to the egg, try not to break the egg, and make sure you don't whisk or stir either. Pour the avocado oil on top.
7. Carefully submerge the immersion blender into the bottom of the jar/glass, and place it right where the egg is. Blend on low power for about 15-20 seconds without moving from where the egg was.
8. Blend until you see that most of the mayo has turned white and pail.
9. Next, slowly move the blender while blending upward without lifting the blender out into the air. Once you reach the top of the oil, slowly move back down to the bottom.
10. Repeat this motion in step 9 until the mayonnaise forms a rich, creamy texture.
11. Chop green chives and cucumbers, and add them into a small bowl.
12. Crack and peel eggs; try peeling the eggs under cold running water for easy shell removal.
13. Add boiled eggs, four tablespoons of mayo, garlic, salt and pepper into the bowl with the chives and cucumber —Mash all together with a fork.
14. Slightly toast bread, build an open face or have a sandwich, and enjoy your creamy, delicious Chive Egg Salad Sandwiches!

Note

- **Store the homemade avocado mayonnaise in an air-tight container/jar in the refrigerator for up to two months.**

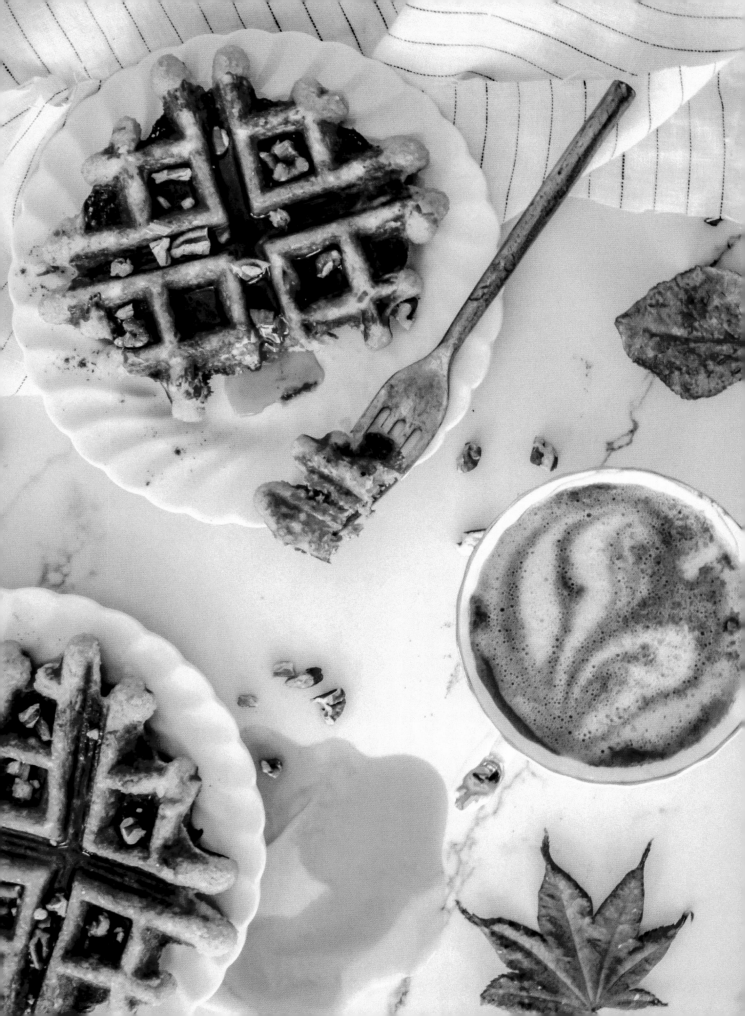

Pumpkin Pie Waffles

prep: *10 min*   **cook:** *15 min*   **cool:** *5 min*   **serves:** *8 medium waffles*

Make these Pumpkin Pie Waffles on a crisp autumn morning with a coffee, and bring that festive joy to your spirit and soul.

Dry ingredients

- 140g *(1¼ cups)* almond flour
- 34g *(1/4 cup)* coconut flour
- 11g *(1 tablespoon)* psyllium husk powder
- 56g *(1/2 cup)* organic collagen *grass-fed*
- 102g *(1/2 cup)* sweetener
   monk fruit, erythritol, xylitol
- 1 teaspoon baking soda
- 1 teaspoon baking powder
- 1/2 teaspoon sea salt

Wet ingredients:

- 2 free-run eggs *room temp*
- 56mL *(1/4 cup)* pumpkin purée *unsweet*
- 118mL *(1/2 cup)* coconut milk *full fat*
- 30mL *(2 tablespoons)* apple cider vinegar

Toppings:

- maple syrup *keto & paleo approved*
- nut butter of choice
   the recipe is found on page 229
- coconut whipped cream
   the recipe is found on page 189

Instructions

1. **Preheat the waffle maker,** and add grass-fed butter *(or avocado/coconut oil if dairy-free)* to grease the pan.
2. In a medium bowl, measure all dry ingredients, whisk together and set aside.
3. Add coconut milk *(full-fat from a can)* in a small bowl and slightly heat up in the microwave for 20-30sec.
4. Add the remainder of the wet ingredients, whisk together, and pour onto the dry ingredients.
5. Using a whisk, mix until well incorporated.
6. Grease the waffle maker with butter or avocado oil.
7. Using a large cookie scoop *(5.4 Tbsp/ 81 ml/ 2.7 oz)*, scoop one heaping spoon into the centre of each waffle grid.
8. Cook waffles for 5-6 minutes and transfers them onto a plate.
9. Add butter or oil to the waffle maker, and repeat until you have no more waffle batter left.
10. **Topping:** Serve with any toppings you desire. My favourite is coconut whipped cream, pecan butter and sugar-free maple syrup.
11. Store leftover french toast in an air-tight container in the fridge for four to five days.

Note

- Be creative; add apple sauce or banana to switch up the flavour from the pumpkin purée.
- If you don't have pumpkin spice, use:
1 teaspoon cinnamon
1/2 teaspoon ginger
1/8 teaspoon cloves
1/8 teaspoon nutmeg

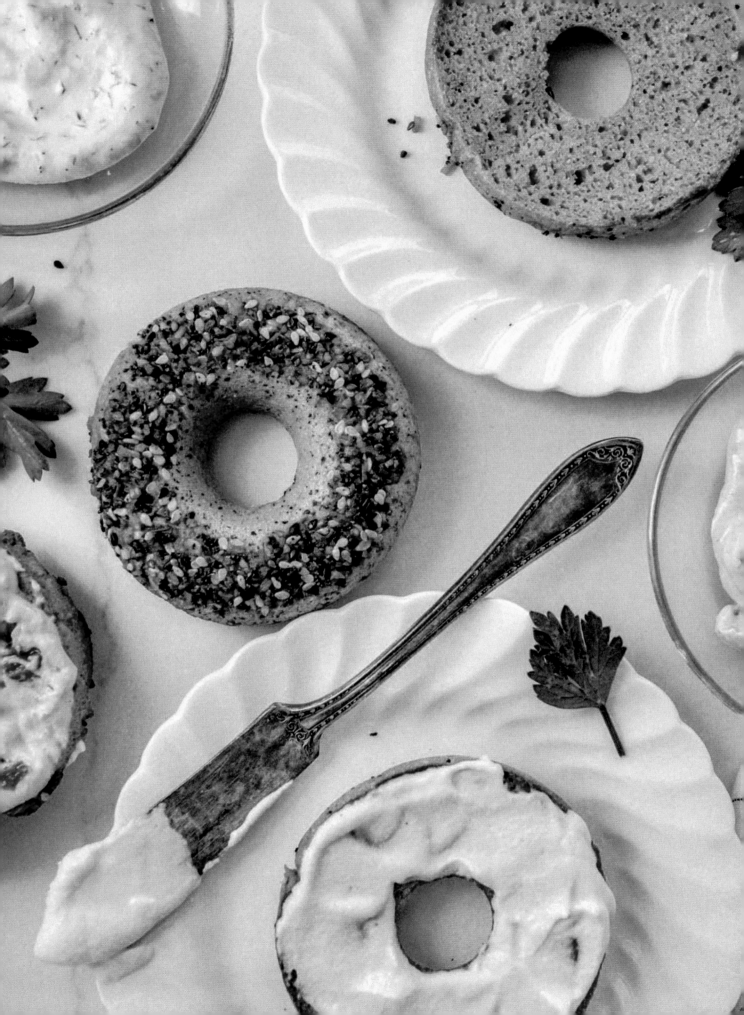

Everything Bagels

prep: *20 min*   **bake:** *20-25 min*   **cool:** *30 min*   **serves:** *19 medium bagels*

*Bread was one of the hardest things to give up when I went on a keto/paleo diet. It became a quest I wouldn't give up until I created a bread that I loved! My **Artisan Sandwich Bread** reminds me of a heavier rye sourdough bread. My favourite way to eat this bread is making avocado toast on-page.*

Dry ingredients
- 140g *(1¼ cups)* almond flour
- 68g *(1/2 cup)* coconut flour
- 42g *(1/4 cup)* arrowroot flour
- 44g *(1/4 cup)* psyllium husk powder
- 56g *(1/2 cup)* organic collagen *grass-fed*
- 20g *(2 tablespoons)* flaxseed meal
- 1 teaspoon baking soda
- 1 teaspoon baking powder
- 2 teaspoons instant yeast
- 2 teaspoons sea salt

Wet ingredients:
- 4 free-run eggs *room temp*
- 3 egg whites *room temp*
- 118mL *(1/2 cup)* warm water
- 56mL *(1/4 cup)* avocado oil
- 15mL *(1 tablespoon)* honey *activates yeast*
- 118mL *(1/2 cup)* apple cider vinegar

Everything Bagel Seasoning:
- 2 tablespoons poppy seeds
- 1 tablespoon white sesame seeds
- 1 tablespoon black sesame seeds
- 1 tablespoon dried minced garlic
- 1 tablespoon dried minced onion
- 2 teaspoons flaky sea salt

Instructions
1. Preheat oven to 350°F/180°C
2. Measure all dry ingredients, whisk them together, and set aside
3. In a medium bowl, measure all dry ingredients, whisk together and set aside.
4. In a separate medium bowl, add all wet ingredients, whisk together, and pour the entire wet ingredients onto the dry ingredients in a separate medium bowl. Using a rubber spatula, mix until well incorporated.
5. Using a rubber spatula, scrape donut dough around the bowl, and use a large cookie scoop to transfer the dough into a piping bag *(you can also you a big ziplock bag)*.
6. Use a silicone donut baking pan with avocado oil to ensure no stick.
7. **Bagle seasoning:** Mix together all the *Everything Bagel Seasoning in a small bowl,* and evenly sprinkle a heaping tablespoon into each donut hole.
8. Cut the bottom of the piping bag & squeeze out the dough just enough to fill halfway up. The bagels are about halfway to the rim of the donut pan.
9. Bake for 20-25 minutes at 350°F/180°C
10. Once the bagels are out of the oven, wait about 10 minutes before flipping them over on a cooling rack. Let the donut cool for an additional 20 minutes.
11. Slice bagels in half with a bread knife, toast, and enjoy some cashew cream cheese **(the recipe is on page 235)** or avocado!
12. Store in a durable zip-lock bag in the fridge for up to two weeks or in the freezer for two months.

Note

- **Arrowroot** *(or tapioca)* **flour is higher in carbs; however, it creates a perfect stretchy texture in bagels.**

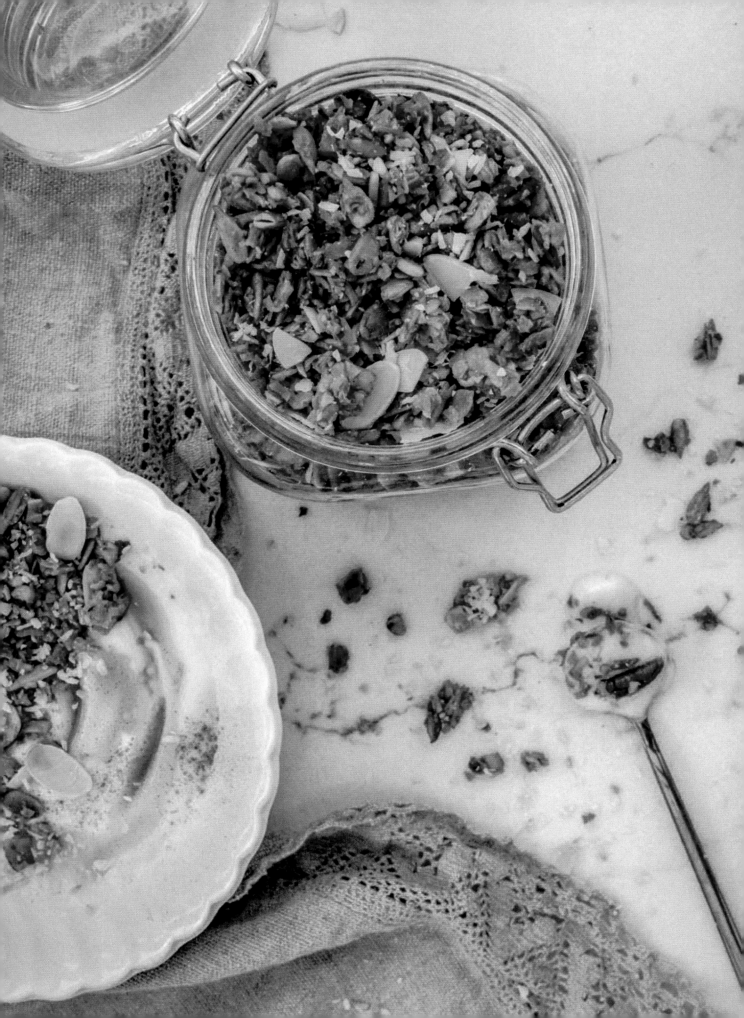

Crunchy Collagen Granola

prep: *20min*　**cook:** *50-60 min*　**cool:** *2 hours*　**serves:** *25 servings*

When I ditched the sugar, grains and went low-carb, I thought I would also have to say goodbye to my love for granola. I tried several recipes and finally created one I adored due to its taste, texture and upgraded with my favourite protein, collagen!

Nut ingredients

- 168g *(2 cups)* coconut flakes *unsweetened*
- 120g *(1 cup)* pumpkin seeds
- 115g *(1/2 cup)* flax seeds
- 160g *(1 cup)* hemp hearts *seeds*
- 220g *(1 1/2 cups)* almond slices
- 220g *(2 cups)* pecans halves
- 46g *(1/2 cup)* organic collagen *grass-fed*
- 205g *(1 cup)* sweetener
  - **xylitol** *works best for this recipe*
- 80g *(1/2 cup)* raisins *optional if on paleo*
- 2 teaspoons cinnamon
- 1 teaspoon sea salt

Wet ingredients

- 30g *(2 tablespoons)* coconut oil *melted*
- 15mL *(1 tablespoon)* blackstrap molasses
- 4 egg whites *room temp*
- 10mL *(2 teaspoons)* pure vanilla extract

Instructions

1. **Preheat oven to 250°F/120°C.** Prep two cookie sheets with parchment paper.
2. On one cookie sheet, toast coconut flakes, flax seeds and hemp hearts for 5-6 minutes.
3. Set aside the other cookie sheet, and toast almonds, pecans, and pumpkin seeds for 8-9 minutes.
4. Mix all dry ingredients (*not the collagen that will go into the wet ingredients*) into a medium bowl, including the toasted nuts, seeds, raisins, cinnamon and sea salt, whisk until combined and set aside.
5. Melt the coconut oil and add the egg whites, molasses, collagen, and vanilla in a stand mixer bowl with a whisk attachment. Whip egg whites mixture until it becomes fluffy. You may also use an electric hand mixer.
6. Add all the dry ingredients to the stand mixer bowl, and switch to a paddle/beater blade attachment.
7. Turn on the mixer to flow at medium speed until well incorporated.
8. Add the sticky wet granola mixture to the two baking sheets. Spread the granola evenly amongst the two cookie sheets.
9. Bake for 50-60 minutes until the granola hardens, checking every 15 minutes. Allow it to cool to room temperature.
10. Break the granola into chunks and store it in an airtight container/jar for two to three weeks.
11. Serve with some creamy Coconut Collagen Yogurt (**the recipe is on page 231**), and you have a high-protein, low-carb breakfast.

Note

- **After the granola is done baking, it will continue to get harder/crunchier while cooling.**
- **The best sweetener to create the desired crunch is xylitol.**

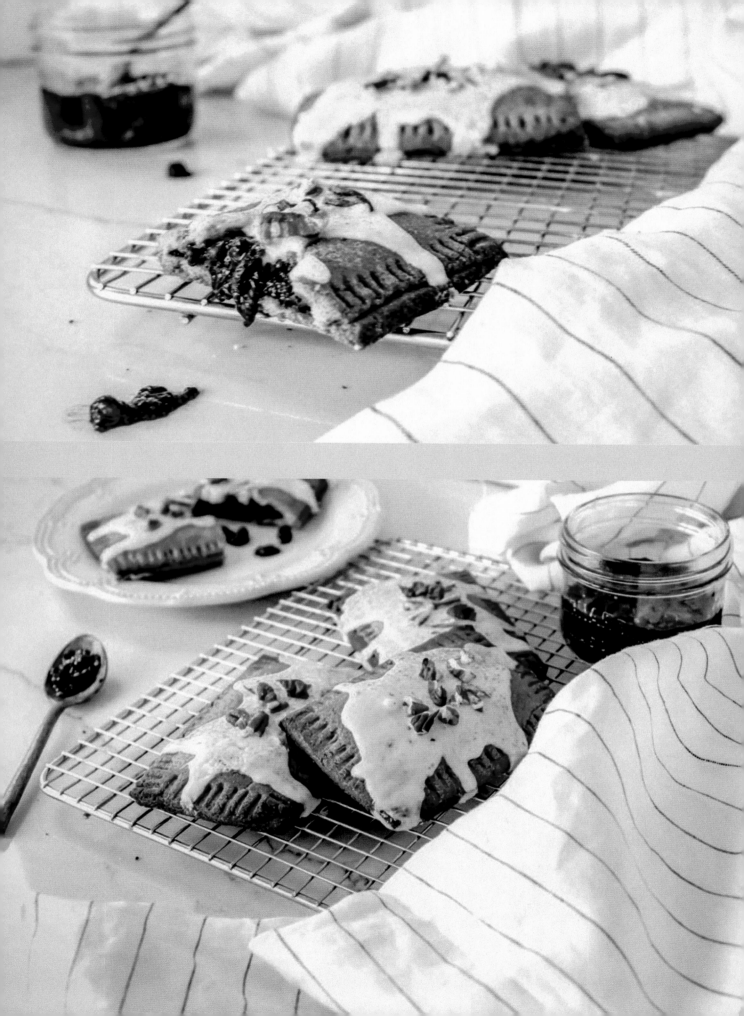

Blueberry Spiced Pop Tarts

prep: *15 min*　**bake:** *10-12 min*　**cool:** *5-10 min*　**serves:** *12 cookies*

Making pop tarts on the weekend fwith your kiddo's always bring a simple childlike joy to the breakfast table.

Crust ingredients

- 112g *(1 cup)* almond flour
- 46g *(1/3 cup)* coconut flour
- 11g *(1 tablespoon)* psyllium husk powder
- 52g *(1/4 cup)* sweetener
    - *monk fruit, erythritol, xylitol*
- 57g *(1/4 cup)* grass-fed butter *chilled*
    - *sub for palm shortening to make* **DF**
- 1 free-run egg *room temp*
- 15mL *(1 tablespoon)* apple cider vinegar
- 1 teaspoon baking soda
- 1 teaspoon sea salt

Filling ingredients:

- 280g *(1 cup)* blueberry jam
    - *recipe on page* **193**

Use any flavour of jam you desire!

Garnish/Glaze

- 60g *(1/2 cup)* powdered sweetener
    - *monk fruit, erythritol, xylitol*
- 30mL *(12 tablespoons)* coconut milk *full fat*
- 1/2 teaspoon cinnamon

Instructions

1. **Crust:** Mix all dry crust ingredients into a bowl, and whisk together.
2. Add chilled cubes of butter & one egg; using your hand, mix the crust dough the old-fashioned way, or use a stand mixer. Mix/knead until it forms a ball.
3. Place dough onto a piece of saran wrap, and shape it into a round sausage shape.
4. Refrigerate for at least 30 min; You can, alternatively, freeze the pie crust at this point and thaw it out as needed *(just as a regular pie crust!).*
5. As your crust dough is hardening in the fridge, ensure the blueberry jam *(or any jam of choice)* is pre-made.
6. Take the dough out of the fridge, and cut it in half, using the first half for the bottom of pop tarts.
7. Roll out the first half of the dough between 2 pieces of wax/parchment paper.
8. Roll the dough out in a long horizontal shape, 13 inches by 5-6 inches.
9. Using a sharp knife, cut the dough's center directly down, then cut the haves in half, leaving you with 4 even rectangular pastry crusts. Cut around the edges to clean them up.
10. Transfer onto prepared parchment pan.
11. **Filling:** Add 2 tablespoons of jam inside the rectangular pastry.
12. Repeat the steps for the second half of the dough.
13. Carefully place the top of the pop tarts and seal the edges shut using a fork.
14. With a sharp knife, cut 3 angled slights on top of the pop tart to allow for breathing.
15. Once pop it in the freezer for 10-15 minutes before baking *(as it will help to keep its shape better and come out flakier).*
16. Bake at 350°F/180°C for 30 minutes.
17. **Garnish:** In a small bowl, add powdered sweetener, full-fat coconut cream, vanilla extract and cinnamon,
18. Cool pop tarts for 10 minutes before adding the glaze. Dust with some cinnamon if you like, and add a few pieces of chopped toasted pecan pieces on top!
19. Store leftover pop tarts in an air-tight container in the fridge for 5-6 days, or freeze for up to 2 months.

Note

- The crust is more fragile than regular gluten pie crust, so you need to work quickly and in a cooler atmosphere, if possible.
- You can patch up any cracks by simply pinching the dough together.

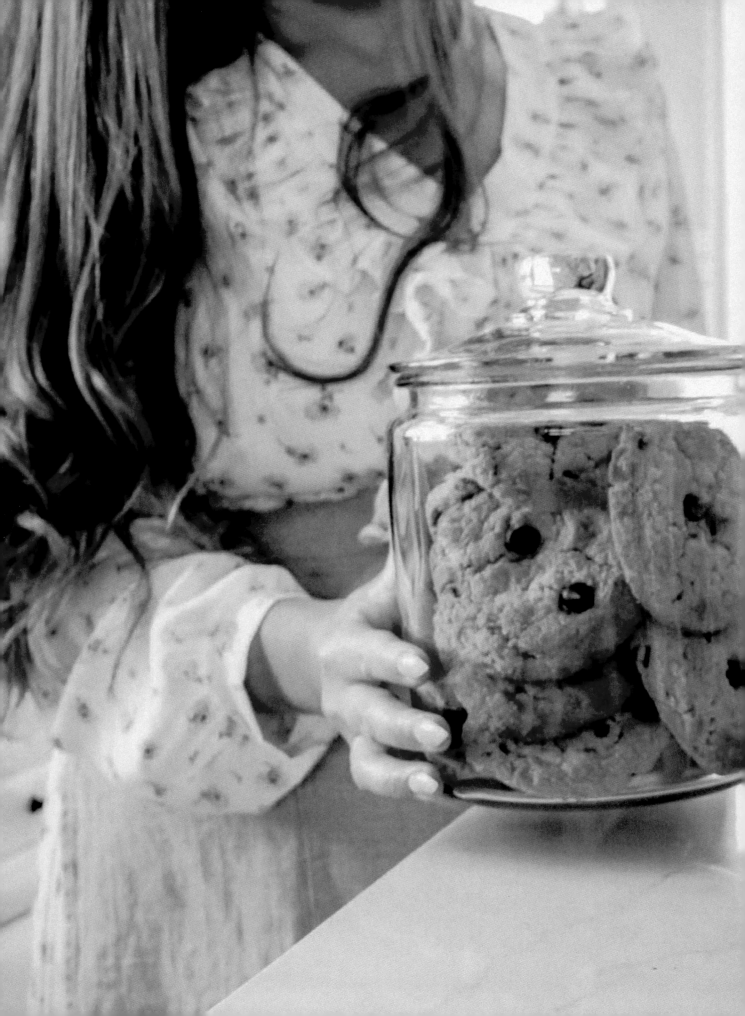

Acknowledgments

I could testify that I could have never dreamed of completing my recipe book in the time I had if it wasn't for my beautiful sweet baby bundle that the Lord blessed me with. I can't wait to bake with you! Baby, I am so excited to gift this book to you and teach you the art of cultivating your God-given creativity rather than just being a consumer and buying your favourite cookies, haha.

Of course, my husband, Tyler! You are my biggest fan and fan my flame each day with your overwhelming gratitude for all that I bake for you. Thank you for believing in me; I love you with my whole being.

To all my customers, friends, and family who were super supportive and excited for me to launch my cookbook! Honestly, your excitement to try my latest creations always motivates me to come up with new recipes!

My beautiful sister in Christ, Ami Ulici. Thank you for taking so much of your valuable time to edit my cookbook. I couldn't think of anyone who would have done such an excellent job! You went over and above to ensure that all the ingredients, instructions, and notes were easy to read and implement. Ami, you made it possible that everyone would enjoy these recipes to their full potential. I am so grateful.

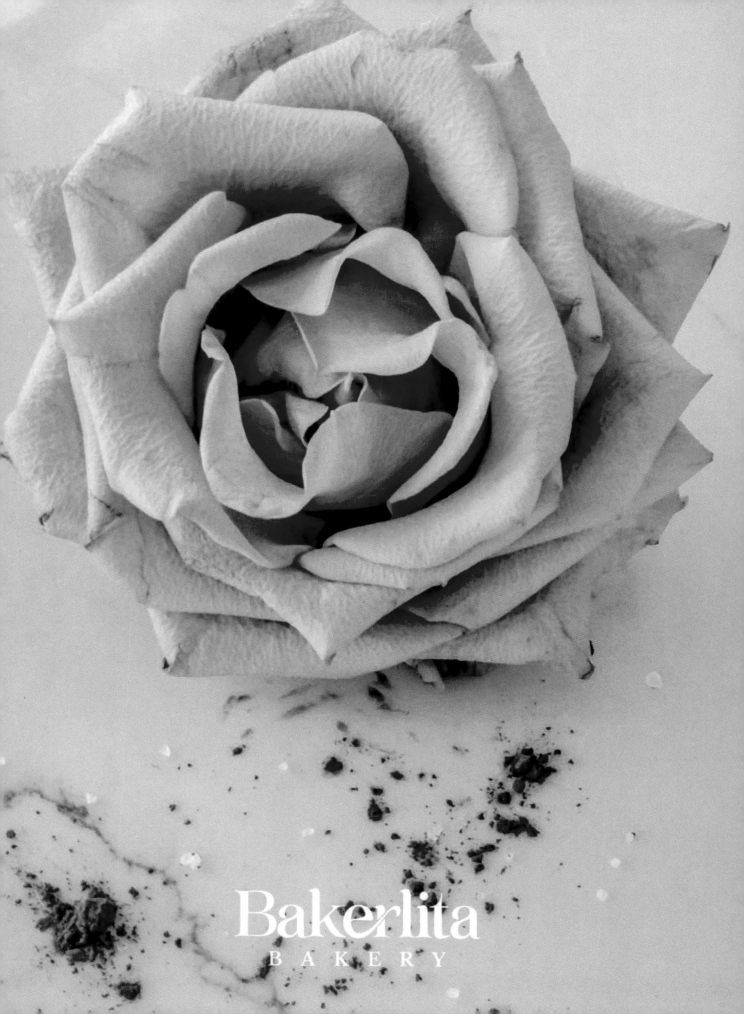

INDEX

G

H

I

J

K

L

M

W

X

Z

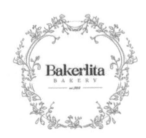

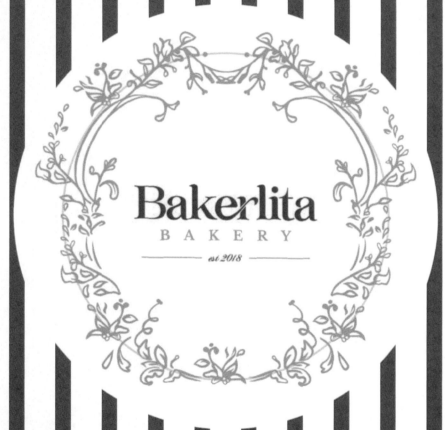

Bakerlita
BAKERY
— est 2018 —

Made in the USA
Monee, IL
08 January 2023

efc08e8c-17be-4a36-a02e-6f5e4dfa6552R01